COMMON PROBLEMS IN
CARDIAC ANESTHESIA

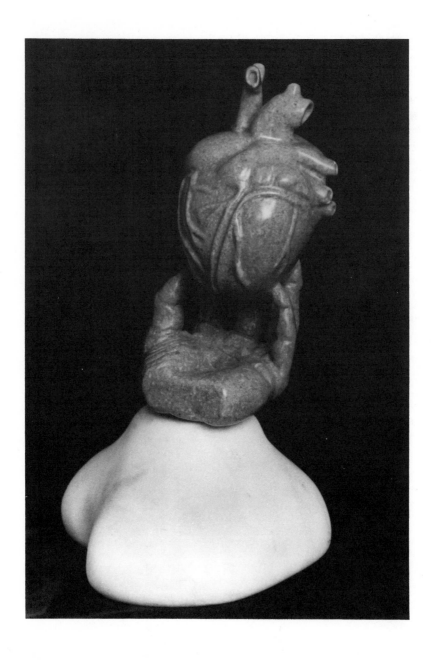

Sculpture in marble by Tim Rider. (Courtesy of Tim Rider.)

COMMON PROBLEMS IN

CARDIAC ANESTHESIA

J. G. REVES, M.D.
Professor of Anesthesiology
Director, Division of Cardiothoracic Anesthesia
Duke University Medical Center
Durham, North Carolina

KENNETH D. HALL, M.D.
Professor of Anesthesiology
Duke University
Director of Blood Gas Laboratory
Duke University Hospitals
Durham, North Carolina

YEAR BOOK MEDICAL PUBLISHERS, INC.
CHICAGO • LONDON • BOCA RATON

1 2 3 4 5 6 7 8 9 0 CK 91 90 89 88 87

Library of Congress Cataloging-in-Publication Data

Common problems in cardiac anesthesia.

  Includes bibliographies and index.
  1. Anesthesia in cardiology.   2.   Heart—Surgery.
3. Heart—Effect of drugs on.   I.   Reves, J. G.
II. Hall, Kenneth D. [DNLM: 1. Anesthesia. 2. Heart—
drug effects. 3. Heart Surgery.   WO 245 C734]
RD87.3.H43C66 1987   617'.967412   86-19065
ISBN 0-8151-7215-X

Sponsoring Editor: David K. Marshall
Manager, Copyediting Services: Frances M. Perveiler
Production Project Manager: Elizabeth J. Dusanic
Proofroom Supervisor: Shirley E. Taylor

CONTRIBUTORS

KEVIN C. ANGERT, M.D.
Assistant Professor of Anesthesia, Bowman Gray School of Medicine of Wake Forest University, Winston-Salem, North Carolina

JOHN L. ATLEE III, M.D.
Professor of Anesthesiology, University of Wisconsin Center for Health Sciences, Madison, Wisconsin

PAUL G. BARASH, M.D.
Professor and Chairman, Yale University School of Medicine; Attending Anesthesiologist, Yale-New Haven Medical Center, New Haven, Connecticut

BYRON C. BLOOR, Ph.D.
Associate Professor, Department of Anesthesiology, UCLA School of Medicine, Los Angeles, California

RICHARD E. BUCKINGHAM, Jr., M.D.
Associate Clinical Professor, University of Washington School of Medicine; Chief, Cardiac Anesthesia Department, Swedish Hospital Medical Center, Seattle, Washington

CHARLES W. BUFFINGTON, M.D.
Associate Professor, University of Washington School of Medicine, Seattle, Washington

GERALD A. BUSHMAN, M.D.
Assistant Professor, University of Arkansas for Medical Sciences, Little Rock, Arkansas

FIONA M. CLEMENTS, M.D.
Assistant Professor of Anesthesiology, Duke University, Durham, North Carolina

JOHN R. COOPER, Jr., M.D.
Clinical Assistant Professor of Anesthesiology, University of Texas Health Science Center at Houston; Attending Anesthesiologist, Texas Heart Institute, Houston, Texas

NARDA CROUGHWELL, C.R.N.A.
Research Coordinator, Division of Cardiothoracic Anesthesia, Duke Medical Center, Durham, North Carolina

NORBERT P. de BRUIJN, M.D.
Assistant Professor of Anesthesiology and Surgery, Duke University Medical Center, Durham, North Carolina

v

JAMES H. DIAZ, M.D.
Associate Professor of Anesthesiology (Clinical), Tulane University School of Medicine; Director of Pediatric Anesthesia, Ochsner Foundation Hospital, New Orleans, Louisiana

NORIG ELLISON, M.D.
Professor of Anesthesia, University of Pennsylvania School of Medicine, Philadelphia, Pennsylvania

FAWZY G. ESTAFANOUS, M.D.
Chairman, Department of Cardio-Thoracic Anesthesia, The Cleveland Clinic, Cleveland, Ohio

JORGE A. ESTRIN, M.D., Ph.D.
Associate Professor, Department of Anesthesiology, University of Minnesota Medical School, Minneapolis, Minnesota

JUDITH A. FABIAN, M.D.
Associate Professor, Medical College of Virginia; Director of Cardiac Anesthesia, McGuire Veterans Hospital, Richmond, Virginia

PAUL FINER, M.D.
Resident in Anesthesiology, Medical College of Georgia, Augusta, Georgia

DONALD C. FINLAYSON, M.D., F.R.C.P.(C.)
Professor of Anesthesiology, Department of Anesthesiology, Emory University School of Medicine; Director, Division of Critical Care Medicine, Department of Anesthesiology, Emory University Hospital, Atlanta, Georgia

JOAN W. FLACKE, M.D.
Professor of Anesthesiology, Department of Anesthesiology, UCLA School of Medicine, Los Angeles, California

WERNER E. FLACKE, M.D.
Professor of Anesthesiology and Pharmacology, Department of Anesthesiology, UCLA School of Medicine, Los Angeles, California

PAOLO FLEZZANI, M.D.
Assistant Professor of Anesthesiology, Duke University, Durham, North Carolina

JOHN F. FRAGOLA, Jr., M.D.
Fellow, Cardiothoracic Anesthesia, Los Angeles County–University of Southern California Medical Center, Los Angeles, California

ANN V. GOVIER, M.D.
Staff Anesthesiologist, Department of Cardiothoracic Anesthesia, The Cleveland Clinic Foundation, Cleveland, Ohio

GLENN P. GRAVLEE, M.D.
Associate Professor, Bowman Gray School of Medicine of Wake Forest University; Director of Cardiothoracic Anesthesia, North Carolina Baptist Hospital, Winston-Salem, North Carolina

WILLIAM J. GREELEY, M.D.
Assistant Professor of Anesthesiology and Pediatrics, Associate in Pediatric Cardiology, Duke University Medical Center, Durham, North Carolina

KENNETH D. HALL, M.D.
Professor of Anesthesiology, Duke University; Director of Blood Gas Laboratory, Duke University Hospitals, Durham, North Carolina

C. E. HENLING, M.D.
Assistant Professor, University of Alabama at Birmingham, Birmingham, Alabama

PAUL R. HICKEY, M.D.
Associate Professor of Anaesthesia, Harvard Medical School; Co-director, Cardiovascular Anesthesia, The Children's Hospital, Boston, Massachusetts

MARK HILBERMAN, M.D.
Clinical Associate Professor of Anesthesia, University of Colorado Health Sciences Center, Denver, Colorado; Anesthesiologist, Boulder Community Hospital, Boulder, Colorado

RUSSELL F. HILL, M.D.
Associate in Anesthesiology, Duke University Medical Center, Durham, North Carolina

ROBERTA L. HINES, M.D.
Assistant Professor of Anesthesiology, Yale University, New Haven, Connecticut

MICHAEL B. HOWIE, M.D.
Associate Professor of Anesthesiology and Pharmacy, The Ohio State University; Director of Cardiovascular Anesthesiology, Ohio State University Hospitals, Columbus, Ohio

DAVID R. JOBES, M.D.
Department of Anesthesia, University of Pennsylvania School of Medicine, Philadelphia, Pennsylvania

WILLIAM E. JOHNSTON, M.D.
Associate Professor of Anesthesiology, Wake Forest University Medical Center; Co-director, Intensive Care Unit, North Carolina Baptist Hospital, Winston-Salem, North Carolina

FRED KAHAN, M.D.
Cardiac Fellow, Mount Sinai School of Medicine, New York, New York

JOEL A. KAPLAN, M.D.
Professor and Chairman, Department of Anesthesiology, Mount Sinai School of Medicine, New York, New York

JOANNES H. KARIS, M.D.
Professor of Anesthesiology, Duke University, Durham, North Carolina

ROBERT A. KATES, M.D.
Associate Professor, Department of Anesthesia, Duke University Medical Center, Durham, North Carolina

STEVEN N. KONSTADT, M.D.
Assistant Professor of Clinical Anesthesiology, Mount Sinai School of Medicine; Assistant Attending, Mount Sinai Hospital, New York, New York

CHARLES J. KOPRIVA, M.D.
Professor of Anesthesiology, Yale School of Medicine, New Haven, Connecticut

CAROL L. LAKE, M.D.
Associate Professor of Anesthesiology, University of Virginia; Clinical Staff, University of Virginia Hospital, Charlottesville, Virginia

WILLIAM A. LELL, M.D.
Vice-Chairman, Department of Anesthesiology, Professor and Director of Cardiovascular Anesthesia, The University of Alabama School of Medicine, Birmingham, Alabama

ALAN LEVINE, M.D.
Fellow, Department of Anesthesiology, University of Washington, Seattle, Washington

JERROLD H. LEVY, M.D.
Assistant Professor of Anesthesiology, Department of Anesthesiology, Division of Cardiothoracic Anesthesia, Emory University Hospital, Atlanta, Georgia

EDWARD LOWENSTEIN, M.D.
Professor of Anaesthesia, Harvard Medical School; Anesthetist, Massachusetts General Hospital, Boston, Massachusetts

ROBERT J. MARINO, M.D.
Section of Cardiovascular Anesthesia, Medical Director, Intensive Care Unit, Ochsner Clinic, New Orleans, Louisiana

JAMES T. MASSAGEE, M.D.
Fellow in Cardiovascular Anesthesia, Duke University Medical Center, Durham, North Carolina

JOHN P. McDERMOTT, M.D.
Department of Anesthesia, University of California at San Francisco, San Francisco, California

R. WILLIAM McINTYRE, M.D.
Assistant Professor of Anesthesiology, Duke University; Attending Anesthesiologist, Duke University Medical Center, Durham, North Carolina

C. CRAIG MOLDENHAUER, M.D.
Assistant Professor, Emory University School of Medicine; Staff Anesthesiologist, Emory University Hospital, Atlanta, Georgia

DENIS R. MOREL, M.D.
Instructor in Anesthesia, Harvard Medical School; Research Fellow in Anesthesia, Massachusetts General Hospital, Boston, Massachusetts

LARS R. NEWSOME, M.D.
Assistant Professor of Anesthesiology, Emory University School of Medicine; Staff Anesthesiologist, Emory University Hospital, Atlanta, Georgia

SUSAN C. NICOLSON, M.D.
Assistant Professor of Anesthesia, University of Pennsylvania School of Medicine; Director, Cardiac Anesthesia, The Children's Hospital of Philadelphia, Philadelphia, Pennsylvania

EDWARD A. NORFLEET, M.D.
Associate Professor and Director of Cardiothoracic Anesthesia, University of North Carolina, Chapel Hill, North Carolina

NANCY A. NUSSMEIR, M.D.
Department of Anesthesia, University of California at Davis, Davis, California

JOSEPH PROFETA, M.D.
Instructor and Senior Clinical Assistant Attending Physician, Department of Anesthesiology, Mount Sinai Hospital, New York, New York

DONALD S. PROUGH, M.D.
Section Head, Critical Care, Associate Professor of Anesthesia and Neurology, Bowman Gray School of Medicine of Wake Forest University; Medical Director, Respiratory Therapy, North Carolina Baptist Hospital, Winston-Salem, North Carolina

RUSSELL C. RAPHAELY, M.D.
Associate Professor of Anesthesia and Pediatrics, University of Pennsylvania School of Medicine; Director, Pediatric Intensive Care Complex, The Children's Hospital of Philadelphia, Philadelphia, Pennsylvania

J. G. REVES, M.D.
Professor of Anesthesiology, Director, Division of Cardiothoracic Anesthesia, Duke University Medical Center, Durham, North Carolina

SANDRA L. ROBERTS, M.D.
Assistant Professor, Department of Anesthesia, University of Iowa College of Medicine, Iowa City, Iowa

ROGER L. ROYSTER, M.D.
Assistant Professor of Anesthesia, Associate in Cardiology, Bowman Gray School of Medicine of Wake Forest University, Winston-Salem, North Carolina

RON RUFF, M.D.
Cardiac Anesthesia Fellow, Duke University Medical Center, Durham, North Carolina

PAUL N. SAMUELSON, M.D.
Professor of Anesthesiology, University of Alabama School of Medicine, Birmingham, Alabama

MICHAEL SCARBROUGH, M.D.
Fellow, Department of Anesthesiology, The University of Alabama School of Medicine, Birmingham, Alabama

JOHN F. SCHWEISS, M.D.
Professor and Chairman of Anesthesiology, St. Louis University School of Medicine; Chief of Anesthesiology, St. Louis University Hospital, St. Louis, Missouri

GEORGE SILVAY, M.D., Ph.D.
Professor of Clinical Anesthesiology, Mount Sinai Medical Center, New York, New York

ROBERT N. SLADEN, M.B., M.R.C.P.(U.K.), F.R.C.P.(C.)
Associate Professor of Anesthesia, Stanford University School of Medicine; Associate Medical Director, Intensive Care, Stanford University Medical Center, Stanford, California

DONALD E. SMITH, M.D.
Clinical Associate Professor, Department of Anesthesiology, Tulane University School of Medicine, New Orleans, Louisiana

THOMAS E. STANLEY III, M.D.
Fellow in Cardiothoracic Anesthesiology, Duke University Medical Center, Durham, North Carolina

NORMAN J. STARR, M.D.
Staff Anesthesiologist, The Cleveland Clinic Foundation, Cleveland, Ohio

M. JEROME STRONG, M.D.
Clinical Professor of Anesthesiology, Department of Anesthesiology, University of California at San Francisco, San Francisco, California

MICHAEL F. SWEENEY, M.D.
Instructor, Department of Pediatrics and Anesthesia, Associate Director of Pediatric Intensive Care, University of Minnesota Medical School, Minneapolis, Minnesota

DANIEL M. THYS, M.D.
Associate Professor of Anesthesiology, Mount Sinai School of Medicine; Director, Division of Cardiothoracic Anesthesia, Mount Sinai Hospital, New York, New York

JOHN H. TINKER, M.D.
Professor and Head, University of Iowa College of Medicine, Iowa City, Iowa

DAVID J. TORPEY, Jr., M.D.
Director, Department of Anesthesiology, Allegheny General Hospital; Clinical Associate Professor of Anesthesiology, University of Pittsburgh School of Medicine, Pittsburgh, Pennsylvania

MARK TRAGER, M.D.
Fellow in Cardiothoracic Anesthesiology, Mount Sinai Medical School, New York, New York

JOHN F. VILJOEN, M.D., F.F.A.R.C.S.
Professor and Chairman of Anesthesiology, University of Southern California; Chief of Anesthesia, Los Angeles County–University of Southern California Medical Center, Los Angeles, California

CAROLYN J. WILKINSON, M.D.
Associate Professor of Anesthesiology, Northwestern Medical School, Chicago, Illinois

K. C. WONG, M.D., Ph.D.
Professor and Chairman, Department of Anesthesiology, Professor of Pharmacology, University of Utah School of Medicine, Salt Lake City, Utah

JOHN A. YOUNGBERG, M.D.
Associate Professor, Department of Anesthesiology, Tulane University School of Medicine, New Orleans, Louisiana

JAMES R. ZAIDAN, M.D.
Associate Professor of Anesthesiology, Emory University School of Medicine; Staff Anesthesiologist, Emory University Hospital, Atlanta, Georgia

FOREWORD

Most anesthetics go well even when administered for cardiac operations. With reasonable planning and anticipation of the most likely complications, major morbidity attributable to anesthesia is low. We tend to credit our knowledge, skills, abundant monitoring, and wisdom in making the right decisions. We tend to forget that most patients respond in predictable fashion and that patients are extraordinarily resilient when protecting their own viability. We therefore learn progressively less from each anesthetic that goes well even when our decisions are not the best.

What of the patient who does not respond in predictable fashion, whose anesthetic management does not go according to plan, and who suffers the unanticipated complication? In the unattainably ideal training program all trainees will have been exposed to all unanticipated responses while attended and will have been instructed in their optimal management. When unattended and faced for the first time with an unpredicted response the ideally trained anesthesiologist would have a ready action plan. Unfortunately, in real life the usual response is confusion, some incredulousness, and much anxiety. Incredulity is probably the most hazardous to the patient. Whatever the outcome a second lesson is usually never necessary. Management of the unanticipated responses provides the great learning opportunities in clinical anesthesia.

I believe Drs. Hall and Reves recognize this limitation of training and practice. All complexities of cardiac anesthesia are not within the experience of all practitioners. From their own broad experience they have collected an exceptional list of common and not so common problems in cardiac anesthesia. Their sense, in my view, is to provide readers with the first experience so that perhaps they will respond when it occurs as if it were the second. Although reading never provides the memorable experience of living through it, reading gives credibility and the important knowledge that it happened before. In this manner hopefully the unanticipated becomes anticipated and the practice of cardiac anesthesia improves.

ARTHUR S. KEATS, M.D.
TEXAS HEART INSTITUTE
HOUSTON, TEXAS

To the patients who have taught us the lessons herein, and to the families of the contributors who have supported the authors by understanding the demands on time for patient care through the years and even for writing the chapters in this book.

PREFACE

The purpose of this book is to expose the reader to a number of common clinical problems and the management of the problems by experienced cardiac anesthetists. The problems are not so common as to occur every day in every patient, but rather are the type of situation one might encounter perhaps once a week in a busy clinical practice.

The cases are grouped into eight parts: (1) technical and monitoring problems, (2) congenital heart disease, (3) acquired valvular heart disease, (4) electrophysiologic dysfunction, (5) ischemic heart disease, (6) pharmacology, (7) coagulation and blood products, and (8) intensive care unit. The organization of each of the 62 chapters is similar: (1) case presentation, (2) analysis of the problem, (3) approach to the problem, and (4) discussion. The intent of this format is to present the case succinctly, have the experienced clinician assess the problem, and then give a preferred course of action. The discussion is intended to give alternative approaches and/or review pertinent literature supporting the management plan.

As with any multiauthored text there is variability in the individual's approach to the book format. The end result is a book with some chapters very short, some long, and some scholarly reviews. Others are "how I do it" chapters ("because I've dealt with this enough to know what to do without referring to any papers"). The intention is to teach by the case-gone-wrong method. This is an effective method of learning in the operating room where we all learn from our mistakes or those of our associates. Not all of the problems in this book are mistakes, however. Some are unexpected events created by an unanticipated pharmacologic or physiologic response of the patient. Regardless of the origin, a number of common problems are collected. This book attempts to teach (and learn) from *reading* rather than *having* each experience in the operating room.

Common Problems in Cardiac Anesthesia is not meant to be a comprehensive text on cardiac anesthesia of which there are an ample number, but rather is designed to educate the clinician who is likely to be confronted with these problems. In addition to the clinician, the book is also for the student, teacher, and researcher in the field of cardiovascular anesthesiology, but readers may have to go to the literature and traditional texts for a comprehensive discussion of the origin of these problems and their treatment.

It is unlikely that all readers will agree with all approaches to these problems—the editors do not. Part of the value of this book is learning what others would do when faced with a common problem. It was in fact, difficult to get some contributors to commit to one single preferred course of action and impossible (if not undesirable) to have a noncontroversial approach to all problems.

The editors thank all the contributors for their work. Their insight, experience, and willingness to manage the cases made the book. Also we are indebted to Maidi Hall for her editing and Laraine Goss for her expert assistance in putting the book together at Duke, and to Susan Harter and Kevin Kelly of Year Book Medical Publishers, Inc., for their help in editing and publishing the book. We are especially grateful to Dr. Arthur Keats for his foreword, which reflects his keen understanding of our purpose. Dr. Keats inspired the concept of this book by telling us once, "It's hard to learn when all goes well."

J. G. REVES, M.D.
KENNETH D. HALL, M.D.

CONTENTS

PART ONE

Technical and Monitoring Problems

1

Inability to Place Radial Arterial Catheter

Recommendations by Michael B. Howie, M.D.

A 44-year-old man scheduled to have a coronary artery bypass arrived at the operating room in a comfortable but slightly apprehensive state. An intravenous catheter was inserted without difficulty prior to placement of a left radial arterial catheter. There was a normal Allen's test bilaterally. With the patient under adequate local anesthesia, several attempts at placing a 20-gauge radial artery catheter failed in both arteries. The patient became more apprehensive and complained of chest pain. Because the patient had a history of labile blood pressure, it was desirable to have arterial monitoring prior to induction, but because of hematomas and/or spasm at each radial artery site, radial arterial catheterization seemed impossible.

ANALYSIS OF THE PROBLEM

The failure to cannulate either radial artery in a patient for whom arterial pressure measurements is mandatory requires either utilization of different radial artery techniques (see below) or choice of a different site.

APPROACH TO THE PROBLEM

In this case a three-staged strategy is recommended. First, a Seldinger technique should be tried in the radial artery with the best possible pulse. If this is unsuccessful, a percutaneous Seldinger approach to a larger (more proximal) artery should be attempted in either the femoral or brachial artery. If this fails, an arterial cutdown and radial catheterization under direct vision must be performed.

DISCUSSION

According to Prys-Roberts and Meloche, "direct continuous monitoring of arterial pressure should no longer be regarded as a complex esoteric measurement, pertinent only to cardiac surgery, an intensive therapy unit or the laboratory."[1] Since 1980 when that statement was made, continuous arterial monitoring either for pressure or for evaluation of blood gases or chemistry has become very common. The increasingly complex surgical procedures performed on patients and the fact that the patients are often at risk within small time periods has made invasive monitoring of arterial blood pressure more acceptable.

An arterial line in surgery is often needed in the following cases:

1. Cardiac surgery

2. Open chest procedures

3. Intracranial operations

4. Major trauma

5. Repeated blood gas estimation

6. Intentional hypotension or pressure control within strict limits

7. Intentional hypothermia

8. Rapid or unpredictable blood pressure changes

9. Inability to measure blood pressure with a cuff[2]

Patients with the following abnormalities may also require an arterial catheter for careful monitoring during surgery or intensive care:

1. Severe acute myocardial infarct

2. Significant acute or chronic pulmonary disease

3. Severe cardiovascular disease

4. Severe metabolic derangement

5. Obesity

6. Dysrhythmias (to ascertain hemodynamic significance)

Intelligent selection of the arterial site is important. In general, the use of the most distal available site for arterial puncture or catheterization reduces the potential for ischemic damage, tissue loss, nerve damage, and air embolism. Compressive neuropathy and other damage caused by bleeding from a needle puncture are less extensive when more distal sites are chosen. The tissue perfused by the radial artery has adequate collateral circulation from the ulnar artery and superficial palmar arch in approximately 90% of the adult population.[3]

Anatomy

The reasons for failure to cannulate the radial artery are for the most part technical. However, we must also consider anatomical findings. In a total series of 750 consecutive upper extremities, McCormack et al. found that the principal arteries of the upper extremities departed from the anatomical normal in respect to origin and course of the arteries in 19% of the limbs, with bilateral occurrence in 6%.[4]

The origin of the radial artery proximal to the intercondylar line formed, by far, the largest group of gross varieties. However, in the radial artery, at the wrist, only 6 specimens out of the 750 had anomalous terminal distribution of the radial artery. Thus, anatomy alone will not account for failure of cannulation. The purpose of this text is first to explain the cannulation techniques and to point out their shortcomings. Then we will demonstrate how the techniques can be improved in the presence of various difficulties.

Before cannulation is attempted, the clinician should possess a thorough knowledge of the normal anatomy of the radial artery at the wrist and its collateral connections to the ulnar artery. The radial artery, a branch of the brachial artery, extends down the anterior radial aspect of the forearm where, after sending a branch to the palm, it disappears deep to the abductor pollicus longus tendon, just beyond the distal end of the radius. From there, it continues across the floor of the anatomical "snuff box" into the dorsum of the hand. At the wrist, the radial artery is palpable in the longitudinal groove formed by the tendon of the flexor carpi radialis medially and the distal radius laterally.[5]

The normal anatomical arrangement of vessels in the hand provides three major connections between the ulnar and radial arteries.[6] The deep and the dorsal arterial arches are primarily fed by the radial, while the superficial palmar arch is usually a continuation of the ulnar linked to the superficial palmar branch of the radial artery. The fingers are predominantly supplied by blood from the superficial palmar arch, via the palmar digital arteries.

Assessment of Collateral Flow

Complete occlusion of the radial artery may exist, despite the presence of a radial pulse, but this considerable "collateral" flow is only possible in the presence of a complete palmar arch. It has been shown that the arch is, in fact, discontinuous in 17.6% of normal individuals,[5] and radial artery occlusion in such cases may lead to greatly reduced blood flow into the isolated segment of the palmar arch, with consequent ischemia of the index and middle fingers.

Allen's test provides a reliable assessment of ulnar collateral blood supply to the hand.[3, 7, 8] The examiner occludes both the radial and the ulnar arteries and instructs the patient to alternately clench and open his hand several times.[9] The patient should then open the hand in the relaxed position; the hand will appear blanched. Pressure over the ulnar artery is then released, and if the ulnar collateral arterial circulation is adequate, the color of the hand will return to normal within a few seconds. Some investigators have recommended that a five-second palmar blush period will indicate adequate collateral flow, with special attention being given to capillary filling of the thumb and thenar eminence.[2] Twelve-second filling time is the maximum. During the Allen's test, the clinician must work to prevent the patient from overextending the wrist; if the wrist is overextended, occlusion of the transpalmar arch under the flexor retinaculum will produce a false abnormal result. An extension of two thirds in a claw-like manner is recommended.[10]

Cannulation Technique

The radial artery, if palpable, has a very high success rate of cannulation by experienced clinicians, if pediatric and emergency procedures and vascular disease of the arm are excluded. Slogoff et al. at the Texas Heart Institute, found that only 83 patients out of 1,699 could not have the radial artery cannulated if the procedures and diseases mentioned above were excluded.[11] They also found that successful nonischemic cannulation could be achieved in patients on whom equivocal Allen tests had been performed. Gardner and associates also found a very high success rate (91.8%) of insertion into the radial artery of choice; an additional 6.7% required catheter insertion at a second site, and 1.5% necessitated insertion at a third site (brachial or femoral).[12]

The failure to cannulate is often a consequence of trauma produced by the initial cannulation attempt. Such trauma may include dissection of the intima, hematoma, and spasms, any of which may make it difficult for the clinician to implement a subsequent procedure. Therefore, the first attempt must be done carefully, under optimal conditions. If the attempt is unsuccessful, then in about 8% of the patients, serious, nearly occlusive spasm occurs.[9] A partial occlusive spasm occurs in 40% of patients.[13] A previous cannulation performed several days before may also change the artery, producing thrombus formation or scarring, with narrowing of the vessel.[14]

To begin cannulation, the clinician should map the radial artery by palpation about 1 in. above the crease of the wrist. At this point the skin is generously infiltrated with 1% plain lidocaine after a Betadine wipe. A short 25-gauge needle is then used to infiltrate lidocaine on both sides of the artery. This extra precaution seems to effectively prevent spasm and also allows time for dispersion of the local anesthetic while full betadine prepping of the area takes place. The wrist should then be positioned in the dorsiflexed position, at an angle of about 50 to 60 degrees on a short arm board with a 2-in. roll of face cloth under the dorsiflexion. The thumb should be taped to the side of the arm board to help fix or stabilize the artery at the wrist.[9] After sterile prepping, gloving, and placing of sterile towels at the site of cannulation, the radial artery should be again palpated for 2 to 3 in.

At this point, the clinician has several cannulation options: the catheter over the needle (CON), the Seldinger technique, or perhaps a combination of both. Whatever technique is chosen, a small nick should first be made over the anticipated site of insertion to facilitate entry of the cannula. The cannula should be 20-gauge, with an inside diameter of 0.7 mm and an outside diameter of 1 mm.[15] Larger cannulas are unnecessary and tend to produce complications because they occupy too much of the arterial lumen. Smaller cannulas should also be avoided since they kink too readily at the skin. The catheter should be made of Teflon which is less thrombogenic. Nontapered catheters are also preferred. In addition, the clinician should inspect the catheter needle unit prior to insertion, observing the distance between the point where the needle bevel ends and the catheter tip begins. This distance is not constant among the various manufacturers, and anything over one eighth of an inch should not be used, since a needle of that length will often reach the back wall of the artery as the cannula enters the lumen.[9]

The catheter should be inserted along the course of the artery at a 20- to 30-degree angle to the surface of the skin. When the artery is entered, as evidenced by a bright red spurt of blood, the angle should be reduced to 10 to 20 degrees and the needle and catheter should be advanced for 2 to 3 mm parallel to the artery. The back wall of the artery should not be penetrated or touched. At the very least, the number of penetrations or arterial punctures should be kept to a minimum, since vessels suffering multiple punctures during cannulation are almost twice as likely to occlude than are those requiring only a single insertion.[16] The cannula is then advanced alone to its hub and secured. If the artery is considered small, maximum pulse volume and lumen size can be obtained by cannulating after a period of occlusion by using a blood pressure cuff held above systolic pressure for two minutes. This procedure causes hyperemia, which should give optimum arterial size for puncture.

Aids to Cannulation

Arterial narrowing and tortuosity coincident with aging and arteriosclerosis occasionally make percutaneous catheterization of the radial artery difficult. [17] Advancement of the catheter inside the vessel lumen may injure the intima, especially in small narrowed vessels. Many times this problem can be overcome by using a guide wire in the arterial cannula. However, some vessels may be so tortuous that not even the thin-wire guide will be able to pass through them. This problem often results in a normal arterial puncture, marked by the spurting of arterial blood. Repeated attempts to pass the catheter fail. To deal with such a situation, Stirt has suggested using the "liquid stylet." [17] This is a steady injection of 1 to 3 ml of sterile saline while advancing the catheter, with aspiration at the end of the insertion to confirm location of the catheter tip in the artery. Stirt postulates that the injected fluid probably temporarily dilates and straightens the narrowed artery. He claims success with the technique and reports few if any complications. However, accurate placement of the initial puncture is essential to avoid intimal dissection which could result from the injection.

Because of its peripheral location, the radial artery may be impalpable due to vasoconstriction from hypotension. [18] In this case, failure to cannulate the narrowed vessel is due to the very small lumen and the immediacy of the back wall. [19] To facilitate entry into the radial artery without damaging the back wall, a clinician may elect to connect the cannula to the transducer system. The needle is then advanced until the arterial pressure curve is displayed on the screen of the monitor. This method seems to work even in cases of shock in which the patient has no palpable pulse. It also reduces considerably the necessity for a cutdown. In these cases, accurate location of the lumen is necessary in order to reduce the probability of puncturing the posterior wall of the artery. Transfixing the artery serves no useful purpose, causes damage, and is another nidus for thrombus formation and a second site of hematoma formation.

A Doppler-flow probe detector may also be used to cannulate when palpation of the radial artery is difficult due to a weak, intermittent, or hypotensive pulse. [20] The flow probe responds to the motion of red blood cells in such a way that the pitch of the signals that are heard is related to the velocity of the motion. Models that eliminate background noise are more efficient because they concentrate on the maximum point of blood flow in the artery. The arterial pathway can be mapped by the use of a transcutaneous Doppler and marking pen. The Doppler detector is held in position while the arterial catheter is directed percutaneously through the skin nick toward the maximum blood flow. As the catheter needle contacts the artery, it narrows the arterial lumen, causing a change in blood flow at that point. This change is then manifested as a change in pitch via the Doppler. The Doppler can also be used for percutaneous evaluation of the palmar arch prior to cannulation of the radial artery. [21] This technique obviates multiple blind sticks or cutdown.

If a grating sensation accompanies the advancement of a catheter into an artery, the catheter tip may be frayed and crimped, with distorted irregular edges. This problem was more common with tapered tips in the past. However, the advancement of any catheter with frayed edges is difficult. The inner needle tip may be in the vessel lumen with a pulsating blood return, yet catheter advancement will be impeded because the distorted edges impinge on the vessel wall. The grating sensation is readily appreciated if the operator grasps the cannula directly by his fingers. [22]

Because of the small size of the artery in children, especially infants, cannulation success is less likely than with adults. [23] But the clinician can improve the chances of successful radial artery cannulation by placing under the slightly dorsiflexed hand a powerful fiberoptic light for transillumination of the wrist. From the ventral side, it is possible to see the radial and ulnar arteries in the lower forearm and the wrist; these appear as dark lines against a bright transilluminated background. The arteries may be differentiated from the veins in this region as follows: the latter move with the skin, whereas the former remain fixed. The aseptic solution used should be clear.

The description we have given of cannulation up to this point has applied to the catheter over needle technique. However, since failure to cannulate the radial artery is usually due to failure of technique, and since the damage caused by multiple cannulation attempts results in vasospasm and hematoma formation, the precision of the Seldinger technique is preferred if a narrow, hardly palpable artery is felt at the onset. With this technique, location is much less traumatic and far easier because only a single needle needs to be placed in the lumen of the artery. The needle is passed at a 20-degree angle through the prepped skin to the maximum flow of blood. With the needle in place as a guide, a small fine scalpel is used to incise in an upward direction at the side of the needle. This prevents "hang up" of the cannula as it passes through the skin. The guide wire is passed very gently down the needle, with the angle reduced to 10 degrees. At the point where the guide wire leaves the needle, the clinician must apply a fine touch in order to ascertain whether the wire moves freely up the artery. The commonest cause of inability to gently advance the guide wire is previously attempted cannulation. The wire will either enter an intimal tear or go directly out the back wall. In either case, the awake patient will experience pain, and the clinician should suspect both conditions if the wire fails to advance freely. Therefore, efficient use of the wire demands this gentle probing.

After the wire is advanced a satisfactory length, the needle is withdrawn and the 6-in. catheter is placed over the guidewire and advanced nearly parallel to the skin. A firm motion at the point of entry into the artery ensures the clean entry of the cannula. Once the cannula is advanced to its hub, the wire is carefully withdrawn. The 6-in. length of the catheter in the Seldinger technique guarantees that the catheter lies in the rigid protected forearm and is less likely to kink. Ultimately, the Seldinger technique permits more precise location, and the guide wire facilitates catheter advancement. At least two extra movements are required in the catheter-over-needle technique, movements that may inadvertently damage the artery and prevent advancement of the catheter.

Alternative Sites

Cannon and Meshier[24] report that certain patients have significant disease profiles that a clinician must consider and that, for these patients, cannulation of a small artery is hazardous. They report a significantly increased risk of thrombosis because of the following: (1) use of dopamine; (2) hypertryglycerides; (3) serum hyperosmolarity; (4) capillary sludging; and (5) hypovolemic state. They maintain that even an Allen's test showing adequate collateral circulation cannot exclude serious consequences in a small artery; a large vessel, such as the femoral, is a preferable site. There are occasions when the radial artery may not be available or is contraindicated as a site for cannulation.[25] These include the presence of preexisting circulatory insufficiency to the hand and fingers as a result of a vasospastic disorder, extensive burns or trauma, infection, multiple punctures, or previous cannulations.

In the above instances, use of the femoral artery is a viable alternative to cannulation of an artery in the arm.[4] Soderstrom et al. found that the morbidity characterized as either minor or major was equal when cannulation of the upper arm arteries was compared to that of the femoral artery.[26] Placement duration was significantly longer for the femoral, and ischemic changes were noted only with use of radial catheters. Russell et al. also found femoral catheterization to be a safe alternative.[27] Their findings revealed that the complication rate for radial artery cannulation was 7.5%, not statistically significantly different from a 6.9% complication rate for femoral artery cannulation. Peripheral vascular disease, greater age, and catheter duration were not associated with a greater number of complications. According to the clinical impression, femoral catheters were also longer lasting and more durable than were radial lines.

Summary

In summary, radial artery cannulation in the modern acute medicine setting allows clinicians to provide better care for their patients. If a 20-gauge Teflon nontapered cannula is carefully used, insertion of an arterial line can be achieved with little difficulty and less morbidity. The most common cause of failure, however, is multiple cannulation attempts or punctures leading to vasospasm, internal damage, hematoma, and distal embolization of air. In case of either a suspected difficulty or an attempt after failed cannulation, the preferred method is the Seldinger technique with gentle, resistance-free passage of a thin wire to guide a 20-gauge cannula. If the percutaneous technique fails, the clinician should rapidly change to a cutdown technique or consider cannulation of a large vessel such as the femoral.

ACKNOWLEDGMENT

The author wishes to thank Mary Tigner for her assistance in the preparation of this manuscript.

REFERENCES

1. Prys-Roberts C, Meloche R: Management of anesthesia in patients with hypertension or ischemic heart disease. *Int Anesthesiol Clin* 1980; 19:181–217.
2. Kaplan JA: *Cardiac Anesthesia.* New York, Grune & Stratton Inc, 1979.
3. Gauer PK, Downs JB: Complications of arterial catheterization. *Respir Care* 1982; 27:435–444.
4. McCormack LJ, Cauldwell EW, Anson BJ: Brachial and antebrachial arterial patterns. *Surg Gynecol Obstet* 1953; 96:43–54.
5. Kaye W: Invasive monitoring techniques: Arterial cannulation, bedside pulmonary artery catheterization, and arterial puncture. *Heart Lung* 1983; 12:395–427.
6. Hamer JD, Mathews ET, Hardman J: Cannulation of the radial artery. *Lancet* 1974; 1:1282.
7. Husum B, Berthelsen P: Allen's test and systolic arterial pressure in the thumb. *Br J Anaesth* 1981; 53:635–637.
8. Allen EV: Thromboangiitis obliterans: Methods of diagnosis of chronic occlusive arterial lesions distal to the wrist with illustrative cases. *Am J Med Sci* 1929; 178:237–244.
9. Blitt CD: Vascular catheterization techniques. *ASA Refresher Course Lectures, No. 136.* Chicago, American Society of Anesthesiologists, 1977.
10. Kamienski RW, Barnes RW: Critique of the Allen test for continuity of the palmar arch assessed by Doppler ultrasound. *Surg Gynecol Obstet* 1976; 142:861–864.

11. Slogoff S, Keats AS, Arlund C: On the safety of radial artery cannulation. *Anesthesiology* 1983; 59:42–47.
12. Gardner RM, Schwartz R, Wong HC, et al: Percutaneous indwelling radial-artery catheters for monitoring cardiovascular function. *N Engl J Med* 1974; 290:1227–1231.
13. Ashbell TS, Kleinert HE, Kutz JE: Vascular injuries about the elbow. *Clin Orthop* 1967; 50:106–127.
14. McCready RA, Hyde GL, Bivins BA, et al: Brachial artery puncture: A definite risk to the hand. *South Med J* 1984; 77:786–789.
15. Lindor: Cardiovascular system. *Int Anesthesiol Clin* 1981; 19:9–29.
16. Davis FM, Stewart JM: Radial artery cannulation: A prospective study in patients undergoing cardiothoracic surgery. *Br J Anaesth* 1980; 52:41–46.
17. Stirt JA: "Liquid stylet" for percutaneous radial artery cannulation. *Can Anaesth Soc J* 1982; 29:492–493.
18. Brown M, Gordon LH, Brown OW, et al: Intravascular monitoring via the axillary artery. *Anaesth Intensive Care* 1984; 13:38–40.
19. Kondo K: Percutaneous radial artery cannulation using a pressure-curve-directed technique. *Anesthesiology* 1984; 61:639–640.
20. Rich JM: Use of the ultrasound stethoscope blood flow detector for cannulation of a weakly palpable radial artery. *Heart Lung* 1984; 13:47–48.
21. Mozersky DJ, Buckley CJ, Hagood CO, et al: Ultrasonic evaluation of the palmar circulation: A useful adjunct to radial artery cannulation. *Am J Surg* 1973; 126:810–812.
22. Talmage EA: Shearing hazard of intra-arterial Teflon catheters. *Anesth Analg* 1976; 55:597–598.
23. Pearse RG: Percutaneous catheterisation of the radial artery in newborn babies using transillumination. *Arch Dis Child* 1978; 53:549–554.
24. Cannon BW, Meshier WT: Extremity amputation following radial artery cannulation in a patient with hyperlipoproteinemia type V. *Anesthesiology* 1982; 56:222–223.
25. Gordon LH, Brown M, Brown OW, et al: Alternative sites for continuous arterial monitoring. *South Med J* 1984; 77:1498–1500.
26. Soderstrom CA, Wasserman DH, Dunham CM, et al: Superiority of the femoral artery for monitoring: A prospective study. *Am J Surg* 1982; 144:309–312.
27. Russell JA, Joel M, Hudson RJ, et al: Prospective evaluation of radial and femoral artery catheterization sites in critically ill adults. *Crit Care Med* 1983; 11:936–939.

2

Damped Arterial Pressure Tracing After Cardiopulmonary Bypass

Recommendations by Charles J. Kopriva, M.D.

A 60-year-old woman underwent coronary artery bypass grafting. Induction and the prebypass period proceeded without any difficulty and the left radial arterial catheter provided a good tracing before and during cardiopulmonary bypass. Immediately after the patient was weaned from bypass without use of vasoconstrictors, the arterial wave form became damped and the mean pressure was 20 mm Hg lower than the pressure transduced with the same system using a 20-gauge metal needle in the thoracic aorta. Repeated attempts at flushing the radial catheter failed to produce a normal pulse contour and one compatible with the central aortic pressure.

ANALYSIS OF THE PROBLEM

Rational management of the cardiac patient in the immediate postcardiopulmonary bypass period depends upon accurate arterial pressures. The most common cannulation site for determination of systemic arterial pressures is the radial artery. Systolic arterial pressure recorded from the radial artery is normally higher than the systolic pressure in the ascending aorta. However, immediately following cardiopulmonary bypass, an inaccurately low systolic arterial pressure recorded from the radial artery has been reported by several investigators and observed in patients in many busy cardiac surgical centers. In this patient, the radial artery pressure waveform was noted to be damped. Many mechanical factors can produce a falsely low systolic arterial pressure and a damped trace.

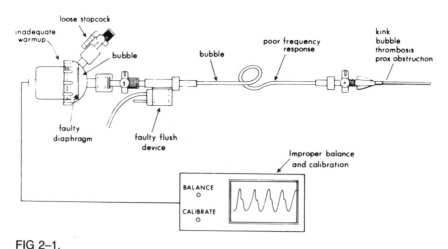

FIG 2–1.
To evaluate potential monitoring malfunction, begin at the patient's monitoring cannula and work back to the oscilloscope and digital readout. (From Barash PG, Kopriva CJ: Anesthesia for cardiac surgery, in Glenn W, et al (eds): *Thoracic and Cardiovascular Surgery*, ed. 4. Norwalk, Conn, Appleton-Century-Crofts, 1983, chap 73. Used by permission.)

A thrombotic narrowing of the radial artery catheter or a bubble within the catheter may be responsible. Bubbles within the monitoring line, in the transducer dome, or within a three-way stopcock may be causal. Blood within the monitoring line may "damp" the tracing. Occasionally, a loose stopcock or a faulty diaphragm on a disposable transducer dome may be the culprit (Figure 2–1). These mechanical factors can be quickly ruled out by astute examination of the monitoring system.

Although mechanical malfunction can produce this error, we have very commonly seen this problem when all components of the monitoring system were functioning properly.[1] Likewise, Stern et al.[2] reported that in 72% of a postbypass study group, the radial artery pressure was lower than the simultaneous aortic pressure. Gravlee et al.[3] reported that 52% of the patients in their immediate postbypass studies had falsely low radial artery pressures. Beker et al.[4] also reported significant inaccuracies in radial artery pressure postbypass. The importance of this problem is obvious. A falsely low systolic arterial pressure recorded from the radial artery will often lead to inappropriate administration of an inotrope or vasopressor. Administration of either of these drugs may increase myocardial oxygen demand and/or increase afterload. Thus, it is important to perceive these inaccuracies when they occur. In the case cited above, the radial artery pressure waveform was obviously damped. However, in many cases, the falsely low radial artery pressure will be accompanied by a *normal radial artery waveform*. Knowledge of this latter fact has persuaded us to measure central aortic pressure directly from the arterial perfusion cannula whenever the radial artery pressure is low enough to warrant some type of therapy.

APPROACH TO THE PROBLEM

As mentioned above, proper treatment will depend upon a high degree of suspicion regarding immediate postbypass radial artery pressures. Whenever radial artery pressure appears to be low enough to warrant therapy, we reflexly measure the pressure from the aortic perfusion cannula. Fortunately, this procedure requires little time and little equipment. Although the measurement is simple, the physician must ensure that there is no air in the line used to measure aortic cannula pressure. Since clearance of all air from the monitoring line will require a little time, it is perhaps best to go back on cardiopulmonary bypass while an air-free monitoring line is prepared. We use a "double-male" connector that can connect directly to the radial artery transducer, thus allowing almost simultaneous measurements of the two pressures. The line is carefully flushed free of air and connected to a three-way stopcock on the aortic perfusion cannula. We prefer not to flush the line while measuring. If the aortic cannula pressure is 3 to 10 mm Hg greater than the radial artery systolic pressure, we know that reversal of the normal pressure relationships exist. In this situation, we prefer to continue monitoring from the aortic cannula for ten minutes following cardiopulmonary bypass. In the majority of published studies, the inaccuracies in radial artery blood pressure monitoring were shown to disappear after approximately ten minutes. Although the mechanism that produces falsely low radial pressures is not known, it is certainly possible that vasoconstriction in the radial or brachial arterial system may contribute. Using this as a working hypothesis, we administer low doses of sodium nitroprusside during the ten-minute period. In the vast majority of cases, this treatment will result in a radial artery pressure equal to or exceeding that of the simultaneous aortic pressure within a matter of a few minutes.

DISCUSSION

Occasionally the outlined approach will not result in accurate radial artery blood pressures. If this approach fails, the physician can continue to measure the arterial pressure from the aortic cannula while a 125-cm heparin-coated wire guide (Amplatz wire guide; Cook, Inc.; Bloomington, Ind) is threaded through the radial catheter up into the axillary artery. The existing indwelling radial catheter is then removed over the wire, and a 65-cm 5F angiographic catheter (Angiographic catheter; Cook, Inc.; Bloomington, Ind) is fed over the wire through the percutaneous radial arteriotomy and up into the axillary or subclavian artery. This procedure can be reasonably accomplished in a few minutes and will give a more central aortic blood pressure. Embolization of clot or air can be a hazard when using these long catheters. Consequently, they must be flushed with very small volumes of flushing solution, preferably 0.5 ml/flush.

Another obvious approach is to cannulate a femoral artery. The femoral artery is usually easy to cannulate, but approximately 0.5% of femoral cannulations will result in ischemia of the leg, requiring embolectomy.[5, 6] Hematomas occur in 8% to 13% of patients after femoral artery cannulation.[7] Because of these potential complications, we prefer the approach outlined above.

REFERENCES

1. Barash PG, Kopriva CJ: Anesthesia for cardiac surgery, in Glenn W, et al (eds): *Thoracic and Cardiovascular Surgery,* ed 4. Norwalk, Conn, Appleton-Century-Crofts, 1983, chap 73, pp 1083–1085.
2. Stern DH, Gerson JI, Allan FB, et al: Can we trust the direct radial artery pressure immediately following cardiopulmonary bypass? *Anesthesiology* 1982; 57:A174.
3. Gravlee GP, Pauca AL, Cordell AR, et al: Comparison of brachial, radial and aortic arterial pressure monitoring during cardiac surgery. *Anesthesiology* 1984; 61:A69.
4. Beker B, LaFontaine E, Lin CY: Accuracy of radial artery pressure monitoring. Abstracts, Fifth Annual Meeting, Society of Cardiovascular Anesthesiologists, 1983, p 198.
5. Colvin MP, Curran JP, Jarvis D: Femoral artery pressure monitoring. *Anaesthesia* 1977; 32:451.
6. Gurman G, Nebler R, Shachar J: The use of alpha-system set for arterial catheterization. *Anaesthesist* 1980; 29:494.
7. Ersoz CJ, Hedden M, Lain L: Prolonged femoral arterial catheterization for intensive care. *Anesth Analg* 1970; 49:160.

3

Ruptured Pulmonary Artery With Swan-Ganz Catheter

Recommendations by Paul G. Barash, M.D.

A 45-year-old woman undergoing mitral valve surgery for mitral stenosis had a history of pulmonary artery hypertension. She had an uneventful placement of a Swan-Ganz catheter prior to induction. At the end of cardiopulmonary bypass, prior to weaning, the pulmonary artery tracings appeared damped and flushing and inflation of the balloon failed to produce acceptable tracings or wedge pressures. Ventilation was impaired by a decrease in compliance and blood was noted in the endotracheal tube.

ANALYSIS OF PROBLEM

Pulmonary artery perforation, probably the most catastrophic complication associated with pulmonary artery catheterization, occurs in approximately 1 in 1,500 patients.[1, 2] Several factors have been identified as placing a patient at greater risk for pulmonary artery perforation. These include: advanced age, hypothermia, pulmonary hypertension. Furthermore, females appear to have a higher incidence of perforation than do males. Although heparinization is not a risk factor, it appears that patients who have received heparin are at a greater risk for larger blood loss and mortality.

APPROACH TO THE PROBLEM

Treatment is supportive in nature. Initially the "good lung" should be protected. If a double lumen endotracheal tube is not available, the ordinary single lumen endotracheal tube should be advanced into the main stem bronchus of the noninvolved lung (usually the left). If the patient has received heparin, reversal with protamine should be accomplished as soon as possible. Massive blood and fluid replacement may be required, and positive end expiratory pressure (PEEP) also has been advocated in an attempt to compress the vascular site of perforation. Following initial resuscitation, diagnostic procedures should be undertaken. These include fiberoptic bronchoscopy and pulmonary wedge angiogram to locate the specific vascular site of bleeding. The importance of determining the exact site of the perforation becomes obvious if surgical intervention (such as lobectomy and pneumonectomy) is required.

DISCUSSION

Causes

Deviation from standard insertion techniques has been noted in a significant number of case reports. This complication is usually associated with distal migration of the catheter and balloon inflation. Pulmonary artery hypertension, by distending smaller pulmonary arteries thus allowing the catheter to wedge in a more distal location, also leads to distal placement. In addition, pulmonary hypertension leads to degenerative changes in the vessel wall such as sclerosis and aneurysmal dilatation. These predispose to vessel rupture. The use of a liquid in the balloon may cause failure of the balloon to deflate. Therefore,

OVERWEDGING

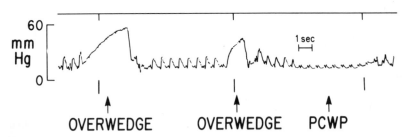

FIG 3–1.
Intraoperative pulmonary artery pressure tracing that demonstrates overwedging patterns observed with balloon inflation. This pattern results from the catheter tip impinging against the vessel wall or balloon herniation over the catheter tip (see Fig 3–2). The pulmonary artery catheter is withdrawn 3 cm and a normal transition from pulmonary artery to capillary wedge pressure is obtained. (From Barash PG, et al: Catheter-induced pulmonary artery perforation: Mechanisms, management and modifications. *J Thorac Cardiovasc Surg* 1981; 82:5. Used by permission.)

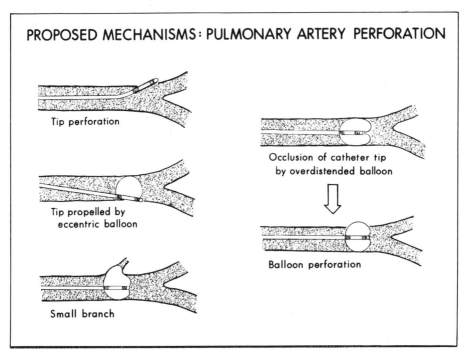

PROPOSED MECHANISMS: PULMONARY ARTERY PERFORATION

Tip perforation

Tip propelled by
eccentric balloon

Small branch

Occlusion of catheter tip
by overdistended balloon

Balloon perforation

FIG 3–2.
Possible mechanisms of pulmonary artery perforation. (From Barash PG, et al: Catheter-induced pulmonary artery perforation. Mechanisms, management and modifications. *J Thorac Cardiovasc Surg* 1981; 82:5. Used by permission.)

only gas (air or CO_2) should be used for balloon inflation. A common technical error is the use of less than 1.5 cc to inflate the balloon. This allows the catheter tip to be placed in a more distal and smaller vessel. Subsequent inflation with 1.5 cc can overdistend and rupture the vessel. The diagnosis of a distal location for the catheter tip may be made by the phenomenon of "overwedging" (Fig 3–1). This results from impingement of the tip of the catheter against the vessel wall or herniation of the balloon over the catheter tip.

Several mechanisms of pulmonary artery perforation have been demonstrated (Fig 3–2). Inflation of the balloon with a distally located catheter results in a direct tearing of the vessel. Balloon inflation can expose the catheter tip and propel the catheter through the arterial wall. The tip of the catheter may also become lodged in a small vascular branch and erode or perforate the vessel. Finally, direct perforation also may occur during insertion.

Prevention

To reduce the incidence of pulmonary artery perforation, guidelines have been suggested for management of the catheter especially in the high-risk group of patients. Balloon inflation should be kept to a minimum. The catheter should be very proximal in location, approximately 4 to 5 cm beyond the pulmonic valve. Some clinicians have advocated withdrawing the catheter to a central venous pressure (CVP) position during cardiopulmonary bypass so that manipulation of the heart will not propel the catheter tip distally during cardiopulmonary bypass.

Diagnosis

The sudden appearance of bright red blood in the airway of a patient who has a pulmonary artery catheter should suggest the diagnosis of pulmonary artery perforation. This episode is usually temporally related to a balloon inflation or catheter manipulation. Hemoptysis also has been associated with flushing the catheter while it is in a wedge position.

REFERENCES

1. Barash PG, Nardi D, Hammond G, et al: Catheter-induced pulmonary artery perforation. Mechanisms, management and modifications. *J Thorac Cardiovasc Surg* 1981; 82:5.
2. Keefer JR, Barash PG: Pulmonary artery catheterization, in Blitt CD (ed): *Monitoring in Anesthesia and Critical Care Medicine*. New York, Churchill Livingstone, Inc, 1985, pp 177–228.

4

Aortic Dissection With Cardiopulmonary Bypass Arterial Cannula

Recommendations by William E. Johnston, M.D.

A 75-year-old man with a history of calcific aortic stenosis was scheduled for aortic valve replacement surgery. The induction, sternotomy, and placement of pump-oxygenator cannulae were uneventful except for the surgeon's noticing that the aortic tissues were abnormally thin and calcified. The aortic purse strings and cannula appeared well placed, but just as cardiopulmonary bypass commenced aortic pump perfusion pressure increased and systemic blood pressure decreased. The aorta appeared acutely dilated.

ANALYSIS OF THE PROBLEM

Acute aortic dissection following cannulation of the ascending aorta is an infrequent but serious complication of cardiac surgery. For proper treatment, the diagnosis must be made early and thus requires a high index of suspicion at the time of cannulation as well as during cardiopulmonary bypass.[1] The evidence is not always as clear as it is in the case presented here; as Benedict and associates have pointed out, with dissection, "the signs of impending disaster may be completely absent until the fatal event has occurred."[2]

APPROACH TO THE PROBLEM

The key to proper management of acute aortic dissection is a rapid diagnosis. Warning signs (whether from antegrade or retrograde dissections) are a sudden unexplained decrease in venous return and in mean arterial pressure, associated with an acute elevation of arterial line pressure, and bluish discoloration and enlargement of the aortic root. Often the last of these signs may easily be confused with bleeding around the aortic cannula, and it is at this point that a high index of suspicion of aortic dissection is most useful.

The patient whose case is discussed here has just sustained a type A aortic dissection with involvement of the ascending aorta and possible extension to the descending aorta.[3] The observed condition of the aortic wall at the time of cannulation should increase the index of suspicion. Typically, this antegrade dissection occurs at the institution of cardiopulmonary bypass, with the dissection process occurring in the direction of blood flow.[1] Cardiopulmonary bypass must be continued—although only after the pump perfusion pressure has been acutely reduced—until another vessel, usually the femoral artery, can be cannulated[1, 4] or until the true aortic lumen can be cannulated at a more distal site on the aortic arch.[5, 6] The aorta is then cross-clamped just below the innominate artery, and cardioplegia is delivered either through an isolated portion of the proximal aortic root or directly into the coronary ostia. Core cooling to 28° C and topical myocardial hypothermia are achieved rapidly. The aorta must be opened to expose the site of intimal disruption, which is then resected and replaced by a tubular graft and the false lumen obliterated with Teflon buttresses. The coronary vessels may require reimplantation if their patency is threatened by the dissecting hematoma.

DISCUSSION

Pathophysiology

For aortic dissection to occur, two factors are necessary: (1) an initiating event, usually an intimal tear and (2) propagation of the dissecting process from hydrodynamic forces.[3] Predisposing factors for dissection are various diseases that weaken the aortic wall, such as cystic medial necrosis, the elastic or medial degeneration associated with aging, atheromatous disease, and poststenotic dilatation.[1]

Death is usually caused by rupture with exsanguination, retrograde dissection causing cardiac tamponade or acute aortic regurgitation, or multiorgan hypoperfusion secondary to luminal narrowing from the progressive dissection process. Despite aggressive treatment, mortality rates of 24% to 60% are reported.[1, 2]

Aortic cannulation can cause the initiating intimal disruption. The number of aortic cross-clamp applications and the ratchet setting at which the clamp is applied can also contribute to direct intimal damage.[1, 7] In one patient reported by Salama and Blesovsky, cross-clamping the aorta a third time caused aortic dissection with shearing of the right coronary artery.[8] In a postmortem study of 45 patients, 5 of 7 aortic dissections had begun at the site of cross-clamping.[7]

The site of cannulation also has an impact on the incidence of aortic dissection. Retrograde aortic dissection secondary to femoral arterial cannulation has occurred in 0.6% to 3.0% of patients,[2, 9–12] which represents a greater incidence than that of antegrade dissection secondary to cannulation of the ascending aorta (0% to 0.1%).[1, 13–15]

Retrograde dissection appears secondary to the trauma of cannulation, particularly that with large cannulae,[15] as well as to the jet of retrograde perfusion against the normal flow of arterial blood.[12] Retrograde dissection also occurs more commonly in patients over 40 years of age, which underscores the significance of atheromatous disease. In one study, the incidence of unsuspected dissection found at autopsy was similar to that of clinically apparent cases,[9] which would suggest that the overall incidence of retrograde dissection may be higher than originally thought. Some authors have recommended aortic arch cannulation in preference to femoral artery cannulation because the former eliminates the possibility of retrograde dissection.[8, 9, 14, 16]

When extent rather than incidence of aortic dissection is considered, hydrodynamic forces have a greater influence than site of cannulation. The most influential of these forces are the blood pressure and the steepness of the pulse wave (or dP/dt); blood viscosity, velocity, and turbulence play lesser roles.[1] A clinical report by Wheat and colleagues in 1965 implicated the acceleration of cardiac output, or "impulse" (a direct function of myocardial contractility) as the most important propagating factor.[17] However, in a later experimental study, Carney and coworkers found mean arterial pressure to be more influential than contractility with respect to the extent of dissection.[18] In dogs with a surgically created pocket in the descending aorta, acute reduction of dP/dt with propranolol, 2 mg/kg, did not lower mean arterial pressure, nor alter the progression of dissection. However, if, in addition to the reduction in dP/dt, the mean systemic pressure were lowered to 90 torr with an infusion of trimethaphan camsylate, the dissection was no longer progressive. Carney et al. concluded that blood pressure control in addition to decreasing dP/dt is essential to limit the extent of dissection. Similar results were found by Moran et al.[19] in whose study infusions of trimethaphan, trimethaphan and propranolol, or nitroprusside and propranolol decreased the extent of dissection from 99% (control) to 24% to 43% ($P < 0.02$). Propranolol, which decreased dP/dt without reducing systolic pressure, or nitroprusside, which decreased systolic pressure while increasing dP/dt, did not limit the dissection process alone.

Additional Considerations

Retrograde Aortic Dissection

If this patient had had a retrograde aortic dissection secondary to femoral arterial cannulation, it could have occurred anytime during bypass. Immediate therapy would then be rapid reduction of the blood pressure to 20 to 30 torr by decreasing pump perfusion and reestablishing antegrade blood flow.[2] In cases of retrograde aortic dissection, if the operation is near completion, the heart may be transfused and bypass discontinued. Otherwise, the aortic arch must be cannulated rapidly and bypass resumed to allow completion of the operation.[15] Gosalbez et al. report one case in which recannulation of the aortic arch was not feasible and they continued the bypass successfully by lowering bypass flow and perfusion pressure, monitoring the patient carefully for signs of central nervous system or renal ischemia, and completing the procedure at maximal speed.[20] With retrograde aortic dissection, extreme care must be taken during coronary artery bypass surgery to ensure that the proximal end of the saphenous vein is sewn to the true aortic lumen or to the right subclavian artery.

Postoperative Care

The morbidity and mortality from aortic dissections result from uncontrollable aortic bleeding and isolated hypoperfusion of major organs, such as the brain,[5, 6, 15, 21, 22] spinal cord,[1] kidneys,[5, 23] and heart.[9, 23] The clinician should watch for the development of aortic valvular insufficiency[2] or cardiac tamponade[23] due to continuation of the dissecting process.

Postoperatively, in this patient, aggressive blood pressure control is necessary to decrease aortic bleeding and the chance of further dissection.[17] An intravenous (IV) drip infusion of trimethaphan camsylate (1 to 2 mg/ml concentration) can be titrated to lower systolic pressure to 100 mm Hg.[17, 18, 24] As a ganglionic blocker with properties of a smooth-muscle relaxant, trimethaphan has the advantage of decreasing both arterial pressure and myocardial contractility. The disadvantages of using trimethaphan include a tendency for tachyphylaxis and the development of mydriasis secondary to parasympathetic inhibition, which makes neurologic assessment difficult. Alternatively, sodium nitroprusside (1 mg/5-ml concentration) can be titrated for blood pressure control. However, since both the force of contraction and the heart rate may increase with nitroprusside,[19, 25] propranolol (1 to 2 mg IV as necessary) must be given as well. Other less commonly used drugs that can be considered are methyldopa, reserpine, and guanethidine.[24]

Summary

As with most perioperative complications, prevention is superior to subsequent management. Aortic arch cannulation appears to have a lower incidence of dissection than femoral arterial cannulation.[8] Effective measures to reduce the incidence of aortic dissection during aortic cannulation include: (1) blood pressure control at the time of cannulation; (2) insertion of the cannula at a right angle to the aorta to prevent dissection of tissue planes, with special caution being taken to locate the tip in the true lumen of the aorta; (3) blood pressure reduction when the aorta cross-clamp is applied or removed; and (4) use of atraumatic clamps with as few applications to the aorta as possible. The anesthesiologist should maintain a high index of suspicion for this rare but potentially disastrous complication of cardiopulmonary bypass.

REFERENCES

1. Litchford B, Okies JE, Sugimura S, et al: Acute aortic dissection from cross-clamp injury. *J Thorac Cardiovasc Surg* 1976; 72:709–713.
2. Benedict JS, Buhl TL, Henney RP: Acute aortic dissection during cardiopulmonary bypass: Successful treatment of three patients. *Arch Surg* 1974; 108:810–813.
3. Wheat MW Jr: Acute dissecting aneurysms of the aorta: Diagnosis and treatment—1979. *Am Heart J* 1980; 99:373–387.
4. Flick WF, Hallermann FJ, Feldt RH, et al: Aneurysm of aortic cannulation site: Successful repair by means of peripheral cannulation, profound hypothermia, and circulatory arrest. *J Thorac Cardiovasc Surg* 1971; 61:419–423.
5. Reinke RT, Harris RD, Klein AJ, et al: Aortoiliac dissection due to aortic cannulation. *Ann Thorac Surg* 1974; 18:295–299.
6. Cooley DA, Wukasch DC, Hallman GL: Acute dissecting ascending aortic aneurysm resulting from coronary arteriography: Successful surgical treatment. *Chest* 1972; 61:317–319.
7. Black LL, McComb RJ, Silver MD: Vascular injury following heart valve replacement. *Ann Thorac Surg* 1973; 16:19–29.
8. Salama FD, Blesovsky A: Complications of cannulation of the ascending aorta for open heart surgery. *Thorax* 1970; 25:604–607.
9. Kay JH, Dykstra PC, Tsuji HK: Retrograde ilioaortic dissection: A complication of common femoral artery perfusion during open heart surgery. *Am J Surg* 1966; 111:464–468.
10. Jones TW, Vetto RR, Winterscheid LC, et al: Arterial complications incident to cannulation in open-heart surgery: With special reference to the femoral artery. *Ann Surg* 1960; 152:969–974.
11. Matar AF, Ross DN: Traumatic arterial dissection in open-heart surgery. *Thorax* 1967; 22:82–87.
12. Bilgutay AM, Garamella JJ, Danyluk M, et al: Retrograde aortic dissection occurring during cardiopulmonary bypass: Successful repair and concomitant subclavian-to-coronary artery vein bypass. *JAMA* 1976; 236:465–468.
13. Salerno TA, Lince DP, White DN, et al: Arch versus femoral artery perfusion during cardiopulmonary bypass. *J Thorac Cardiovasc Surg* 1978; 76:681–684.
14. Roe BB, Kelly PB: Perfusion through the ascending aorta: Experience with 410 cases. *Ann Thorac Surg* 1969; 7:238–241.

15. Carey JS, Skow JR, Scott C: Retrograde aortic dissection during cardiopulmonary bypass: "Nonoperative" management. *Ann Thorac Surg* 1977; 24:44–48.
16. Lefrak EA, Howell JF: Successful surgical management of acute retrograde dissection of the aorta during coronary artery bypass. *J Thorac Cardiovasc Surg* 1972; 63:149–153.
17. Wheat MW Jr, Palmer RF, Bartley TD, et al: Treatment of dissecting aneurysms of the aorta without surgery. *J Thorac Cardiovasc Surg* 1965; 50:364–373.
18. Carney WI Jr, Rheinlander HF, Cleveland RJ: Control of acute aortic dissection. *Surgery* 1975; 78:114–120.
19. Moran JF, Derkac WM, Conkle DM: Pharmacologic control of acute aortic dissection in hypertensive dogs. *Surg Forum* 1978; 29:231–236.
20. Gosalbez F, Cofiño JL, Naya JL, et al: Retrograde aortic dissection, letter. *Ann Thorac Surg* 1979; 28:608.
21. Michaels I, Sheehan J: EEG changes due to unsuspected aortic dissection during cardiopulmonary bypass. *Anesth Analg* 1984; 63:946–948.
22. Elliott DP, Roe BB: Aortic dissection during cardiopulmonary bypass. *J Thorac Cardiovasc Surg* 1965; 50:357–363.
23. Miller DC, Mitchell RS, Oyer PE, et al: Independent determinants of operative mortality for patients with aortic dissections. *Circulation* 1984; 70(suppl I): I153–I164.
24. Wheat MW Jr: Current status of medical therapy of acute dissecting aneurysms of the aorta. *World J Surg* 1980; 4:563–569.
25. Bolooki H: Management of aortic dissection. *J Fla Med Assoc* 1979; 66:1064–1069.

5

Increased Central Venous Pressure During Cardiopulmonary Bypass

Recommendations by Russell F. Hill, M.D.

A 52-year-old man was just placed on cardiopulmonary bypass after customary placement of the aortic cannula and a Sarns single venous cannula in the right atrium. There was a fall in the arterial and pulmonary arterial pressures and a rapid fall in the pump oxygenator venous reservoir volume. The central venous pressure recorded from the right atrium read zero, but there was obvious venous engorgement in the face and neck.

ANALYSIS OF THE PROBLEM

Collection of deoxygenated venous blood from the patient and delivery to the pump oxygenator are essential functions of any cardiopulmonary bypass circuit. Access to the venous system is gained peripherally when the femoral vein is used or centrally when the right atrium is cannulated after sternotomy. In procedures involving the right side of the heart, cannulation of both the superior and inferior venae cavae is necessary to accomplish "total" cardiopulmonary bypass. The right side of the heart is isolated from the venous circulation by tapes encircling the cannulae so that caval blood is diverted from the right atrium. In procedures not involving the right side of the heart, requiring partial bypass, both cavae may be cannulated with or without tapes. Alternatively, the right atrium alone or the right atrium and the inferior vena cava are cannulated by using a single two-stage cavoatrial catheter.[1,2] A 1980 survey of cardiac surgeons performing coronary revascularization revealed a prefer-

27

ence for single atrial cannulation by 50.5%, separate cannulation of the cavae without tapes by 35.4% and with tapes by 24.1%.[3]

At the onset of bypass, blood drains from the patient through the venous cannula and connecting tubing to the oxygenator by gravity flow. Assuming adequate patient elevation, blood flows freely with very little pressure gradient along the pathway.

Impairment of venous drainage may have several causes. The common causes of mechanical obstruction are failure to remove a venous line clamp, a kink, or air-lock due to large air bubbles in the venous line.[4] Incorrect positioning of cannulae may impede venous flow. For example, when two cannulae are used, the superior vena cava (SVC) cannula can be placed in the azygous vein or, if advanced too far cephalad, in the innominate vein. The inferior caval cannula may be inadvertently positioned into the hepatic vein.[5] With single cannulation, the tip of an atrial cannula, or the large stage port of a two-stage cavoatrial cannula should be positioned near the coronary sinus at the junction of the inferior vena cava and the right atrium.[2]

Obstruction of venous drainage can be detected by observing a change in the level of blood-prime mixture in the pump venous reservoir. The level should remain fairly constant over any short time interval. A rapid decline in reservoir volume suggests that more blood is being delivered to the patient than is returning to the pump, most likely due to an obstruction. This problem is associated with an increase in venous pressure distal to the site of cannulation. Increased venous pressure can be detected with a continuously transduced catheter placed with its tip in the superior vena cava. Right atrial pressure is often significantly lower than SVC pressure during bypass.[6] Monitoring pressure in the right atrium, as is done through the proximal port of a pulmonary artery catheter, may not detect pressure elevation in the SVC and therefore underestimate venous obstruction. Finlayson and Kaplan recommend routine monitoring of SVC pressure while the patient is on bypass.[7] Reduced drainage from the SVC can result in venous engorgement of the head and neck, which is detected by visual inspection. Lack of drainage from the right side of the heart may result in dilatation of the left ventricle, which is detected by direct inspection of the heart or by an increase in pulmonary artery or left atrial pressures if these are being monitored.

APPROACH TO THE PROBLEM

Bypass management of a patient who demonstrates obvious venous engorgement of the upper body because of reduced venous return to the oxygenator requires immediate identification and correction of the obstruction. The operating team is informed of the problem. The venous line is inspected for kinks, clamps, or large bubbles and, if present, they are removed. The venous cannula is meticulously checked and, if necessary, repositioned to ensure proper flow from both cavae. Only after adequate venous return is established with recovery of volume in the venous reservoir of the oxygenator is bypass continued.

DISCUSSION

Obstruction of venous return to the pump-oxygenator reservoir that is unrecognized or not corrected can result in serious complications. Cerebral blood flow in the normal brain is maintained over a wide range of cerebral perfusion pressure (mean arterial pressure minus cerebral venous pressure) by autoregulation. When cerebral perfusion pressure is reduced to about 40 mm Hg, brain tissue perfusion fails.[8] A prolonged increase in superior vena cava pressure, by decreasing cerebral perfusion pressure below the lower limit of autoregulatory compensation, may lead to ischemic injury of the normothermic brain. Elevated hydrostatic pressure within the cerebral capillaries in addition to low oncotic pressure associated with hemodilution may cause cerebral edema as described by Starling's law of capillary-interstitial fluid exchange.

Inadequate drainage from the right side of the heart can result in elevation of right and left ventricular wall tension by increasing both ventricular pressure and dimension. Excess wall tension leads to lower myocardial perfusion pressure, higher energy demands, and possible myocardial ischemia.

In summary, when properly positioned, both single and double cannulas provide adequate venous return during bypass in most cases. It is the responsibility of the anesthesiologist, perfusionist, and surgeon to ensure proper venous drainage. Constant observation of the pump-oxygenator venous reservoir level, frequent inspection of the patient's heart and head, and reliable monitoring of superior vena cava pressure will result in early diagnosis of impaired venous return. Immediate correction of any obstruction is necessary to prevent complications from this potential problem during cardiopulmonary bypass.

REFERENCES

1. Cooley DA: *Techniques in Cardiac Surgery*. Philadelphia, WB Saunders Co, 1984.
2. Doty OB: *Cardiac Surgery*. Chicago, Year Book Medical Publishers Inc, 1985.
3. Miller DW Jr, Ivey TD, Bailey WW, et al: The practice of coronary artery bypass surgery in 1980. *J Thorac Cardiovasc Surg* 1981; 81:423–427.
4. Branthwaite MA: Extracorporeal circulation and associated techniques, in Branthwaite MA: *Anesthesia for Cardiac Surgery*. Oxford, England, Blackwell Scientific Publications, 1980, pp 148–170.

5. Taylor PC, Effler DB: Management of cannulation for cardiopulmonary bypass in patients with adult-acquired heart disease. *Surg Clin North Am* 1975; 55:1205–1215.
6. Bennett EV Jr, Fewel JG, Ybarra J, et al: Comparison of flow differences among venous cannulas. *Ann Thorac Surg* 1983; 36:59–65.
7. Finlayson DC, Kaplan JA: Cardiopulmonary bypass in Kaplan JA (ed): *Cardiac Anesthesia*. New York, Grune & Stratton, 1979, pp 393–440.
8. Lassen NA: Control of cerebral circulation in health and disease. *Circ Res* 1974; 34:749–760.

6

Low Perfusion Pressure
With the Onset of
Cardiopulmonary Bypass

Recommendations by Ann V. Govier, M.D.

A 65-year-old man in good general health except for severe coronary artery disease underwent coronary artery bypass grafting. On physical examination he had bilateral carotid bruits but no history of neurologic events. Preoperative noninvasive vascular studies revealed no significant carotid occlusive disease. Induction and sternotomy were uneventful but, with the onset of coronary artery bypass, the perfusion pressure dropped to 30 mm Hg, despite a pump perfusion flow of 2.2 L/minute/m^2 at 28° C.

ANALYSIS OF PROBLEM

Systemic perfusion pressure is markedly reduced in this patient with a history of atherosclerotic cardiovascular disease and the preoperative finding of bilateral carotid bruits. A decision must be made regarding the presumed adequacy of cerebral perfusion in this patient.

APPROACH TO THE PROBLEM

Since it is known by noninvasive studies that this patient does not have significant carotid disease, I do not believe therapy with a vasoconstrictor is necessary. The hypothermia (28° C) and perfusion flow (2.2 L/minute/m^2) should provide adequate cerebral and other organ perfusion despite the lowered perfusion pressure.

DISCUSSION

The development of cardiopulmonary bypass (CPB) has been essential to the remarkable improvements in the surgical management of cardiac diseases. Although advances in technique and equipment have substantially reduced morbidity and mortality related to CPB, unpredictable permanent and transient central nervous system complications continue to occur. The exact causes of central nervous system injury following uncomplicated open-heart surgery are not known.

Early studies by Tufo et al.[1] in 1970 and Stockard et al.[2] in 1973 concluded that mean arterial pressure (MAP) during CPB needed to be maintained at greater than 50 mm Hg to avoid postoperative disorders of cerebral function, presumably due to inadequate cerebral blood flow (CBF). However, Kolkka and Hilberman[3] in 1980 and Slogoff et al.[4] in 1982 were unable to confirm the relationship between postoperative cerebral dysfunction and perfusion pressure less than 50 mm Hg during hypothermic CPB.

Important questions related to this case presentation are as follows: does perfusion pressure correlate with CBF; does cerebral autoregulation exist on CPB, and what is the significance of carotid bruits?

Pathophysiology of Cerebral Circulation

Major Cerebral Blood Supply

Perfusion of the normal brain is supplied primarily by the carotid and vertebral arteries. Normally, the majority of the CBF is supplied through the carotid arteries. The left carotid and left subclavian arteries are direct branches of the aortic arch. The right carotid and right subclavian arteries arise from the innominate branch of the aorta. The vertebral arteries are given off by the subclavian arteries.

Under normal physiologic conditions, perfusion of the normal brain is maintained by two intrinsic characteristics: the adequate provision of anastomotic channels or collaterals and the inherent ability of the cerebral vasculature to autoregulate over a wide range of perfusion pressures.

The major arteries to the brain communicate with each other through the arterial anastomosis that forms the circle of Willis. The circle of Willis connects the vertebral and internal carotid arteries to each other and to the vessels of the contralateral side. Under physiologic conditions, the adequacy of the collateral circulation is dependent primarily on the circle of Willis and this is one of the more important sources of collateral blood supply in patients with occlusive disease of the carotid artery. However, anastomotic channels also exist between the external carotid and vertebral arteries (the occipital artery) and the external and internal carotid arteries (the superficial temporal and ophthalmic arteries). In addition to the anastomotic vessels at the base of the brain, there is fairly extensive anastomosis of pial vessels that contribute to collateral blood flow. Under normal conditions, flow does not cross over within the circle of Willis. If flow is decreased and thus pressure decreased in one carotid system, crossover flow through the communicating arteries will divert blood to the compromised region.

A major extrinsic physiologic factor contributing to the overall perfusion of the brain is the cerebral perfusion pressure. Cerebral perfusion pressure (CPP) is the difference between the mean arterial blood pressure (MAP) and the intracranial pressure (ICP): CPP = MAP − ICP. Since in the normal person the ICP does not vary markedly (normal range: 10 to 15 mm Hg while supine),[5] the MAP is the major factor affecting CPP. In normothermic, normotensive, awake man, a decrease of perfusion pressure less than 50 mm Hg is associated with decreases in CBF and the potential for cerebral ischemia exists.

Regulation of Cerebral Blood Flow

Physiologic control of cerebral circulation is maintained by an interaction of a number of responses including autoregulation or myogenic, metabolic, chemical, and possibly neurogenic vascular responses.

Autoregulation, often referred to as myogenic control, is the ability of a vascular bed to alter its resistance in response to a pressure change whereby the flow remains relatively constant (Fig 6–1). In normotensive, normothermic hu-

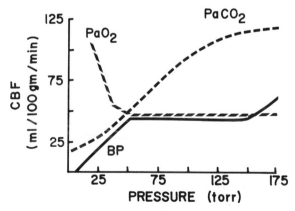

FIG 6–1.
Relationship between cerebral blood flow (CBF) and mean arterial pressure (BP), arterial carbon dioxide ($PaCO_2$) and oxygen tension (PaO_2). When one variable is altered, the other two variables remain stable at normal values. (From Shapiro HM: Anesthesia effects upon cerebral blood flow, cerebral metabolism, electroencephalogram, and evoked potentials, in Miller RD (ed): *Anesthesia*, ed 2. New York, Churchill Livingstone, vol 2, 1986. Used by permission.)

man beings with normal cerebrovascular status, autoregulation maintains CBF near a constant value over a wide range of cerebral perfusion pressures (50 to 150 mm Hg). The exact mechanism for autoregulation is not completely understood; however, it is not dependent on the autonomic nervous system. Of importance is that autoregulation may be impaired by anesthetic agents, trauma, hypoxia, chronic hypertension, known cerebrovascular disease, and other abnormal states.

The brain has a high rate of aerobic metabolism and thus depends on continuous blood flow for proper functioning. Metabolic control of CBF refers to the close association between the level of oxidative metabolism in brain tissue and blood flow. As the metabolic rate increases or the relative supply of oxygen within areas of the brain decreases, release of local metabolites occurs resulting in regional vasodilatation. It is believed that an increase of the hydrogen ion concentration rather than a decrease in oxygen is considered the major metabolic factor coupling flow and metabolism.

Cerebral blood flow and metabolism are well known to be temperature dependent. Hypothermia lowers the cerebral metabolic oxygen requirement. With decreasing temperature, there is an exponential decrease in cerebral metabolic rate of oxygen ($CMRO_2$), which is approximately matched by a decrease in cerebral blood flow. Hypothermia is an important factor in the metabolic control of CBF and probably the most effective procedure with which to depress metabolic activity.

Chemical control of CBF is mediated by alteration of arterial oxygen (PaO_2) and carbon dioxide tension ($PaCO_2$) (Fig 6–1). One of the most potent physiologic determinants of CBF is the tension of CO_2 in the arterial blood. A near linear relationship exists between CBF and $PaCO_2$: there is a 4% rise in CBF for each 1 mm Hg increase in $PaCO_2$ between a $PaCO_2$ of 20 to 80 mm Hg.[6] Above 80 mm Hg a near maximal vasodilatation occurs and little further increase in CBF is observed. In awake, normothermic man, the decrease in CBF with hypocapnia is also limited and minimal flow is reached at about 20 mm Hg of $PaCO_2$. Moderate changes in arterial oxygen tension (PaO_2) do not measurably influence CBF. However, with a marked arterial hypoxia (PaO_2 less than 50 mm Hg), CBF does increase.[7]

The precise role of neurogenic control is still highly controversial. Both adrenergic and cholinergic nerves innervate extracranial and intracranial blood vessels.[8] The size of pial vessels can be notably affected by stimulation of these nerves. However, the response of these vessels to stimuli such as hypoxia and hypercapnia appears to be similar whether the nervous pathways are intact or not. Neurogenic control is probably not of major importance under normal circumstances but may play a significant role under nonphysiologic states.

Pharmacology (Effect of Anesthesia)

Many anesthetic agents are known to influence CBF and cerebral metabolism ($CMRO_2$). However, there is no obvious common denominator that characterizes the effects of anesthetics on CBF and $CMRO_2$.

Inhalational Agents

The inhalational anesthetics appear to increase CBF while reducing $CMRO_2$. This apparent disassociation or uncoupling of the flow and metabolism does not occur with the intravenous anesthetics. Volatile anesthetic agents and other drugs with the capacity to produce cerebrovascular dilatation can modify and even abolish autoregulation. High doses of volatile anesthetic agents can cause a total loss of autoregulation, i.e., CBF becomes blood-pressure dependent (Fig 6–2). The increase in CBF and decrease in $CMRO_2$ are progressive (but not linearly related) with increasing concentrations of halothane, enflurane, and isoflurane, with the major effect ocurring at or below 1 minimum alveolar concentration (MAC).

Increasing doses of halothane progressively increase CBF, which in turn increases cerebral blood volume and ICP. Among the volatile anesthetics, halothane appears to be the most potent of the cerebral vasodilators. A majority of the studies indicate about a 25% reduction in $CMRO_2$ at approximately 1% inspired halothane.[9]

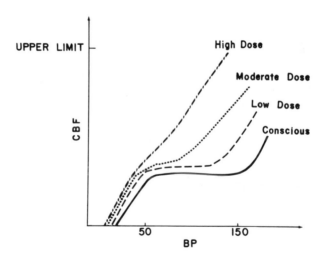

FIG 6–2.
The effects of an increasing dose of a volatile anesthetic agent on cerebrovascular autoregulation. (From Shapiro HM: Anesthesia effects upon cerebral blood flow, cerebral metabolism, electroencephalogram, and evoked potentials, in Miller RD (ed): *Anesthesia,* ed 2. New York, Churchill Livingstone, vol 2, 1986. Used by permission.)

Enflurane is a weaker cerebral vasodilator than halothane but is the most potent depressant of $CMRO_2$ (25 to 35% decrease at 1 MAC^9). Enflurane in high concentrations can cause generalized seizures, which in turn cause a marked increase in CBF and brain metabolism.[10]

Isoflurane increases CBF and ICP while decreasing the cerebral metabolic rate. Hyperventilation instituted simultaneously with isoflurane may be adequate to block the increase in the ICP.

The effect of nitrous oxide on both CBF and $CMRO_2$ in man has not been clearly established. The weight of evidence does suggest that it will cause a slight decrease in $CMRO_2$ with a modest increase in CBF.[11]

Intravenous Anesthetics

Intravenous anesthetics differ significantly from inhalational agents in regard to their effects on CBF and $CMRO_2$.

Among all anesthetics, barbiturates are recognized to be the most potent depressants of $CMRO_2$. The metabolic depression with barbiturates affects primarily the cells' energy requirements for neurophysiologic function rather than the requirements to maintain cellular integrity.[10] Barbiturates do not appear to uncouple the normal relationship between CBF and cerebral metabolic rate, thus as $CMRO_2$ falls so does the CBF. Hence, because barbiturates reduce CBF and cerebral blood volume, they can also lower ICP significantly. Due to a greater decrease in MAP than ICP, a reduction in cerebral perfusion pressure may be seen with barbiturates.

Studies in man have not thoroughly examined the effects of narcotics on CBF and $CMRO_2$. It has been demonstrated in normal man that morphine-nitrous oxide anesthesia causes minimal decrease in CBF (with normocapnia) and moderate decreases in $CMRO_2$.[12] Fentanyl has been shown in normal man not to significantly influence CBF or $CMRO_2$ with normocapnia maintained.[13]

Diazepam, midazolam, and lorazepam cause a modest decrease in CBF and $CMRO_2$, theoretically decreasing intracranial pressure when it is elevated.

The effects of neuroleptics on human CBF and $CMRO_2$ have not been carefully studied. In dogs, droperidol was shown to markedly decrease CBF (40%) without a concomitant decrease in $CMRO_2$.[14] When droperidol was combined with fentanyl, the CBF decrease was approximately the same, but was accompanied by a 15 to 20% decrease in $CMRO_2$.

Induction doses of etomidate (0.2 to 0.3 mg/kg) decrease the CBF and therefore ICP. Whereas a reduction of cerebral perfusion pressure is often seen with thiopentone, etomidate is known to have no significant influence on either blood pressure or cerebral perfusion pressure.

Among the intravenous anesthetic agents, ketamine is unique in its ability to activate cerebral function during anesthesia for surgical procedures. Associated with this activation is approximately a 50% increase in CBF and less than a 20% increase in overall $CMRO_2$. A potent vasodilator, ketamine causes an increase in ICP in normal man. The increase in the MAP by ketamine does not compensate for this increase in ICP, consequently the overall cerebral perfusion pressure is reduced.

Whether in combination or alone, little is known regarding the mechanisms whereby the anesthetics actually alter the CBF and $CMRO_2$. The basis for the regulation and control of CBF in unanesthetized man is complex and in many areas still controversial. Anesthetics introduce new complexities that continue to defy our understanding.

Nonanesthetic Drugs—Vasoactive Agents

Systemic vasoactive drugs can alter cerebrovascular resistance or may indirectly change CBF by shifting brain metabolic rates. The effects of systemically administered α and β receptor agonists or antagonists on cerebral circulation have not been clearly established. The weight of evidence suggests that, as a group, they have little or no effect unless their systemic effects result in a blood pressure change sufficient to exceed the limits of autoregulation. Clinical doses of the vasoactive drugs do not appear to cross the blood brain barrier when administered intravenously; however, they can profoundly influence the cerebral circulation when they are given to correct arterial hypotension. When administered to treat hypotension, epinephrine, norepinephrine, angiotensin, and isoproterenol can restore cerebral perfusion pressure, which in turn will increase CBF.

Cerebral and systemic vasodilators can directly reduce cerebrovascular resistance. Nitroprusside and nitroglycerin are potent vascular muscle relaxants and can increase total CBF provided the arterial blood pressure has not been significantly reduced. An increase in CBF may lead to an increase in ICP in some situations.

Ganglionic blockers such as trimethaphan, used for the induction of hypotension, are presently considered to have no direct cerebrovascular effects.

The muscle relaxants probably have little or no effect on either CBF or $CMRO_2$. Studies have shown that they do not cross the blood brain barrier, alter cerebral function, or change the EEG. One exception may be curare, which has been reported to transiently increase ICP.[15] The effects of curare are probably due to its releasing of histamine and the resulting increase in CBF.

Anesthetic Management

Preoperative Evaluation

In general, preoperative anesthetic evaluation of a patient provides a guide for the anesthetic management, intraoperative monitoring, supportive techniques, and postoperative care. In addition to the usual review for major considerations and gathering of anesthetic information, two special concerns for this case presentation must be addressed preoperatively. The first concern is to understand the type and the extent of the patient's cardiac disease. It is important to understand the effects of the heart disease on other organ systems, as well as the effects of other systemic diseases upon the cardiovascular system. The second important consideration preoperatively, specifically in the case of this patient, is the significance of the bilateral carotid bruits and the influence, if any, on the anesthetic management during CPB.

The clinical management is well established for a patient with a symptomatic carotid bruit who is scheduled for a cardiac operation. Angiography is mandatory and, if a correctable lesion is found, a carotid endarterectomy (either prior to or at the time of the cardiac operation) is advised to prevent neurologic damage.[16] However, many patients with carotid artery lesions are asymptomatic and the disease is manifested only by a cervical bruit. Because a cervical bruit does not always correlate with severe carotid occlusive disease, noninvasive screening techniques have often been advocated to define the extent of carotid obstruction and whether the need for cerebral angiogram and possible carotid endarterectomy exists.[17]

In this case presentation, noninvasive screening preoperatively has revealed no significant carotid occlusive disease. The consideration for management of a patient with known carotid occlusive disease during CPB will be discussed later.

Intraoperative Management

When the clinician knows the characteristic of the specific cardiac disease and the hemodynamic status of the patient, any one of a combination of anesthetic drugs can be selected based on both their anesthetic properties and their hemodynamic effects. Anesthesiologists should accomplish two goals in the anesthetic management of patients undergoing coronary revascularization: (1) amnesia and analgesia should be provided and (2) the balanced myocardial oxygen supply-and-demand ratio should be either maintained or improved with the anesthetic technique.

Having chosen an anesthetic that achieves the above goals, intraoperative management of this case centers upon management of low perfusion pressure with the onset of CPB. Major anesthetic principles include the following: (1) maintain an adequate pump perfusion flow; (2) maintain hypothermia thus lowering the cerebral metabolic oxygen requirement; (3) maintain a normal $PaCO_2$; (4) avoid arterial hypoxia; and (5) do not administer vasopressors.

Cerebral Perfusion During Cardiopulmonary Bypass

Patients Without Carotid Disease

In a lightly anesthetized, normothermic, normotensive man without cerebrovascular disease, the critical CBF has been shown to be approximately 18 to 20 ml/100 gm/minute.[18] At CBF below this level, ischemic EEG changes have been demonstrated. However, the critical CBF is not known for humans undergoing hypothermic CPB with general anesthesia. Extracorporeal circulation is a condition that exposes a living body to an entirely nonphysiologic environment. The organ systems may respond differently to the environment brought about by the nonphysiologic condition of extracorporeal circulation.

Govier et al.[19] studied the factors that influence regional CBF during nonpulsatile hypothermic CPB. There was a significant decrease in regional CBF (55%) during CPB, with nasopharyngeal temperature and $PaCO_2$ being the only two significant factors influencing CBF. Importantly, there was no association of regional CBF with MAP, a finding consistent with preserved autoregulation (Fig 6–3). In fact, during hypothermic CPB, the lower limit of autoregulation

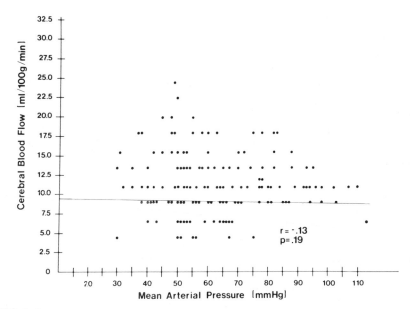

FIG 6–3.
Cerebral blood flow vs. mean arterial pressure during cardiopulmonary bypass. The line represents an average regression line over all patients. There are 44 hidden observations, i.e., data points superimposed on each other.

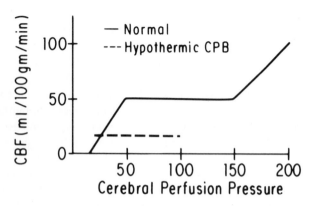

FIG 6–4.
Intact cerebrovascular autoregulation in normotensive, normothermic human beings and in patients during hypothermic cardiopulmonary bypass (CPB).

appears to be as low as 30 mm Hg (Fig 6–4). This is in contrast to the normotensive, normothermic human beings with a normal cerebrovascular status, in whom autoregulation maintains a constant CBF between 50 and 150 mm Hg. Most likely the reason for the extension of this lower limit of autoregulation is that less CBF is required in the hypothermic state due to the significant decrease in cerebral metabolic oxygen requirement.

It is now known that pharmacologic treatment of arterial pressures between 30 and 110 mm Hg is not necessary to ensure constant cerebral blood flow in normotensive patients with normal cerebrovascular status. The previously held belief that the perfusion pressure should be maintained at a level greater than 50 mm Hg during CPB for cerebral protection cannot be defended solely on the premise that below this level CBF falls. In addition, the effects of the vasopressors on other organ systems, especially the renal system, are not known in man during CPB and nonpulsatile flow. It is possible that the vasopressors may actually interfere with renal perfusion to a greater degree than a lower perfusion pressure and further compromise the renal system. Thus, in this case presentation, no vasopressors should be given during the onset of CPB with a pump perfusion flow of 2.2 L/minute/m^2 at 28° C.

Freeman et al.[20] did not find a relationship between postoperative cognitive dysfunction and age, duration of CPB, or lowered CBF during bypass. These results were consistent with a report by Fish et al.[21] and Slogoff et al.[4] The lowered perfusion pressures which were observed during hypothermic nonpulsatile CPB did not prove to be significantly associated with postoperative cerebral dysfunction. This supports the hypothesis of many investigators that emboli may be the primary cause of persistent postbypass cognitive dysfunction.

It is known that in normothermic, awake man chronic hypertension shifts the entire autoregulation curve to the right. [18] As a result of this shift, the brain is better protected at high cerebral perfusion pressure but may be more vulnerable to ischemia at low cerebral perfusion pressure. A variety of intracranial disorders may impair autoregulation. Additional studies are needed to address the impact of both cerebrovascular disease and hypertension on CBF during hypothermic CPB. If cerebral autoregulation is disordered during bypass, regardless of the cause, it is possible that hypotension and associated decreased cerebral perfusion could produce central nervous system ischemic injury.

Patients With Carotid Disease

The second issue to be discussed is the management of this case if the patient had significant carotid disease. As mentioned earlier, there have been no studies performed on human beings during hypothermic nonpulsatile CPB that assess the influence of significant carotid disease or cerebrovascular disease on CBF and autoregulation. Therefore, it cannot be said with any certainty where the perfusion pressure should be maintained during CPB. However, it is known that there is no relationship between incidence of perioperative strokes and the presence of high-grade stenosis. Reports of Barnes et al. [22] and Turnipseed et al. [23] could not relate the incidence of perioperative strokes to the presence of high-grade carotid stenosis. Turnipseed et al. found no direct relationship between bruits, severity of disease, and the incidence of perioperative strokes. Of importance is that their study included patients with antecedent neurologic symptoms as well as patients that were asymptomatic.

Summary

It appears that CBF is independent of perfusion pressure in a range from 30 to 110 mm Hg during hypothermic nonpulsatile CPB in patients with normal cerebral circulation. In this case presentation, with the maintenance of cerebral autoregulation during hypothermic CPB, there is no indication to pharmacologically treat a perfusion pressure of 30 mm Hg.

REFERENCES

1. Tufo HM, Ostfeld AM, Shekelle R: Central nervous system dysfunction following open-heart surgery. *JAMA* 1970; 212:1333.
2. Stockard JJ, Bickford RG, Schauble JF: Pressure-dependent cerebral ischemia during cardiopulmonary bypass. *Neurology* 1973; 23:521.
3. Kolkka R, Hilberman M: Neurologic dysfunction following cardiac operation with low flow, low pressure CPB. *J Thorac Cardiovasc Surg* 1980; 79:432.
4. Slogoff S, Girgis KZ, Keats AS: Etiologic factors in neuropsychiatric complications associated with CPB. *Anesth Analg* 1982; 61:903.

5. Shapiro H: Neurosurgical anesthesia and intracranial hypertension, in Miller R (ed): *Anesthesia.* New York, Churchill Livingstone Inc, 1981, pp 1079–1132.

6. Lassen NA, Christensen MS: Physiology of cerebral blood flow. *Br J Anaesth* 1976; 48:719.

7. McDowall DG: Interrelationships between blood oxygen tensions and cerebral blood flow, in Payne JP and Hill DW (eds): *Oxygen Measurements in Blood and Tissues.* London, Churchill, 1966, p 205.

8. Frost E: Ischemic cerebrovascular disease, in Newfield P, Cottrell J (eds): *Handbook of Neuroanesthesia: Clinical and Physiologic Essentials.* Boston, Little Brown & Co, 1983, pp 209–224.

9. Smith AL, Wolman H: Cerebral blood flow and metabolism: Effects of anesthetic drugs and techniques. *Anesthesiology* 1972; 36:378.

10. Shapiro H: Anesthesia effects upon cerebral blood flow, cerebral metabolism, and the electroencephalogram, in Miller R (ed): *Anesthesia. New York, Churchill Livingstone* Inc, 1981, pp 795–824.

11. Michenfelder JD: The cerebral circulation, in Prys-Roberts P (ed): *The Circulation in Anaesthesia.* Oxford, England, Blackwell, 1980, pp 209–225.

12. Jobes DR, Kennell E, Bitner R, et al: Effects of morphine-nitrous oxide anesthesia on cerebral autoregulation. *Anesthesiology* 1975; 42:30.

13. Sari A, Okuda Y, Takeshita H: The effects of thalamonal on cerebral circulation and oxygen consumption in man. *Br J Anaesth* 1972; 44:330.

14 Michenfelder JD, Theye RA: Effects of fentanyl, droperidol and innovar on canine cerebral metabolism and blood flow. *Br J Anaesth 1971; 43:630.*

15. Tarkkanen L, Laitiner L, Johansson G: Effect of d-tubocurarine on intracranial pressure and thalamic electrical impedence. *Anesthesiology* 1974; 40:247.

16. Okies JE, MacManus Q, Starr A: Myocardial revascularization and carotid endarterectomy: A combined approach. *Ann Thorac Surg* 1977; 23:560–563.

17. Balderman SC, Gutierrez IZ, Makula P, et al: Noninvasive screening for asymptomatic carotid artery disease prior to cardiac operation. *J Thorac Cardiovasc Surg* 1983; 85:427–433.

18. Michenfelder J: The cerebral circulation, in Prys-Roberts C (ed): *The Circulation in Anesthesia.* Oxford, England, Blackwell, 1980, pp 209–225.

19. Govier AV, Reves JG, McKay RD, et al: Factors and their influence on regional cerebral blood flow during nonpulsatile cardiopulmonary bypass. *Ann Thorac Surg* 1984; 38:592.

20. Freeman AM, Folk DG, Sokol R, et al: Cognitive function after coronary bypass surgery: Effect of decreased cerebral blood flow. *Am J Psychiatry* 1985; 142:110.

21. Fish KJ, Helms K, Sarnquist FH, et al: Neuropsychological dysfunction after coronary artery surgery (abstract). *Anesthesiology* 1982; 57:A55.

22. Barnes RW, Liebman PR, Marszalek PB, et al: The natural history of asymptomatic carotid disease in patients undergoing cardiovascular surgery. *Surgery* 1981; 90:1075.

23. Turnipseed WD, Berkoff HA, Belzer FO: Postoperative stroke in cardiac and peripheral vascular disease. *Ann Surg* 1980; 192:365.

7

Cardiopulmonary Bypass Oxygenator Failure

Recommendations by James T. Massagee, M.D.

A 55-year-old man underwent cardiopulmonary bypass for replacement of a stenotic aortic valve. The induction and sternotomy were uneventful. Five minutes after cardiopulmonary bypass was instituted, dark blood was observed by the anesthesiologists in the aortic cannula. An immediate blood gas sampling of the arterial perfusion line revealed an unacceptably low PaO_2.

ANALYSIS OF THE PROBLEM

Dark blood in the arterial cannula constitutes an emergency. Early recognition is crucial to the correction of a potentially devastating problem during cardiopulmonary bypass (CPB). This requires an understanding of the oxygenator equipment and a systematic diagnostic approach. The anesthesiologist should consider three sources as possible causes of arterial inflow desaturation: (1) the gas supply system, (2) the oxygenator, and (3) patient characteristics or pathophysiology.

APPROACH TO THE PROBLEM

When "dark blood" appears in the arterial cannula shortly after the institution of cardiopulmonary bypass, action must be prompt. The cardiac anesthesiologist and perfusionist should have a checklist of observations and immediate actions to perform, thereby correcting the problem and averting patient injury. The following is a guide for use when oxygenator failure occurs:

1. Immediately obtain blood sample for arterial blood gas analysis.

2. Simultaneously instruct the perfusionist to increase O_2 gas flows and determine adequacy of mechanical pump flow.

3. Begin a careful inspection of the gas circuits: gas sources (oxygen and carbon dioxide), all connections, tubing, as well as the gas line filter and vaporizer, up to the circuits' entrance into the oxygenator.

4. Inspect the oxygenator for appropriate blood levels, adequacy of "foaming" if a bubbler is in use (though this does not guarantee adequate O_2 flows); examine the shell for leaks or cracks.

5. Have surgeons or assistants check arterial and venous lines for appropriate patient connections.

6. Ensure adequacy of muscle relaxation, patient temperature, and level of anesthesia.

7. Repeat blood gas analysis.

Secondary considerations at the start of cardiopulmonary bypass include:

8. Continue ventilating the patient's lungs until apparent "arterialized" blood is observed in the aortic cannula.

9. If the heart is still beating, just after the initiation of cardiopulmonary bypass consider allowing it to eject blood through the pulmonary circulation for additional oxygenation.

DISCUSSION

Background

The successful application of extracorporeal circulation (ECC) during open-heart surgery has contributed significantly to the low operative risk. Still, there exist significant potential hazards to the patient whose oxygenation relies upon the complex technology and bioengineering features of extracorporeal blood oxygenators. Additionally, the cardiac anesthesiologist is in the position of having to relinquish control of oxygenation, CO_2 elimination, and systemic perfusion to the cardiopulmonary bypass perfusionists. A list of the potential problems associated with the use of ECC has been published elsewhere.[1, 2] When an accident or failure occurs immediate action must be taken and the perfusionist and anesthesiologist must be in close, rapid communication. The cardiac anesthesiologist, therefore, needs to be familiar with the oxygenator unit and have an awareness for the potential modes of failure.

Little information is available on the incidence of failures or mishaps during extracorporeal circulation.[3] There are no prospective analyses. Yet, most perfusionists can relate one or several instances of failures or accidents while performing cardiopulmonary bypass. The incidence of desaturated blood appearing in the aortic cannula is unknown. Some indication is provided by a questionnaire sent to 1,700 cardiac surgeons in the United States and Canada requesting information on the safety and accidents related to the use of pump oxygenators during the six-year period from 1972 through 1977.[4] Three hundred forty-nine respondents who performed nearly 375,000 operations using a pump oxygenator during this period identified 1,419 "accidents." Among the 1,419 accidents, oxygenator failure accounted for 124; six incidents among 1,419 accidents were associated with permanent injuries and two deaths. A final question addressed "miscellaneous accidents" that occurred that were not covered in the questionnaire. Of 71 miscellaneous accidents, 16 were cases in which oxygenator leaks occurred. No details on the type of leak or mode of oxygenator failure were given, thus the potential for and real incidence of arterial desaturation is unknown. There are three general causes discussed below.

Causes of Arterial Desaturation

The Gas Supply Circuit

There are only a few reports of hypoxemia due to leaks in the gas supply system, though this probably represents an underreporting of true occurrence. In 1980 Schwartz et al.[5] reported one such complication due to leakage of gases from a gas line filter. Gas line filters are used to reduce the potential bacterial or particulate contamination of medical gases.[6] In this instance, a break in the gas line filter created an oxygen leak resulting in inadequate oxygen flow and hypoxemia. Yet, the leak was not so great as to eliminate visible bubbling within the oxygenator. Removal of the filter immediately corrected the problem. Several cracks were subsequently found in the filter's housing, resulting in a change in design by the manufacturer and the institution of an oxygen pressure test prior to distribution.

In another incident reported by Gravelee et al.[7] the use of a disposable bubble oxygenator was associated with the need for very high ratios of gas to blood flow to maintain adequate arterial oxygenation. In all three cases hypoxemia shortly after the institution of cardiopulmonary bypass was recognized by dark blood in the arterial line. Initial PaO_2 was less than 100 in all three; with a PaO_2 of 47 in one case. In two of the three occurrences, a leak was discovered in an inline vaporizer. When the vaporizer was removed, oxygenation improved. One of the vaporizers was found to have worn gaskets and O-rings; the other had a loosened male to female friction seal adapter as the cause of the gas leak. The third case involved a leak in a gas line filter. The authors of this report now routinely test the integrity of the gas circuit by placing an aneroid manometer in series with the gas supply tubing and testing for leaks with the vaporizer in both the on and off positions. In a fourth case the O_2 and CO_2 lines were reversed at the flowmeters giving 95% CO_2 and 5% O_2. This was immediately recognized and the lines reversed.

Figure 7–1 illustrates a typical gas supply circuit. Gas is supplied from a wall source or tanks. The diagram illustrates the multiple connections, including the vaporizer and gas line filter, that all pose potential sources of gas leakage. The perfusionist should routinely check the integrity of this circuit and its connections during pump set up and again just prior to instituting CPB.

Human error is another cause of inadequate or no gas flow during cardiopulmonary bypass. In one occurrence dark blood appeared in the aortic cannula at the onset of CPB while a membrane oxygenator was in use. A quick check of the gas supply circuit revealed no apparent leaks and oxygenator failure was assumed. The membrane oxygenator was replaced without improvement of color in the arterial circuit. A second scan of the gas supply system then revealed that the gas source had been connected to the wrong flowmeters. Some cardiopulmonary bypass machines are equipped with separate flowmeters for use with a bubble oxygenator and an additional oxygen:air mixer for use with the membrane oxygenator. In this instance the gas source had been mistakenly connected to the flowmeters for use with a bubbler. When this was corrected, arterial line saturation improved immediately.

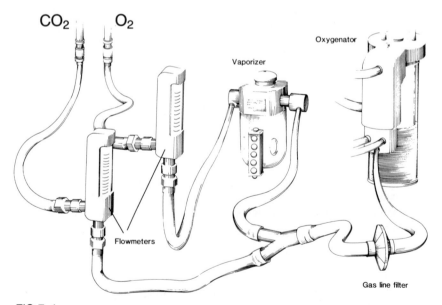

FIG 7–1.
A typical gas supply circuit including flowmeters, vaporizer, and gas line filter used in conjunction with a cardiopulmonary bypass unit.

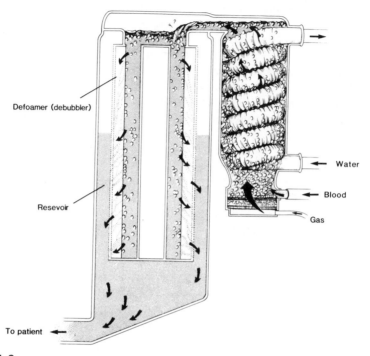

Defoamer (debubbler)

Resevoir

To patient ←

← Water

← Blood

← Gas

FIG 7–2.
Cross-sectional diagram illustrating the functional components of a typical bubble oxygenator.

The Oxygenator

Of the 124 "oxygenator failures" noted by Stoney et al.[4] in his questionnaire, no specific details were provided. However, oxygenator failure accounted for 8.7% of accidents. Of all the potential and technical difficulties inherent to extracorporeal circulation, the exchange of gases is simplest to perform. Oxygen is exposed directly, as in a bubble oxygenator, or through a gas-permeable membrane. Exchange typically proceeds rapidly as the rate-limiting step becomes the thickness of the blood film between gas bubble or surfaces or between the gas membrane surface. Thus, the efficiency of an oxygenator is determined by its ability to exchange gases.[8]

A typical bubble oxygenator in use at this institution (Duke University Medical Center) is the Shiley-100 oxygenator (Fig 7–2). This is a very efficient gas exchanger capable of low gas:blood flow ratios. The Shiley-100 can be used with oxygen:blood flow ratios of as low as 0.6 and yield acceptable levels of PaO_2.[9] This generally provides a margin of safety when gas:blood ratios are maintained near unity. However, too low a gas flow can lead to unsaturated hemoglobin leaving the oxygenator, an increase in the arteriovenous difference, and arterial desaturation.[8] Maintaining appropriate O_2 gas flow relative to mechanical pump flow or simply increasing gas flows can remedy this potential problem.

An appreciation of factors that increase gas exchange efficiency will enable one to understand potential causes of poor gas exchange. In Figure 7–2, gas enters the oxygenator and must pass through a diffuser (or sparger) that creates bubbles of appropriately small diameter to pass into the blood. The oxygen transfer efficiency is related to the size of the bubbles.[10] The bubble and blood mixture pass through a porous sponge where mixing occurs and exchange takes place. As seen in the schematic, they then enter the oxygenating chamber where the helical shape of the heat exchanger prolongs contact of blood and bubbles thus enhancing exchange. A good deal of the gas exchange continues to occur in the debubbling portion of the oxygenator. This is surrounded by a reservoir which, if allowed to become too full, will reduce the area available for gas-blood interaction and will decrease exchange efficiency.[11]

Oxygenators in use today are efficient and dependable. The perfusionist should have examined the unit prior to bypass for structural integrity and the absence of leaks during priming. Close continued observation during the course of cardiopulmonary bypass will allow assessment of the adequacy of volume in the reservoir and the degree of bubbling if a bubble oxygenator is in use.

Patient Characteristics or Pathophysiology

With the usual conduct of extracorporeal circulation, patient characteristics or pathophysiology should, in general, not be responsible for the appearance of dark blood in the arterial cannula. However, variations in patient physiology can influence oxygen demand and transfer. As previously noted, overfilling the reservoir of a bubbler can reduce the area available for gas exchange. Situations in which this might occur are those in patients whose blood volumes are large (as in the very large patient or the patient with congestive heart failure whose blood volume is greater than normal). Additionally, overzealous use of α-adrenergic agents resulting in peripheral vasoconstriction would have the same result by translocating volume from the patient to the oxygenator.[11] Patients with low cardiac output and significantly reduced venous saturation may stress the oxygenator beyond its oxygenation capacity at the initiation of bypass. Finally, instances in which oxygen consumption by the patient is increased out of proportion to delivery may lead to a decrease in the mixed venous saturation and desaturation in the arterial circuit. Examples include increases in patients' body temperature, light anesthesia, and muscle activity due to inadequate relaxation.[8, 11] These remain unlikely mechanisms for the appearance of dark blood in the aortic cannula shortly after the institution of cardiopulmonary bypass. Indeed, the vigilant anesthesiologist and perfusionist should be able to correct such problems by appropriate increases in mechanical pump flow and gas flows or by the administration of muscle relaxants well before any harm could come to the patient.

Summary

At present, it is not routine to have in-line monitors of PaO_2 or percent saturation in the arterial circuit. The perfusionist, like the anesthesiologist, depends on vigilance and experience to monitor proper function of the oxygenator. Despite the mechanical complexities, extracorporeal circulation has proved to be relatively safe and dependable. When a relatively rare occurrence such as "dark blood in the arterial cannula" manifests, a systematic and efficient approach (as outlined above) will likely uncover the problem and allow correction before patient morbidity occurs.

REFERENCES

1. Mortensen JD: Safety and efficacy of extracorporeal blood oxygenators: A review. *Med Instrum* 1978; 12:128–132.
2. Utah Biomedical Test Laboratory: *Final Report: Safety and efficacy of blood oxygenators: Project Summary*, TR166–004. Silver Spring, Md, FDA Bureau of Medical Devices, 1976, vol 1.
3. Final Report: Safety and efficacy of blood oxygenators. Volume III: Literature Review. *Utah Biomedical Test Laboratory* TR166–004. Silver Spring, MD, FDA Bureau of Medical Devices, 30 April 1976.
4. Stoney WS, Alford WC, Currus GR, et al: Air embolism and other accidents using pump oxygenators. *Ann Thorac Surg* 1980; 29:336–340.
5. Schwartz AJ, Howse J, Ellison N, et al: The gas line filter: A cause of hypoxia. *Anesth Analg* 1980; 59:617–18.
6. Mortensen JD, Hurd G, Hill G: Bacterial contamination of oxygen used clinically: Importance and one method of control. *Chest* 1962; 42:567–572.
7. Gravelee GP, Wong AB, Charles DJ: Hypoxemia during cardiopulmonary bypass from leaks in the gas supply system. *Anesth Analg* 1985; 64:649–650.
8. Bartlett RH, Gazzaniga AB: Physiology and pathophysiology of extracorporeal circulation in Ionescu MI (ed): *Techniques in Extracorporeal Circulation*, ed 2. London, Butterworths, 1981, pp 1–43.
9. Björk VO, Bergdahl L, Wussow C: Gas flow in relation to blood flow in oxygenators: An evaluation of the new Shiley bubble oxygenator. *Scand J Thorac Cardiovasc Surg* 1977; 11:81–84.
10. Hammond GL, Bowley WW: Bubble mechanics and oxygen transfer. *J Thorac Cardiovasc Surg* 1976; 71:422–428.
11. Finlayson DC, Kaplan JA: Cardiopulmonary bypass in Kaplan JA (ed): *Cardiac Anesthesia*. New York, Grune & Stratton Inc, 1979, pp 401–410.

8

Ventricular Tachycardia, Ventricular Fibrillation With Insertion of Pulmonary Artery Catheter

Recommendations by John A. Youngberg, M.D., and Donald E. Smith, M.D.

A 50-year-old, 70-kg man with severe coronary artery disease and history of ventricular arrhythmias was scheduled for coronary artery bypass surgery. Preinduction and monitoring instrumentation went well except for multiple premature ventricular contractions (PVCs). After administration of 70 mg of lidocaine, the Swan-Ganz pulmonary artery catheter was floated into the heart while the patient was awake. At this time a short run of ventricular tachycardia preceded ventricular fibrillation.

ANALYSIS OF THE PROBLEM

This is a life-threatening complication of monitoring. Diagnosis and prompt therapy are essential.

APPROACH TO THE PROBLEM

The pulmonary artery (PA) catheter should be drawn back into the superior vena cava immediately and a precordial thump should be delivered. The fist should be closed and the blow delivered from a height of 8 to 12 in. above the sternum. This maneuver will generate 4 to 5 watt/second of energy. Depending on the result of this maneuver, we follow the flow chart (Fig 8–1).

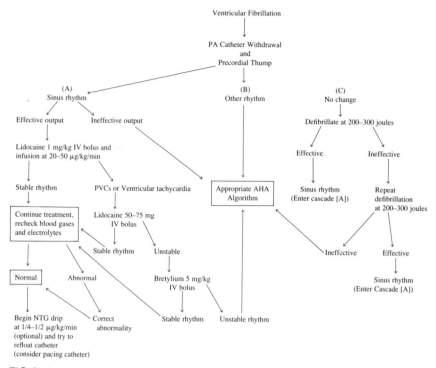

FIG 8–1.
Flow chart used to determine course of action in the event of ventricular fibrillation with insertion of PA catheter. *IV* = intravenous; *PVCs* = premature ventricular contractions; *NTG* = nitroglycerine; *AHA* = American Heart Association.

If the patient had responded to the precordial thump and/or defibrillation, we would attempt reflotation of the catheter after rechecking results of blood gas and electrolyte studies and initiating lidocaine and nitroglycerin therapy. If more extensive therapy was required to treat the ventricular fibrillation, we would consider proceeding without a PA catheter if the operation was judged to be emergent or urgent. Conversely, if more involved therapy had been required and the procedure was not urgent or emergent, we would recommend treatment with antiarrhythmics prior to another attempt at catheter insertion.

DISCUSSION

Background

Pulmonary artery catheters (PAC) are frequently used to assist in the care of critically surgical or medical ill patients.[1–4] As in other hospitals, we employ pulmonary artery catheters in essentially all adult open-heart procedures. The thermodilution pulmonary artery catheter allows for both direct and indirect assessment of right and left ventricular function, measurement of pulmonary and systemic vascular resistances, and determination of the need for fluid replacement. Additionally, mixed venous blood samples can be obtained for measurement of arterial-mixed venous oxygen content differences so that pulmonary shunt fractions can be calculated. Newer catheters also provide a port for direct right ventricular pressure measurement, an extra central venous port, and fiberoptics for continuous mixed venous oxygen saturation. A PAC is not without potential hazard. Numerous complications have been reported including pneumothorax; hematoma; air embolism; thrombosis; perforation of subclavian, pulmonary, or carotid arteries; arrhythmias; neurologic damage; cardiac perforation; and mediastinal infiltration.[5-10]

Arrhythmias are one of the most common complications reported. The reported incidence of premature ventricular contractions (PVCs) has ranged from 12% to 72%.[11-13] Ventricular tachycardia has been reported in up to 33% of patients and ventricular fibrillation has also been reported.[6, 12, 14] Right bundle-branch block (RBBB) has been reported with passage of a PAC or with balloon inflation alone and complete heart block has developed in patients with preexisting left bundle-branch block (LBBB).[11, 12, 14-17] Left fascicular blocks have also been reported following insertion of a PAC.[18] Arrhythmias occur most frequently during insertion of the catheter but may also occur with displacement of the catheter tip from the pulmonary artery to the pulmonary outflow tract and during withdrawal of the catheter.[19, 20]

The production of arrhythmias is most likely the result of mechanical stimulation of the endocardium or conduction pathways. Damage to or stimulation of the bundle of His may occur during insertion of a PAC.[18] In some patients ventricular tachycardia can be induced by atrial stimulation.[21] Right bundle-branch block can be produced by stimulation of the coronary sinus or cardiac perforation.[22] The right main bundle is located only 0.5 to 1 mm below the right-sided septal endocardium during its course from the His bundle to the moderator band in the right ventricle, making it accessible to catheter trauma.[23]

Various risk factors have been identified as predisposing to the development of ventricular arrhythmias, including acidosis (pH< 7.2), hypoxia (PaO$_2$ < 60 mm Hg), electrolyte imbalance (K$^+$ < 3.5 mEq/L and Ca^{++} < 8.0 mg/dl), and myocardial ischemia or infarction.[11] Added to this list would be a history of arrhythmias, especially ventricular arrhythmias.

The balloon on the catheter tip is designed with three objectives: (1) to assist in flotation of the catheter; (2) to enable a pulmonary capillary wedge pressure to be obtained; and (3) to extend beyond the tip of the catheter when inflated making the catheter less irritating to the conduction system and perforation less likely. It is clear that the PAC is still capable of producing arrhythmias even with a properly inflated balloon that extends beyond the catheter tip when inflated. It has been suggested that a loop of catheter rather than the tip is the source of irritation in some patients.[24] The incidence of arrhythmias has also been shown to increase with an increase in catheterization time (time to pass the catheter through the heart and into the pulmonary artery).[11] Most arrhythmias are of short duration and self-limiting or can be abated by either advancing or withdrawing the catheter.[12]

During withdrawal, some authors recommend that the balloon be maintained at 50% inflation volume to lessen incidence of arrhythmias.[19] Most authors recommend the use of lidocaine to treat ventricular arrhythmias that occur during catheter insertion, whereas the use of lidocaine prophylactically is more controversial.[19, 25, 26]

Case Discussion

This patient is an example of patients at increased risk of developing ventricular arrhythmias during PAC insertion because of his history of ventricular arrhythmias and ischemia. Assessment of oxygenation, acid-base status, and electrolyte balance is indicated prior to catheter insertion. The patient should receive supplemental oxygen during PAC placement. This patient might have benefited from both a lidocaine and a nitroglycerin infusion prior to and during catheter passage. It has also been suggested that increased circulating catecholamine levels may contribute to the development of ventricular arrhythmias.[25] For that reason we usually sedate our adult patients with a combination of morphine sulphate (0.05 to 0.10 mg/kg) and scopolamine (0.2 to 0.3 mg) given intramuscularly and diazepam (0.05 to 0.10 mg/kg) given orally prior to PAC insertion.

Care should be exercised during catheter insertion. The most direct route requiring the least catheter manipulation (such as the right internal jugular vein) should be utilized and care should be taken not to advance either the dilator or guide wire into the right atrium or ventricle. On visualization with fluoroscopy, the catheter can be seen moving forward with the current of blood. The catheter tip moves most rapidly when it is expelled through the outflow tract of the right ventricle (RV), and most arrhythmias occur at that time.[12, 26] Most arrhythmias have been attributed to stimulation caused by the catheter tip; however, it has been suggested that a loop of catheter could also cause trauma.[24] Each time the catheter strikes the endocardial surface it can potentially cause a premature depolarization. A persistent arrhythmia will reduce cardiac output and blood pressure. In the awake or sedated patient, this reduction in blood pressure may cause nausea, vomiting, loss of consciousness, loss of airway reflexes, or aspiration. Acute hypoxia metabolically impairs cardiac tissue by altering all membrane physiology, increasing sympathetic tone, reducing myocardial contractility, and enhancing arrhythmogenicity. The balloon should be fully inflated during insertion and the catheter should be advanced quickly with close attention to wave form and insertion distance to avoid coiling.

Patients with right ventricular infarcts may be more susceptible to ventricular fibrillation during PAC placement.[27] Most catheter-induced ventricular arrhythmias are self-limiting and of short duration or respond to a precordial thump, intravenous lidocaine administration, and/or defibrillation.[28] Neither advancing nor withdrawing the PAC guarantees that the PVCs or arrhythmia will abate.[12]

The first line of therapy in the treatment of arrhythmias caused by insertion of a PAC is either passage of the PAC into the pulmonary artery (PA) or its removal from the RV.[12, 26, 29] Further treatment includes the precordial thump,[28] direct current cardioversion or defibrillation,[11] and cardiac drug therapy.[12, 26, 28, 29] Lidocaine is the most commonly used drug for ventricular arrhythmias in this setting.[11, 12, 26, 28, 29] Although the prophylactic use of lidocaine, 1 mg/kg, by bolus intravenous administration prior to catheter insertion is controversial, we recommend its use 60 to 90 seconds prior to catheter passage through the cardiac chambers in patients with a history of arrhythmias.[12, 19, 24–26] We also recommend the use of a nitroglycerin drip prior to and during catheter insertion to promote subendocardial blood flow, thereby lessening the irritability in patients with significant coronary disease.

It is unlikely that mechanical depolarization of cardiac tissue can be entirely blocked by levels of antiarrhythmic drugs that would allow normal cardiac conduction and junction.[26] With the catheter tip in the RV, a mechanically triggered form of ventricular premature depolarizations (VPDs) can occur that usually terminates with removal or repositioning of the PAC. Antiarrhythmic drugs may prevent the premature depolarizations caused by a catheter from starting self-sustained ventricular tachyarrhythmias.

Of the arrhythmias that occur during PAC insertion, the most common are isolated premature ventricular depolarizations, then coupled ventricular depolarizations; then short runs of ventricular tachycardia. Sustained ventricular tachycardia (VT) or ventricular fibrillation are less common.[11, 12, 26, 28, 29]

Ventricular tachyarrhythmias require specific conditions to exist in a critical mass of tissue in order to occur or to be self-sustaining. Patients without these predisposing conditions are unlikely to develop any sustained ventricular arrhythmias. This accounts for the large numbers of patients with only transient arrhythmias during instrumentation.

Especially in patients with cardiac disease, the physiologic stress of hypoxia, hypercarbia, anxiety, pain, etc. may increase the critical mass of metabolically impaired tissue and increase the likelihood for the development of arrhythmias.[30]

Mechanisms of Ventricular Tachyarrhythmias

In order to gain a greater understanding of the use of antiarrhythmic therapy, it is necessary to have an understanding of the electrophysiologic basis of ventricular arrhythmias. Despite the complexity of cellular electrophysiologic mechanisms responsible for cardiac arrhythmias,[31] the old simple concept[32] that "arrhythmias result from abnormalities of impulse initiation and/or impulse conduction" is probably still applicable to the majority of clinical arrhythmias.[33-35]

Impulse Initiation

Two forms of impulse initiation may be involved in the genesis of cardiac arrhythmias: "automatic activity" and "triggered activity." Automatic activity is described as spontaneous diastolic (phase 4) depolarization. As the membrane potential (V_m), or maximum diastolic potential (MDP) as it is termed in automatic fibers, declines to the threshold potential as a result of the spontaneous diastolic depolarization, an action potential occurs. Automaticity arising in Purkinje fibers can be called "normal automaticity" or a "normal automatic mechanism"[31, 36] in that the site normally possesses spontaneous diastolic depolarization. Having slower rates, the Purkinje fibers are usually overdrive-suppressed by the higher rate of the sinoatrial (SA) node. Spontaneous diastolic depolarization occurring in metabolically impaired, partially depolarized, cardiac tissue is considered an abnormal automatic mechanism or "abnormal automaticity," because it arises from normally nonautomatic as well as automatic cardiac cells.[31, 36] Ventricular muscle fibers normally do not exhibit automaticity; however, if the membrane potential of these fibers is experimentally maintained at approximately -60mV, spontaneous diastolic depolarization and automatic impulse initiation may occur.[37-39] Similarly, if myocardial fibers become partially depolarized to approximately -60mV because of ischemia or infarction, phase 4 depolarization may occur.[40, 41]

It is still doubtful whether the ectopic foci arising from abnormal automaticity actually contribute to the genesis of clinical tachyarrhythmias. If the action potentials generated at low levels of resting V_m or MDP occur via slow-inward calcium currents as those in slow response fibers (e.g., sinus node), then it is unlikely that they will be generated at extremely fast rates.[42] On the other hand, when the membrane potential is depressed by metabolic impairment, slow conduction and unidirectional block tends to occur, increasing the probability for a reentry mechanism to develop as will be discussed later. Reentry, rather than abnormal automaticity, is more likely to be the mechanism for the genesis of cardiac tachyarrhythmias.

The other form of impulse initiation is "triggered activity,"[31, 33, 42] which has been discussed by some authors under the heading "abnormal automaticity."[43, 44]

"Delayed afterdepolarizations" are secondary depolarizations that occur after full repolarization of a previous action potential. A delayed afterdepolarization can reach threshold and give rise to a single extrasystole that may have a delayed afterdepolarization leading to further depolarization. This is currently regarded as the mechanism for many cardiac arrhythmias including some VPDs and VT caused by digitalis toxicity.[42, 45]

Impulse Conduction

Abnormal impulse conduction may result in arrhythmias by either of two mechanisms: (1) failure of impulse propagation, or (2) reentry.[31, 46]

Reentry is probably the mechanism responsible for the great majority of tachyarrhythmias.[31, 35, 43, 46–48] Reentry is a reexcitation caused by continuous propagation of the same impulse for one or more cardiac cycles. Two prerequisite conditions for the reentry to occur are: (1) slow conduction and (2) unidirectional block, which will be discussed later.

Prior to a discussion of reentry, two important properties relating to impulse conduction need to be understood; one is "conduction velocity," and the other is "effective refractory period." Antiarrhythmic drugs abolish reentry by affecting conduction velocity and/or the effective refractory period in or around reentrant circuit.

"Conduction velocity" (CV) is the speed of impulse propagation through the cardiac fibers. It is dependent upon the maximal rate of depolarization during phase O ($\dot{V}_{max}$ or upstroke velocity) and the amplitude of the action potential.[43, 49] Furthermore, the $\dot{V}_{max}$ and the amplitude of an action potential are determined by the level of membrane potential (V_m) at the instant of excitation, i.e., the resting V_m. The lower the magnitude of resting V_m (less negative), the lower will be the $\dot{V}_{max}$ and the amplitude of an action potential when it occurs, because more sodium channels will be deactivated at lower levels (less negative) of resting V_m.[43, 49] Therefore, in cardiac fibers with partially depolarized cell membranes (lower levels of resting V_m), the impulses will be conducted more slowly.

In ventricular muscle and Purkinje fibers in areas of ischemia and infarction,[50–53] the resting membrane potentials have been found to be less negative than those of cells from normal hearts. Thus, in a metabolically impaired region, the rate of depolarization ($\dot{V}_{max}$), the amplitude of an action potential, and the conduction velocity of an impulse are decreased. It has been demonstrated that in a bundle of cardiac fibers stimulated at either end the conduction velocity is slowed in both directions as the $\dot{V}_{max}$ and amplitude of the action potential decreases. At a critical degree of depression of $\dot{V}_{max}$, conduction may fail in one direction but proceed slowly in the opposite direction.[54] This slowed conduction with a unidirectional block is the situation that predisposes to a reentry mechanism. Further depression of $\dot{V}_{max}$ of the action potential usually results in a bidirectional block.

"Effective refractory period" (ERP) may be defined as the time interval from the onset of an action potential until the fiber is able to conduct another action potential.[49, 55] The earliest propagated action potential elicited defines the end of the ERP. However, the action potentials generated prior to complete repolarization are characterized by slow rates of depolarizations (low $\dot{V}_{max}$) and low action potential amplitudes, and are conducted slowly. Once the membrane potential has returned to its normal V_m, $-90mV$, the action potential regains its normal characteristics. It is apparent that the timing of the ERP closely parallels the action potential duration (APD).

When effective refractory periods of adjacent groups of cardiac fibers differ markedly ("dispersion of refractoriness"), a unique condition for slow conduction and unidirectional block and, thus, for reentry exists.[33, 35, 36]

Disease states may affect the ERP and APD greatly. In ventricular muscle and Purkinje fibers, the APD and ERP are shortened acutely after the onset of ischemia but markedly prolonged in chronic ischemia.[40, 51, 53, 56] Thus, there is a great dispersion of refractoriness between normal and diseased cardiac fibers, and a properly timed premature impulse may induce unidirectional block and reentry.

Reentry is probably the cause of ventricular tachycardia, flutter, and fibrillation.[31, 35, 43, 47, 48] The concept of reentry has been well described and established since 1928 by Schmitt and Erlanger.[57] As mentioned previously, two conditions are essential for reentry to occur, slow conduction and unidirectional block.

Reentry over a finite pathway is called "ordered reentry" and over randomly changing pathways is called "random reentry."[31] Ordered reentry in the ventricle causes ventricular flutter or tachycardia. Random reentry in the ventricles causes ventricular fibrillation.[31, 47, 48]

Autonomic Influences on the His-Purkinje System and Ventricular Myocardium

His-Purkinje fibers.—Acetylcholine has been shown to have some effects on the activity of His-Purkinje fibers; however, vagal innervation of the His-Purkinje system and ventricles is not considered to be functionally important.[58, 59] Catecholamines have more pronounced effects on cardiac Purkinje fibers; they increase automaticity and decrease both the action potential duration and the effective refractory period.[60, 61]

Ventricles.—Acetylcholine has negligible effect on the cardiac electrophysiology of normal ventricular muscle.[59, 62]

Catecholamines.—The principal effect of catecholamines on ventricular muscle fibers is to increase the slow calcium inward current which causes an increased amplitude and duration of the AP plateau phase and the accelerated repolarization phase. Catecholamines have minimal effects on the resting membrane potential, the rate of depolarization ($\dot{V}_{max}$), and the amplitude of the action potential, and, thus, the conduction velocity in normal His-Purkinje and ventricular fibers. However, when the fibers are partially depolarized as a result of disease, catecholamines may increase the resting membrane potential, thereby improving conduction.[63]

The increase in influx of Ca^{++} is responsible for the increased inotropy. The overall cardiac electrophysiologic actions of vagal and sympathetic responses are summarized in Table 8–1.

Selection of Pharmacologic Antiarrhythmic Agents for the Treatment of Arrhythmias During PAC Insertion

Selection criteria[30] can be reasonably approached by considering that the drug should be able to be administered intravenously and should have rapid onset and clearance for the sake of control. Of the currently approved drugs, this leaves for class I_A, procainamide; class I_B, lidocaine; class II, propranolol; and class III, bretylium. Class IV, calcium-channel blockers, and class V, digitalis,[30] are not useful for ventricular arrhythmias. The other criteria are electrophysiologic effects, autonomic effects, and adverse reactions.

TABLE 8–1.

Cardiac Electrophysiologic Actions of Vagal and Sympathetic Stimulation

ACTIONS*	VAGAL†	SYMPATHETIC†
His-Purkinje fibers		
Automaticity	↓	⬆ (large)
CV	—	↑ (small)
ERP (or APD)	—	⬇ (large)
Ventricle		
CVP	—	↑
ERP	—	↓

*CV = conduction velocity; ERP = effective refractory period; APD = action potential duration.
†Large arrows = significant effect; small arrows = minor effect; dashes = minimal effect.

Electrophysiologic Effects.—The electrophysiologic effects of antiarrhythmic agents are summarized below (Table 8–2).

Class I$_A$ (procainamide).—The effects of class I$_A$ drugs are related to sodium (Na) channel blockade. Procainamide decreases Purkinje fiber automaticity. Ventricular myocardial fibers normally do not possess automaticity. Procainamide reduces membrane excitability. In other words, the threshold potential at which depolarization of the Purkinje or ventricular muscle fiber will depolarize becomes less negative.

Procainamide also decreases membrane responsiveness, which means the

TABLE 8–2.

Cardiac Electrophysiologic Actions of Antiarrhythmic Drugs*†

	CLASS I		CLASS II	CLASS III	CLASS IV	CLASS V
	QUINIDINE PROCAINAMIDE DISOPYRAMIDE	LIDOCAINE PHENYTOIN	β-BLOCKERS PROPANOLOL	BRETYLIUM	CALCIUM CHANNEL BLOCKERS VERAPAMIL	DIGITALIS
AUTOMATICITY						
Ectopic foci, e.g., Purkinje fibers	↓	↓	↓	—	—	⇧
Triggered activity, e.g., delayed after depolarization	—	↓	↓	—	↓	⇧
CONDUCTION						
His-Purkinje fibers						
CV	↓	↓	—	—	—	⇩
ERP	↑	↓	↑	↑	—	⇩
Ventricles						
CV	↓	↓	—	—	—	⇩
ERP	↑	↓	—	↑	—	⇩

*The *arrows* represent significant electrophysiologic effects. The *dashes* represent minor or minimal electrophysiologic effects. In the column under class V, the *empty arrows* represent direct membrane effects of toxic concentrations of digitalis, and the solid arrows represent vagal effects at therapeutic concentration.

†Adapted from Weng JT, et al: *J. Thorac Surg* 1986; 41:106–112.

rate of depolarization or $\dot{V}_{max}$ is decreased. Membrane responsiveness is a major determinant of conduction velocity, thus procainamide decreases conduction velocity. Procainamide increases the ERP and APD; specifically the ERP is increased greater than the APD. Thus, the ERP/APD increases and the chance for premature conduction decreases.

Class I_B (lidocaine).—The effects of lidocaine are also considered to be related to Na-channel blockade. Lidocaine decreases automaticity of Purkinje fibers. Lidocaine has no effect on membrane excitability (threshold potential). It decreases membrane responsiveness (the $\dot{V}_{max}$ for a given V_m) at normal extracellular levels of K^+. Thus, at normal levels of extracellular K^+, lidocaine reduces the conduction velocity in Purkinje and ventricular muscle fibers. At low resting membrane potentials, it not only depresses $\dot{V}_{max}$ but it totally blocks membrane depolarization at V_m less negative than $-65mV$. In other words, lidocaine markedly inhibits conduction of impulses through partially depolarized, metabolically impaired ventricular or Purkinje fibers. Lidocaine, in contrast to procainamide, shortens the ERP and APD, probably caused by enhanced potassium efflux during the plateau phase of the action potential. The ERP is decreased less than the APD; therefore, the ERP/APD is increased.

Class II (propranolol).—Propranolol decreases the automaticity of Purkinje fibers by β-blockade, especially in the presence of increased catecholamine effect. It has no effect on excitability (threshold potential) except in very high doses at which it has a mild direct sodium channel blocking effect similar to lidocaine. It likewise has no effect on Purkinje muscle fiber, membrane responsiveness, or conduction velocity, except for a mild negative effect at toxic doses.

At therapeutic doses, the β-blockade effect of propranolol may reverse the effects (decreased ERP and APD) of catecholamines and thus increase the ERP and APD of Purkinje fibers. Less effect is seen in ventricular muscle fibers.

Class III (bretylium).—Bretylium has no effect on Purkinje fiber automaticity other than a possible mild increase during the transient release of norepinephrine. Neither does it affect membrane excitability, membrane responsiveness, or conduction velocity. Its antiarrhythmic action lies in its ability to uniformly increase ERP and APD in such a way that the ERP/APD ratio remains the same. It reduces the dispersion of refractoriness of the fibers.

Autonomic Effects.—The autonomic effects can be summarized as follows:

Class I_A.—Procainamide possesses a mild to moderate vagolytic effect and a mild α-sympathomimetic blocking effect.

Class I_B.—Lidocaine has no autonomic effects.

Class II.—Propranolol acts primarily by β-blockade.

Class III.—Bretylium causes a mild initial release, then subsequent inhibition of release of endogenous catecholamines.

Major Adverse Effects After Acute Intravenous Administration.—Major adverse effects are listed below.

Class I_A.—Procainamide can cause dose-related depression of myocardial contractility, vasodilation by α-adrenergic blockade, and increase heart rate by direct vagolytic and baroreceptor reflex mechanisms in low doses and bradycardia and arrhythmias in high doses. Procainamide can cause nausea and vomiting if rapidly administered to the awake patient, especially in the presence of hypotension. Procainamide (60%) and its active metabolite, N-acetylprocainamide, are cleared in the urine.

Class I_B.—Excessive serum levels of lidocaine are associated with adverse CNS effects, mild cardiac depression and vasodilatation in a dose-related manner. Lidocaine is rapidly cleared by the liver.

Class II.—Propranolol has many adverse effects that are related to β-blockade. These include bradycardia, atrioventricular block, decreased inotropy (especially in patients who require enhanced sympathetic tone for compensation), increased airway resistance in bronchospastic patients, and glucose intolerance and enhanced insulin sensitivity in diabetics.

Class III.—Bretylium, as discussed, causes initial hypertension followed by hypotension which may be accompanied by nausea and vomiting.

Summary

Lidocaine is dramatically effective against almost all ventricular arrhythmias—even those related to digitalis toxicity—is free of autonomic effects, has relatively mild CNS and cardiovascular side effects, and is rapidly cleared by the liver. It has the greatest therapeutic index and is most familiar to medical personnel. It has been used prophylactically with marginal success with freedom of side effects. In arrhythmias refractory to lidocaine, bretylium or procainamide are reasonable second choices. Propranolol should be reserved for special circumstances (such as massive catecholamine overdose) and then should be used cautiously.

Pulmonary artery catheters are useful tools in the assessment of critically ill patients and can be employed relatively safely with adequate preparation and familiarity with the treatment of sequelae.

REFERENCES

1. Swan HJC, Ganz W, Forrester J, et al: Catheterization of the heart in man with use of a flow directed balloon tipped catheter. *N Engl J Med* 1971; 283:447.
2. Civetta JM, Gabel JC: Flow directed pulmonary artery catheterization in surgical patient. *Ann Surg* 1972; 176:753.
3. Swan HJC: The role of hemodynamic monitoring in the management of the critically ill. *Crit Care Med* 1975; 3:83.
4. Swan HJC: Balloon flotation catheters: Their use in hemodynamic monitoring in clinical practice. *JAMA* 1975; 233:865.
5. Pace NL: A critique of flow-directed pulmonary arterial catheterization. *Anesthesiology* 1977; 47:455.
6. Katz JD, Cronau LH, Mandel SD, et al: Pulmonary artery flow guided catheters in the perioperative period: Indications and complications: An analysis of 340 consecutive insertions. *Crit Care Med* 1976; 4:99.
7. Daily PO, Griepp RB, Shumway NE: Percutaneous internal jugular vein cannulation. *Arch Surg* 1970; 101:534.
8. Blitt CD, Wright WA, Petty WC, et al: Central venous catheterization via the external jugular vein: A technique employing the J-wire. *JAMA* 1974; 229:817.
9. Carlon GC, Howland WS, Kahn RC, et al: Unusual complications during pulmonary artery catheterization. *Crit Care Med* 1978; 6:364.
10. Briscoe CE, Bushman JA, McDonald WI: Extensive neurological damage after cannulation of internal jugular vein. *Br Med J* 1974; 1:314.
11. Sprung CL, Jacobs LJ, Caralais JJ, et al: Ventricular arrhythmias during Swan-Ganz catheterization of the critically ill. *Chest* 1981; 79:413.
12. Shah KB, Rao TLK, Laughlin S, et al: A review of pulmonary artery catheterization in 6,245 patients. *Anesthesiology* 1984; 61:271.
13. Kumar V, Komatsu T, Masiello J, et al: Incidence of complications during Swan-Ganz catheter insertion performed by trainees. *Anesthesiology* 1983; 59:A473.
14. Cairns JA, Holder D: Ventricular fibrillation due to passage of a Swan-Ganz catheter, letter. *Am J Cardiol* 1975; 35:589.
15. Strasberg B, Berkowitz CE, Rosen KM: Right bundle branch block reflecting balloon inflation of Swan-Ganz catheter. *Chest* 1982; 81:368.
16. Thomson IR, Dalton BC, Lappas DG, et al: Right bundle branch block and complete heart block by Swan-Ganz catheter. *Anesthesiology* 1979; 51:359.
17. Abernathy WS: Complete heart block caused by the Swan-Ganz catheter. *Chest* 1974; 65:349.
18. Castellanos A, Ramirez AV, Mayorga-Cortes A, et al: Left fascicular blocks during right-heart catheterization using the Swan-Ganz catheter. *Circulation* 1981; 64:1271.

19. Nichols WW, Nichols MA, Barbour H: Complications associated with balloon-tipped flow directed catheters. *Heart Lung* 1979; 8:503.

20. Shimm DS, Rigsby L: Ventricular tachycardia associated with removal of a Swan-Ganz catheter. *Postgrad Med* 1980; 67:291.

21. German LD, Packer DL, Bardy GH, et al: Ventricular tachycardia induced by atrial stimulation in patients without symptomatic cardiac disease. *Am J Cardiol* 1983; 52:1202.

22. Abernathy WS, Crevey BJ: Right bundle branch block during transvenous ventricular pacing. *Am Heart J* 1975; 90:774.

23. Massing GK, James TN: Anatomical configuration of the His bundle and bundle branches in the human heart. *Circulation* 1976; 53:609.

24. Luck JC, Engel TR: Transient right bundle branch block with Swan-Ganz catheterization. *Am Heart J* 1976; 92:263.

25. Shaw TJ: The Swan-Ganz pulmonary artery catheter. *Anaesthesia* 1979; 34:651.

26. Salmenpera M, Peltola K, Rosenberg P: Does prophylactic lidocaine control cardiac arrhythmias associated with pulmonary artery catheterization? *Anesthesiology* 1982; 56:212.

27. Sclarovsky S, Zafrir N, Strasberg B, et al: Ventricular fibrillation complicating temporary ventricular pacing in acute myocardial infarction: Significance of right ventricular infarction. *Am J Cardiol* 1981; 48:1160.

28. Sprung CL, Pozen RG, Rozanski JL, et al: Advanced ventricular arrhythmias during bedside pulmonary artery catheterization. *Am J Med* 1982; 72:203.

29. Iberti TJ, Benjamin E, Gruppi L, et al: Ventricular arrhythmias during pulmonary artery catheterization in the intensive care unit. *Am J Med* 1985; 78:451.

30. Weng JT, Smith DE, Moulder PV: Antiarrhythmic drugs: The electrophysiologic basis of their clinical usage. *Ann Thorac Surg* 1986; 106–112.

31. Hoffman BF, Rosen MR: Cellular mechanisms for cardiac arrhythmias. *Circ Res* 1981; 49:1.

32. Hoffman BF, Cranefield PF: Physiologic basis of cardiac arrhythmias. *Am J Med* 1964; 37:670.

33. Gadsby DC, Wit AL: Normal and abnormal electrophysiology of cardiac cells in Mandel WJ (ed): *Cardiac Arrhythmias—Their Mechanisms, Diagnosis and Management*. Philadelphia, JB Lippincott Co, 1980, pp 55–82.

34. Wit AL, Rosen MR, Hoffman BF: Electrophysiology and pharmacology of cardiac arrhythmias. II. Relationship of normal and abnormal electrical activity of cardiac fibers to the genesis of arrhythmias: A. Automaticity. *Am Heart J* 1974; 88:515.

35. Wit AL, Rosen MR, Hoffman BF: Electrophysiology and pharmacology of cardiac arrhythmias: II. Relationship of normal and abnormal electrical activity of cardiac fibers to the genesis of arrhythmias: B. Re-entry, *Am Heart J* 1974; 88:664.

36. Boyden PA, Wit AL: Pharmacology of the antiarrhythmic drugs, in Rosen MR, Hoffman BF (eds): *Cardiac Therapy*. Boston, Martinus Nijhoff Publishers, 1983, pp 171–234.

37. Brown HF, Noble SJ: Membrane currents underlying delayed rectification and pacemaker activity in frog atrial muscle. *J Physiol* (London) 1969; 204:717.

38. Imanishi S, Surawicz B: Automatic activity in depolarized guinea pig ventricular myocardium: Characteristics and mechanism. *Circ Res* 1976; 39:751.

39. Katzung BO, Morgenstern JA: Effects of extracellular potassium on ventricular automaticity and evidence for a pacemaker current in mammalian ventricular myocardium. *Circ Res* 1977; 40:105.

40. Lazzara R, El-Sherif M, Scherlag BJ: Electrophysiological properties of canine Purkinje cells in one-day-old myocardial infarction. *Circ Res* 1973; 33:722.

41. Spear J, Horowitz L, Hodess A, et al: Cellular electrophysiology of human myocardial infarction: I. Abnormalities of cellular activation. *Circulation* 1979; 59:247.

42. Cranefield PF: Action potentials, afterpotentials and arrhythmias. *Circ Res* 1977; 41:415.

43. Bigger JT Jr: Mechanisms and diagnosis of arrhythmias, in Braunwald E (ed): *Heart Disease: A Textbook of Cardiovascular Medicine*. Philadelphia, WB Saunders Co, 1980, pp 630–690.

44. Bigger JT Jr, Hoffman BF: Antiarrhythmic drugs, in Gilman AG, Goodman LA, Gilman A (eds): *The Pharmacological Basis of Therapeutics*. New York, MacMillan Publishing Co Inc, 1980, pp 761–792.

45. Ferrier GR: Digitalis arrhythmias: Role of oscillatory afterpotentials. *Prog Cardiovasc Dis* 1977; 19:459.

46. Hoffman BF, Rosen MR, Wit AL: Electrophysiology and pharmacology of cardiac arrhythmias: III. The causes and treatment of cardiac arrhythmias. *Am Heart J* 1975; Part A 89:115, Part B 89:253.

47. Gallagher JJ: Mechanisms of arrhythmias and conduction abnormalities, in Hurst JW, et al (eds): *The Heart*, ed 5. New York, McGraw-Hill Book Co, 1982, pp 489–518.

48. Zipes DP: Genesis of cardiac arrhythmias: Electrophysiological considerations, in Braunwald E (ed): *Heart Disease: A Textbook of Cardiovascular Medicine*, ed 2. Philadelphia, WB Saunders, 1984, pp 605–647.

49. Berne RM, Levy MN: Electrical activity of the heart, in Berne RM, Levy MN (eds): *Cardiovascular Physiology*, ed 4. St Louis, CV Mosby Co, 1981, pp 5–51.

50. Downar E, Janse MJ, Durrer D: The effect of acute coronary artery occlusion on subepicardial transmembrane potentials in the intact porcine heart. *Circulation* 1977; 56:217.

51. Friedman PL, Stewart JR, Fenoglio JJ Jr, et al: Survival of subendocardial Purkinje fibers after extensive myocardial infarction in dogs: In vitro and in vivo correlations. *Circ Res* 1973; 33:597.

52. Gilmour RF Jr, Heger JJ, Prystowsky EN, et al: Cellular electrophysiologic abnormalities of diseased human ventricular myocardium. *Am J Cardiol* 1983; 51:137.

53. Lazzara R, El-Sherif N., Scherlag BJ: Early and late effects of coronary artery occlusion on canine Purkinje fibers. *Circ Res* 1974; 35:391.

54. Cranefield PF, Wit AL, Hoffman BF: Genesis of cardiac arrhythmias. *Circulation* 1973; 47:190.

55. Rosen MR, Wit Al, Hoffman BF: Electrophysiology and pharmacology of cardiac arrhythmias: I. Cellular electrophysiology of the mammalian heart. *Am Heart J* 1974; 88:380.

56. McDonald DP, MacLeod DP: Anoxia-recovery cycle in ventricular muscle: Action potential duration, contractility and ATP content. *Pflugers Arch* 1971; 325:305.

57. Schmitt FO, Erlanger J: Directional differences in the conduction of the impulse through heart muscle and their possible relation to extrasystolic and fibrillary contractions. *Am J Physiol* 1928; 87:326.

58 Hoffman BF, Bigger JT Jr: Digitalis and allied cardiac glycosides in Gilman AG, Goodman LS, Gilman A (eds): *The Pharmacological Basis of Therapeutics,* ed 6. New York, Macmillan Publishing Co Inc, 1980, pp 729–760.

59. Levy MN, Martin PJ: Neural control of the heart, in *Handbook of Physiology.* Bethesda, Md, American Physiology Society 1979, vol 1, pp 581–620.

60. Bailey JC, Watanabe AM, Besch HR Jr, et al: Acetylcholine antagonism of the electrophysiological effects of isoproterenol on canine cardiac Purkinje fibers. *Circ Res* 1979; 44:378.

61. Rosen MR, Hordof AJ, Ilvento JP, et al: Effects of adrenergic amines on electrophysiological properties and automaticity of neonatal and adult canine Purkinje fibers. *Circ Res* 1977; 40:390.

62. Levy MN: Neural control of cardiac rhythm and contraction, in Rosen MR, Hoffman BF (eds): *Cardiac Therapy.* Boston, Martinus Nijhoff, 1983, pp 73–94.

63. Wit AL, Hoffman BF, Rosen MR: Electrophysiology and pharmacology of cardiac arrhythmias: IX. Cardiac electrophysiologic effects of beta adrenergic receptor stimulation and blockade. *Am Heart J* 1975; part A, 90:521; Part B, 90:665; Part C, 90:795.

9

Delayed Rewarming During Cardiopulmonary Bypass

Recommendations by Glenn P. Gravlee, M.D.

A 52-year-old man weighing 130 kg (body surface area 2.7 m^2) underwent cardiopulmonary bypass grafting. Seven distal and three proximal vein graft anastomoses were performed during a total cardiopulmonary bypass time of 2 hours and 45 minutes, with the ascending aorta cross-clamped for 100 minutes while systemic perfusate temperature was 26° C. During rewarming, esophageal temperature and nasopharyngeal temperatures lagged behind blood temperature only slightly; however, the rectal thermistor displayed a reading of 30° C when the nasopharyngeal temperature reached 37° C. The upper limit of perfusion flow for this patient was 2.2 L/minute/m^2. The perfusionist, surgeon, and anesthesiologist disagreed about discontinuing cardiopulmonary bypass.

ANALYSIS OF THE PROBLEM

This patient presents the operating team with everyday problems carried to an extreme. He falls on the tail of the "bell-shaped curve" in body size, number of distal coronary artery bypass grafts performed, aortic cross-clamp duration, and duration of hypothermia. Systemic hypothermia during myocardial revascularization protects the patient in several ways.[1] By decreasing systemic oxygen utilization (MVO$_2$), hypothermia allows adequate systemic perfusion at reduced blood flows and extends the safe period for complete circulatory arrest. Reduced systemic blood flows enhance myocardial protection by reducing washout of protective cardioplegic solutions via noncoronary collateral flow. Systemic hypothermia also facilitates myocardial protection by reducing the temperature gradient between the myocardium and surrounding mediastinal tissues during cold cardioplegic arrest. Although systemic hypothermia attenuates some problems, it creates others. When should rewarming begin? What is the maximum safe water-to-blood temperature gradient? What is a suitable end point for rewarming? This latter question particularly elicits disagreements among practitioners of surgery, anesthesiology, and perfusion technology.

Temperatures measured with cooling and rewarming during cardiopulmonary bypass (CPB) reflect the perfusion of the monitoring site. This physiology bears a strong resemblance to models used by Eger to explain uptake and distribution of anesthetic drugs.[2] The vessel-rich group contains the least body mass, but receives the greatest blood flow. These organs (brain, lungs, heart, intestines, liver, kidneys, endocrines), sometimes termed the body "core," therefore warm and cool quickly in response to induced changes in arterial blood temperature. Temperatures measured in the esophagus, nasopharynx, or adjacent to the tympanic membrane best represent perfusion of the vessel-rich group. Next in line is the muscle group, normally representing the majority of body mass while extracting a small fraction (18%) of resting systemic blood flow. Intramuscular and rectal temperature probes reflect perfusion to the muscle group, despite the rectum's obvious connection to more proximal conduits belonging to the vessel-rich group. Finally come the fat and vessel-poor groups, consisting primarily of bone, subcutaneous tissues, and skin. Skin temperature best represents the perfusion of these tissues, variously monitored on the great toe, forearm, or thumb.[3, 4]

Just as would be predicted, the rapidity of temperature descent during the "core cooling" used with CPB depends upon the temperature monitoring site. Changes in temperature usually manifest in the following order: (1) arterial/venous blood; (2) urinary bladder; (3) esophagus; (4) nasopharynx or tympanic membrane; (5) rectum; (6) muscle; (7) skin.[3, 5–7] Figures 9–1 and 9–2 demonstrate most of this progression during systemic cooling and warming. Prolonging systemic hypothermia to accommodate sustained myocardial cardioplegic arrest progressively distributes hypothermia to poorly perfused tissues. The obese patient maintained at 26° C for 100 minutes accumulates a staggering caloric deficit (I will leave the calculations to those possessing a propensity for mathematics). Reawakening an obese patient following several hours of receiving methoxyflurane at the 1.3 MAC (minimal alveolar concentration) poses an anesthetic analogy. Although a light plane of surgical analgesia with adequate respiration might ensue fairly rapidly, mental alertness would lag far behind. Continued seepage of sequestered anesthetic from poorly perfused tissues into the blood stream accounts for this sequence.

In much the same manner, separating from CPB before achieving adequate peripheral rewarming will result in substantial core recooling, sometimes called hypothermic rebound or "afterdrop." Gradual equilibration of the vari-

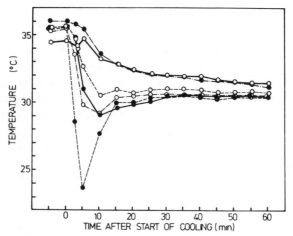

FIG 9–1.
Mean temperatures during cooling and hypothermia: ● – – – – ●, arterial; ○ —.—.— ○, mixed venous; ● ———— ●, esophageal; ○ – – – – ○, nasopharyngeal; ● —.—.— ●, rectal; ○ ———— ○, deltoid. (From Davis FM, et al: *Br J Anaesth* 1977; 49:1130. Used by permission.)

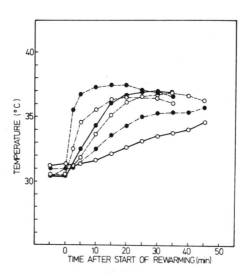

FIG 9–2.
Mean temperatures during rewarming. Symbols as in Figure 9–1. (From Davis FM, et al: *Br J Anaesth* 1977; 49:1130. Used by permission.)

ous temperature gradients in the body explains this process. In this obese patient, separation from CPB at a rectal temperature of 30° C would likely engender an esophageal temperature afterdrop to 32° C or below. Evolving over the first two hours following CPB, this rebound hypothermia predisposes to electrolyte disturbances, ventricular arrhythmias, unfavorable hemodynamic alterations, and greatly increased oxygen consumption (by shivering).[8–11] The hemodynamic consequences include increased systemic vascular resistance and decreased cardiac index.[12] Although the clinician can treat these physiologic disturbances successfully, many hours will elapse before this large patient will rewarm sufficiently to simplify postoperative management. The efficiency of core rewarming during CPB far exceeds that offered by other modalities such as radiant heat, heated inspired gases, and warmed intravenous fluids.

When it rains it pours, so we must also manage with a limited CPB perfusion flow capacity in this patient. Many oxygenators approach an upper limit of effective oxygen transfer in a total blood flow range of 6 to 7 L/minute.[13] Both bubble and membrane oxygenators have maximum recommended blood flows known as rated flow, defined as the maximum blood flow at which the oxygenator can produce 95% oxygen saturation while receiving a normal mixed venous inflow (hematocrit reading 40%, O_2 saturation 65%). A 6.0-L flow limit achieves a perfusion index of 2.2 in this patient. While most clinicians consider a 2.2 L/minute/m^2 flow index adequate during CPB, such flows fail to induce adequate rewarming in the presence of prolonged hypothermia at 26° C. Stanley and Jackson argue that perfusion flows often exceeding 3.0 L/minute/m^2 should be routinely employed during CPB to prevent a peripheral oxygen debt from accumulating lactic acid.[14]

APPROACH TO THE PROBLEM

I believe that this patient should remain on CPB until achieving a rectal temperature of 35° C. Rewarming to a higher rectal temperature would prove impractical because of excessive prolongation of CPB, which increases the risk of neurologic, renal, and coagulation disturbances.[15–17] Limiting perfusion flow to 2.2 L/minute/m^2 would probably achieve this goal in 30 to 45 minutes, but I suggest taking several steps to hasten rewarming.

First, I recommend using sodium nitroprusside prophylactically to reduce mean arterial pressure to 40 to 50 mm Hg at the maximum perfusion flow. Noback and Tinker showed that routine use of sodium nitroprusside during rewarming increases the rate of temperature rise, presumably by facilitating capillary perfusion to vessel-poor hypothermic areas.[18]

Second, I would place this patient on partial CPB and pulmonary ventilation as soon as the myocardium achieved a vigorous appearance with a satisfactory intrinsic or paced rhythm. My goal would be to maintain the highest achievable level of perfusion flow that permits a partial CPB pulse pressure exceeding 30 mm Hg. Gradually occluding venous return to the oxygenator should accomplish this. Physiologic arterial pulsatility generated by the patient's left ventricle will likely speed the rewarming process by improving capillary blood flow.[19] Because the patient's heart and lungs will contribute to systemic oxygen delivery, this approach may increase total oxygen delivery (total systemic blood flow × arterial oxygen content) while decreasing oxygenator blood flow. If the heart overdistends before achieving a suitable pulse pressure, I would abandon this approach and return to full cardiopulmonary bypass until the heart became more vigorous.

Third, I prefer attaining a hematocrit value between 25% and 30% for this patient while rewarming proceeds. Physicians at most medical centers use hemodilution for patients during hypothermia to a 20% to 25% hematocrit reading to facilitate blood flow. Maintaining this reduced hematocrit value during rewarming ordinarily incurs no additional risk.[20] In this patient, however, CPB proceeds at the limit of the oxygenator's O_2-delivery capacity; plus partial CPB mandates that the patient's lungs contribute to systemic oxygen delivery. Under these circumstances, increasing red blood cell mass offers an increased oxygen-carrying capacity for any given PaO_2. One proviso: increasing the red blood cell mass may decrease the PaO_2 by transferring (in effect) some dissolved oxygen onto hemoglobin. This should cause little concern unless the PaO_2 during complete cardiopulmonary bypass is below 100 mm Hg. I would achieve the desired hematocrit level by transfusing packed red blood cells if the oxygenator reservoir volume were low, but would utilize ultrafiltration instead if the reservoir volume were high.

Finally, I would scrupulously maintain deep anesthesia in this patient, to keep oxygen consumption as low as possible. In view of proportionate increases in oxygen consumption during rewarming, deep narcotic anesthesia will considerably reduce MVO_2.[21] Maintaining complete suppression of the twitch response to peripheral motor nerve stimulation will minimize subclinical muscle activity, further reducing total body oxygen consumption.[22] These anesthetic maneuvers will also minimize the adverse metabolic and hemodynamic consequences of the temperature afterdrop that will inevitably occur after terminating systemic rewarming at a 35° C rectal temperature.

DISCUSSION

The rewarming end point selected following hypothermic CPB varies from hospital to hospital. Different practices coexist even within my own institution. We utilize rectal temperature as a primary guide to adequate rewarming. With restoration of rectal temperature to 37° C, we seldom observe an afterdrop in esophageal or blood temperature to below 36° C unless the thorax remains open for more than an hour. When discontinuing CPB in patients with an esophageal temperature of 38° C and a rectal temperature of 34° C to 35° C, the esophageal and blood temperatures frequently drop below 35° C before beginning a delayed postoperative ascent. Occasionally we disregard a slowly rising rectal temperature if other clinical signs (perspiration, warm deltoid muscles) indicate complete rewarming. In the absence of clinical signs signaling adequate rewarming of peripheral tissues, failing to heed a slowly rising rectal temperature usually results in excessive hypothermic afterdrops. Muravchick and colleagues recommend utilizing a skin temperature exceeding 30° C as an index for sufficient rewarming.[3] Although I have not utilized that monitoring site during cardiac procedures, I suspect that restoring skin temperature to 32° C constitutes a better rewarming end point.

It could be argued that moderate hypothermia (33° C to 35° C) after CPB entails little risk if properly managed. By reducing oxygen consumption approximately 7% per degree centigrade, the periphery should require less work from the possibly compromised myocardium. The clinician must pay particular attention to maintaining an anesthetized state with complete neuromuscular blockade to avert the increased oxygen consumption induced by muscle shivering. Such muscle activity may increase total body oxygen demands beyond the heart's capacity to increase peripheral oxygen delivery. Despite taking these precautions, hypothermia usually increases systemic vascular resistance (SVR), thus placing an increased afterload on a heart that often cannot compensate adequately for that stress. Compromised left ventricular function exists in obese patients even in the absence of coronary artery disease, an elevated SVR, or the added insult presented by CPB.[23]

Although vasodilators can effectively counteract the increased SVR and maintain cardiac performance, the hemodynamic vicissitudes of the early postoperative period appear proportionate to the magnitude of the hypothermic afterdrop. As resumed rewarming proceeds over the first several hours, the increased SVR erratically converts to a vasodilated state when the temperature "overshoots" to 39° C several hours later. This necessitates frequent readjustments in vasoactive drug dosages and fluid administration. Additionally Sladen documented that ventilation requirements vary directly with body temperature.[24] If hypothermic patients are placed on usual ventilator settings when they first enter the postoperative recovery area unacceptable hypocarbia occurs. During rewarming and "overshoot," the minute ventilation should be increased accordingly to prevent hypercarbia. I believe that rewarming to a rectal temperature above 36° C simplifies postoperative management by reducing the temperature afterdrop, thereby diminishing the frequency and magnitude of these physiologic disturbances. However, the clinician must temper the urge to fully rewarm with an appreciation for the adverse consequences of prolonged CPB. I favor relaxing these temperature rewarming criteria when CPB exceeds two hours, after allowing sufficient time for postischemic myocardial reperfusion.

Because most available bubble and membrane oxygenators perform quite well, the clinician can easily forget that they possess upper limits for safe oxygen delivery. When dealing with patients having body surface areas exceeding 2.2 m^2, it behooves the perfusionist to select an oxygenator with a rated flow exceeding 6 L/minute. With some trepidation, we occasionally exceed oxygenator rated flows, finding that this can be safely accomplished if the perfusionist closely monitors PaO$_2$ and mixed venous oxygen saturation. Monitoring venous oxygen saturation continuously with an in-line oximeter greatly facilitates that capability. Although most oxygenators will oxygenate the blood adequately somewhat above the rated flow, common sense dictates selection of a unit possessing a predetermined high-flow capacity when perfusing larger patients.

Some would disagree with the selection of partial CPB to elicit pulsatile flow. Reports conflict with regard to the utility of pulsatility to enhance rewarming. Williams and co-authors demonstrated its value in children,[25] yet Singh and colleagues found no advantage to its use in adults.[26] The latter authors also reported absence of the expected hemodynamic accompaniments to pulsatile CPB, notably a normal SVR. Systemic vascular resistance rises progressively during nonpulsatile CPB, while pulsatile CPB normally diminishes that trend. Observing Singh's pulsatile assist waveform makes one suspect that their pulsatile flow pattern was insufficiently physiologic to "fool" the peripheral vascular bed. The contour of a generated pulsatile wave is as important as the presence of a pulse pressure.[19] It's not easy to fool Mother Nature, but pulsatile flow generated by the left ventricle during partial CPB might do the trick.

Summary

This patient challenges the entire surgical team. As is so often the case in the practice of anesthesiology, understanding the fundamentals of respiratory and circulatory physiology should lead the clinician to appropriate therapeutic actions during CPB.

REFERENCES

1. Reitz BA, Ream AK: Uses of hypothermia in cardiovascular surgery, in Ream AK, Fogdall RP (eds): *Acute Cardiovascular Management.* Philadelphia, JB Lippincott Co, 1982, pp 830–851.

2. Eger EI II: *Anesthetic Uptake and Action*. Baltimore, William & Wilkins Co, 1974, pp 88–89.
3. Muravchick S, Conrad DP, Vargas A: Peripheral temperature monitoring during cardiopulmonary bypass operation. *Ann Thorac Surg* 1980; 29:36.
4. Henning RJ, Wiener F, Valdes S, et al: Measurement of toe temperature for assessing the severity of acute circulatory failure. *Surg Gynecol Obstet* 1979; 149:1.
5. Davis FM, Parimelazhagan KN, Harris EA: Thermal balance during cardiopulmonary bypass with moderate hypothermia in man. *Br J Anaesth* 1977; 49:1127.
6. Lilly JK, Boland JP, Zekan S: Urinary bladder temperature monitoring: A new index of body core temperature. *Crit Care Med* 1980; 8:742.
7. Azar I: Rectal temperature is best indicator of adequate rewarming during cardiopulmonary bypass. *Anesthesiology* 1981; 55:189.
8. Moyer JH, Morris G, DeBakey ME: Hypothermia: I. Effect on renal hemodynamics and on excretion of water and electrolytes in dog and man. *Ann Surg* 1957; 145:26.
9. Black PR, Devanter SV, Cohn LH: Effects of hypothermia on systemic and organ system metabolism and function. *J Surg Res* 1976; 20:49.
10. Brock L, Skinner JM, Manders JT: Observations on peripheral and central temperatures with particular reference to the occurrence of vasoconstriction. *Br J Surg* 1975; 62:589.
11. Vandam LD, Burnap TK: Hypothermia. *N Engl J Med* 1959; 261:546.
12. Czer L, Hamer A, Murphy F, et al: Transient hemodynamic dysfunction after myocardial revascularization. *J Thorac Cardiovasc Surg* 1983; 86:226.
13. Bartlett RH, Gazzaniga AB: Physiology and pathophysiology of extracorporeal circulation, in Ionescu MI (ed): *Technique in Extracorporeal Circulation*. London, Butterworths, 1981, pp 3–43.
14. Stanley TH, Jackson J: The influence of blood flow and arterial blood pressure during cardiopulmonary bypass on deltoid muscle gas tensions and body temperature after bypass. *Can Anaesth Soc J* 1979; 26:277.
15. Utley JR: Renal effects of cardiopulmonary bypass, in Utley JR (ed): *Pathophysiology and Techniques of Cardiopulmonary Bypass*. Baltimore, Williams & Wilkins Co, 1982, vol 1, pp 40–54.
16. Aberg T, Kihlgren M: Cerebral protection during open-heart surgery. *Thorax* 1977; 32:525.
17. Sotaniemi KA, Juolasmaa A, Hokkanen ET: Neuropsychologic outcome after open-heart surgery. *Arch Neurol* 1981; 38:2.
18. Noback CR, Tinker JH: Hypothermia after cardiopulmonary bypass in man: Amelioration by nitroprusside-induced vasodilation during rewarming. *Anesthesiology* 1980; 53:277.
19. Hickey PR, Buckley MJ, Philbin DM: Pulsatile and nonpulsatile cardiopulmonary bypass: Review of a counterproductive controversy. *Ann Thorac Surg* 1983; 36:720.
20. Moores WY: Oxygen delivery during cardiopulmonary bypass, in Utley JR (ed): *Pathophysiology and Techniques of Cardiopulmonary Bypass*. Baltimore, Williams & Wilkins Co, 1982, vol 1, pp. 1–11.
21. Reiz S, Balfors E, Haggmark S, et al: Myocardial oxygen consumption and

coronary haemodynamics during fentanyl-droperidol-nitrous oxide anaesthesia in patients with ischaemic heart disease. *Acta Anaesthesiol Scand* 1981; 25:286.

22. Lowenstein E: personal communication.
23. DeDivitiis O, Fazio S, Petitto M: Obesity and cardiac function. *Circulation* 1981; 64:477.
24. Sladen RN: Temperature and ventilation after hypothermic cardiopulmonary bypass. *Anesth Analg* 1985; 64:816.
25. Williams GD, Seifen AB, Lawson NW, et al: Pulsatile perfusion versus conventional high-flow nonpusatile perfusion for rapid core cooling and rewarding of infants for circulatory arrest in cardiac operation. *J Thorac Cardiovasc Surg* 1979; 78:667.
26. Singh RKK, Barratt-Boyes BG, Harris EA: Does pulsatile flow improve perfusion during hypothermic cardiopulmonary bypass? *J Thorac Cardiovasc Surg* 1980; 79:827.

10

Air in the Aortic Perfusion Cannula at Conclusion of Cardiopulmonary Bypass

Recommendations by John R. Cooper, Jr., M.D.

A 60-year-old man with aortic value disease and coronary artery disease underwent an uneventful aortic valve replacement and coronary artery bypass operation. Immediately after cessation of cardiopulmonary bypass, air was observed in the aortic perfusion cannula, and in the vein graft to the left anterior descending coronary artery. The blood pressure was 90/80mm Hg, heart rate 80 beats per minute, PAWP 16, and cardiac index 1.8 L/min/m^2. The left ventricle appeared dilated.

ANALYSIS OF THE PROBLEM

This patient presents low cardiac output after aortic value replacement and aortocoronary bypass with low pulse pressure, relatively high pulmonary artery wedge pressure (PAWP), and low cardiac index. There are many causes of low cardiac output after weaning from bypass but air in the aorta perfusion cannula (Fig 10–1) and in the left anterior descending vein graft requires that the most obvious cause, coronary air embolism, be considered first.

Coronary air emboli derive from air introduced into the left side of the heart by one of several mechanisms, most commonly from deliberate opening of the left side of the heart or aorta for valve replacement, resection of ventricular aneurysm, or repair of the ascending aorta. Air may also be introduced by placement of left-sided heart vents into the left atrium, ventricular apex, or aortic root, or additionally from suction of these vents during the procedure.

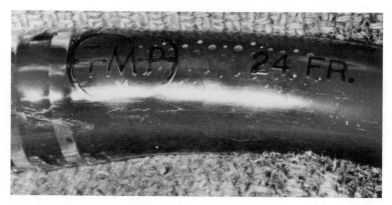

FIG 10–1.
Air in aortic perfusion cannula after mitral valve replacement in a 26-year-old woman.

Accidents during extracorporeal circulation, such as reversal of arterial and venous or vent tubing, can lead to massive air embolism. During coronary artery bypass procedures, air may be introduced directly into the coronary grafts when the distal anastomoses are performed first. Flushing the vein with a fluid-filled syringe to check the distal suture line can result in injection of air if there are bubbles in the syringe. Air may also be sucked retrograde through the coronary arteriotomy by a left ventricular vent.

In most cases, air in the coronary arteries produces a mechanical block of blood flow with resulting myocardial ischemia, dysfunction, and dysrhythmias. Air bubbles will lodge in a coronary artery or vein graft with a diameter equal to their own and can persist unless dislodged or until the gas is absorbed, which occurs slowly. Obstruction of coronary flow by air usually produces marked ST-segment elevation on electrocardiogram (ECG) and, characteristically, the degree of elevation is not constant and will fall rapidly with dislodgement of the embolus (Fig 10–2). The ST elevation may not be present in all leads, but will most likely be in those reflecting the right coronary artery distribution (II,III,aVF). There may also be reciprocal ST depression in other leads (see Fig 10–2). The right coronary artery is more often affected because its orifice is superior in the supine position. Therefore, ejected air is more likely to enter it. Vein grafts are usually anastamosed to the anterior ascending aorta, so air may enter any or all of them.

APPROACH TO THE PROBLEM

Assuming coronary air is the cause of low output, the objective of therapy is to raise the perfusion pressure to force the bubbles through to the venous side and/or to increase myocardial contractility. This is most readily accomplished with a single dose of epinephrine. Five or ten micrograms given intravenously will often suffice. The increased perfusion pressure from increased cardiac output and increased systemic vascular resistance will tend to force the bubbles through the coronary circulation. Increased contractility will disrupt the

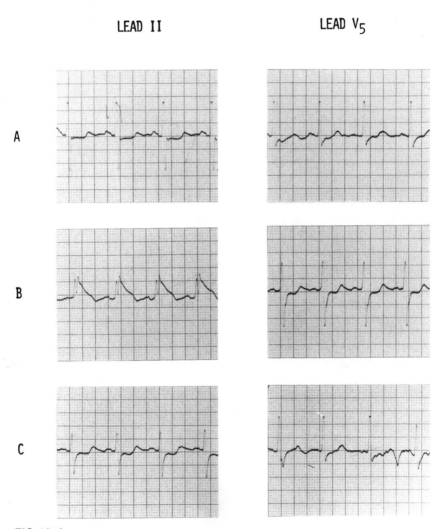

LEAD II   **LEAD V₅**

A

B

C

FIG 10–2.
Electrocardiograms in a 56-year-old woman having aortic valve resection. *A,* preinduction. *B,* five minutes after cross-clamp removal; note ST elevation in II, reciprocal ST depression in V₅. *C,* five minutes after *B;* changes have resolved.

adhesive frictional forces between the bubbles and the vessel wall and may break larger bubbles into smaller ones. Both of these actions will enhance forward movement.

If cardiac contractility is already vigorous but with low output and ST-segment elevation, which is often a finding after repair of congenital defects in children, phenylephrine (Neo-Synephrine) in doses of 25 to 50 μg intravenously would be a preferred alternative to epinephrine. If perfusion pressure is already high but contractility is poor or heart block is present, then isoproterenol (4 to 10μg) may be effective. Heart block under these circumstances may be from an embolus in the right coronary artery affecting flow to the conduction system and a temporary pacemaker will be needed if the isoproterenol does not increase heart rate.

When the vasopressor is given, this patient should also be placed in head-down position. This may prevent any remaining left ventricular air from being embolized to the cerebral circulation. The rationale is that since air is buoyant, it will tend to remain uppermost. Therefore, air ejected into the aorta will remain on the anterior surface of the arch and go up the descending aorta instead of down into the carotid arteries.

When bubbles are seen in a coronary graft, as in this case, the surgeon can vent the air from the vein graft or artery using a small (usually 25-gauge) needle. Such small needle holes rarely bleed postoperatively.

With multiple air emboli, the myocardium may not respond with increased contractility and perfusion pressure because the epinephrine does not reach the cardiac receptors. In this event, cardiopulmonary bypass must be reinstituted after removal of the air present in the aortic cannula by disconnection, flushing, and reconnection. After return to bypass, partial clamping of the ascending aorta distal to the aortic perfusion cannula can be performed. The maneuver forces a large volume of perfusate at high pressure through the coronary circulation and will usually push air bubbles through. Failure of this maneuver, failure of additional doses of epinephrine or isoproterenol, and failure of ST segments to decrease toward normal suggests air embolism is not the cause of the low cardiac output and other diagnoses should be entertained.

DISCUSSION

Alternative Therapy

The goals of increasing perfusion pressure and increasing contractility to dislodge emboli are the mainstays of therapy, short of placing the patient in a hyperbaric chamber, which is not practical in most circumstances. Obviously the circulation must be supported while these goals are achieved by whatever means are deemed appropriate. A different sequence could be used for the therapy illustrated above. A return to cardiopulmonary bypass first, before additional pharmacologic therapy, might be considered safest especially if the patient's cardiac output were falling rapidly. Other vasopressors could also be used, such as dobutamine or dopamine, as long as an increased perfusion pressure and increased contractility result.

Biophysical Factors

Gas, when mixed with a colloidal solution such as blood, will form bubbles that are composed of an inner gas phase and an outer membrane of proteins, lipids, and platelets. This membrane stabilizes the bubble, with greater membrane thickness conferring greater stability. Once formed, bubbles may react with themselves—producing foam, coalescing into bubbles of larger size, or fracturing into microbubbles. When a bubble lodges in a vessel, friction between the vessel wall and bubble capsule will retard movement. The bubble will still respond to hydraulic forces but they must overcome the friction and the resistance of the bubble's capsule to deformation. The bubble will tend to shrink but the rate will depend on La Place forces influencing surface tension, and on the composition of the gaseous phase, with oxygen bubbles shrinking faster than air bubbles.[1] Without intervention, the natural history of bubble emboli is initial obstruction followed by gradual decrease in size and slow distal movement.[2]

Cerebral Emboli

The other organ system primarily affected by left-sided air emboli is the brain. Cerebral damage from secondary ischemia has been well documented, but the degree of damage is often very difficult to predict from clinical events. Though death or a vegetative state can result, several cases of massive emboli have been documented that resolved with little if any sequelae.[3] Conversely, relatively small amounts of air such as in the case presented have been judged responsible for postoperative neurologic damage.[4] The factors that govern the extent of damage are not clear, though the clinical course is often one of rapid, sometimes dramatic, improvement. In cases such as the one illustrated here, appropriate preventive measures (see below) should reduce the chances of significant cerebral air embolization (see Chapter 23). It should also be recognized that particulate embolization from thrombi, calcium, or atheromatous debris may be a significant contributor to neurologic sequelae, especially when the left side of the heart is opened.

Emboli Prophylaxis

Careful evacuation of air before discontinuation of bypass provides the best opportunity for prevention. If left-sided air is likely, the patient should be placed in head-down position before the aortic cross clamp is removed. This position should be maintained for several minutes after left ventricular ejection starts, as bubbles have been echocardiographically detected as being expelled for five minutes and longer after bypass was discontinued.[4,5] The usefulness of this maneuver in terms of outcome has never been documented but seems logical and otherwise harmless. Surgical procedures to prevent or remove air emboli include: closing the left-sided heart vent under blood; venting air from the left ventricle and ascending aorta, or both; manual massage of the ventricles and coronaries; partial clamping of the distal ascending aorta for coronary perfusion; and needle venting of vein grafts. Despite all efforts to evacuate air from the left side of the heart, it is impossible, as has been shown experimentally, to evacuate all the air without chemically altering the surface tension of the surrounding fluid.[5] Some ejection of air is therefore inevitable and should be expected.

As noted above, air has been detected leaving the left side of the heart for several minutes after cardiac contraction restarts. It is unknown though how long air that is not ejected may remain trapped in the left atrium or left ventricle. Air emboli persisting hours postoperatively are difficult to document, but occasional cases of transient ST elevation in patients after cardiac surgery with rapid resolution of these ECG changes could represent air. Cases of patients who suffer hypotension or cardiovascular collapse after a change of position (such as sitting up for a chest x-ray) could also represent release of trapped air from the left-sided chambers.

Coronary air embolism may not manifest itself as clearly as in the illustrated case. There may be no visible air in the aortic cannula, coronary grafts, or coronary arteries themselves. The ST segment elevation, even in isolated leads, may be secondary to a particulate embolus or a myocardial infarction from another cause. Indeed, the diagnosis of air embolus may be made in retrospect, after observing a rapidly changing ECG configuration and improvement with vasopressor therapy. Air emboli must be included in any differential diagnosis when difficult weaning from bypass with low cardiac output is encountered.

REFERENCES

1. Butler BD: Biophysical aspects of gas bubbles in blood. *Med Instrum* 1985; 19:59–62.
2. Virtue RW, Wagner WW, Swanson GD: Fate of gas emboli in the dog. *Anesthesiology* 1982; 59:A72.
3. Mills NH, Ochsner JO: Massive air embolism during cardiopulmonary bypass. *J Thorac Cardiovasc Surg* 1980; 80:708–717.
4. Rodigas PC, Meyer FJ, Hoasler GB, et al: Intraoperative 2-dimensional echocar-

diography: Ejection of microbubbles from the left ventricle after cardiac surgery. *Am J Cardiol* 1982; 50:1130–1132.

5. Oka Y, Moriwaki KM, Hong Y, et al: Detection of air emboli in the left heart by M mode transesophageal echocardiography following cardiopulmony bypass. *Anesthesiology* 1985; 63:109–113.

6. Padula RT, Eisenstat TE, Bronstein MH, et al: Intracardiac air following cardiotomy: Location, causative factors, and a method for removal. *J Thorac Cardiovasc Surg* 1971; 62:736–742.

11

Intraoperative Pacemaker Failure

Recommendations by James R. Zaidan, M.D.

An emergency transvenous atrioventricular (AV) sequential pacemaker was placed in a 70-year-old man with coronary artery disease who developed third-degree heart block during an acute myocardial infarction two days prior to coronary artery bypass surgery. The patient was monitored with ECG, arterial line, and a nonpacing Swan-Ganz catheter. During induction of anesthesia, his temporary pacemaker, which had been maintaining a paced heart rate of 72 beats per minute with adequate cardiac outputs, failed to capture the atrium and ventricle. The heart rate fell to 40 beats per minute, and there was a decrease in cardiac output and blood pressure.

ANALYSIS OF THE PROBLEM

This is a case of pacemaker failure in a patient whose cardiac output is dependent on maintaining a heart rate greater than 50 beats per minute.

APPROACH TO THE PROBLEM

In the event of pacemaker failure, the following steps should be taken.

1. Assure an inspiratory oxygen concentration of 1.0.

2. Quickly check all pacemaker connections.

3. Observe the on-off switch. If the pacer is on, but the light does not work, then the battery is low. The flashing light on the pacemaker generator fails before the generator's output stops. Change the pacemaker or the battery inside the pacemaker.

4. Increase the ventricular current output. In a sequential pacemaker, also decrease the atrial output. It is better to lose the atrial kick than ventricular contraction.

5. Begin cardiopulmonary resuscitation (CPR) if blood pressure cannot be maintained with the slower rate.

6. Use isoproterenol to increase the ventricular rate.

DISCUSSION

Patients occasionally require pacemakers for heart block associated with acute myocardial infarction. Sometimes these patients also require emergency coronary artery surgery. The anesthesiologist, therefore, must make medical judgments concerning monitoring, anesthetic techniques, and intraoperative care. This section will discuss the pathophysiology of heart block, the preanesthetic evaluation, monitoring, and the possible causes and treatment of intraoperative pacing failure.

Pathophysiology

High-degree heart block occasionally occurs after an acute myocardial infarction.[1,2] When it occurs, heart block requires immediate treatment, because it causes a profound decrease in cardiac output and blood pressure.

Inferior myocardial infarctions are associated with first-degree and second-degree Mobitz type I (Wenckebach) block.[3] Cardiologists will not place a temporary pacing electrode in these patients, because the block generally does not proceed to complete heart block. Patients with an acute anterior myocardial infarction, however, can develop second-degree Mobitz type II that quickly proceeds to third-degree block.[3] Cardiologists insert temporary electrodes when patients develop any degree of block after an acute anterior myocardial infarction.

Pacing increases heart rate but does not reverse the underlying cause of the block. The type of pacing is important. A patient with a heart rate of 35 beats per minute benefits from ventricular pacing at 75 beats per minute. The cardiac output does not necessarily increase further with a greater increase in heart rate.[4] Ventricular pacing at 100 beats per minute could sufficiently decrease diastolic filling time to worsen myocardial ischemia. Pacing techniques that maintain a normal atrioventricular (AV) contraction sequence increase cardiac output above the cardiac output associated with ventricular pacing.[4-6] Although atrial pacing effectively reverses bradycardia in the presence of intact AV conduction, atrial pacing cannot treat bradycardia when the AV node is sufficiently ischemic to stop AV conduction at higher pacing rates. In this situation and in the presence of third-degree block, atrial pacing cannot facilitate ventricular contraction. Sequential pacing, a technique that stimulates first the atrium, then the ventricle after an adjustable PR interval, should replace atrial pacing when AV conduction is abnormal. Sequential pacing allows manipulation of the heart rate and of the PR interval to achieve the highest possible cardiac output.

Preanesthetic Evaluation

Evaluate the patient with the understanding that the requirement for a pacemaker implies more advanced coronary artery disease. Otherwise, proceed as you would for any other cardiac surgical procedure, noting the extent and location of the coronary lesions and left ventricular function. Auscultate for carotid, subclavian, and femoral arterial bruits, and determine if the patient has an element of congestive failure. Evaluate the airway.

Laboratory evaluation does not have to be extensive. Follow your usual guidelines for determination of electrolytes and hemoglobin. A portable chest x-ray film generally adds little to your knowledge of the patient.

Pacemaker evaluation assumes secondary importance to evaluation of the patient. Ensure that each pacemaker impulse is followed by ventricular contraction by palpating a peripheral pulse and correlating the pulse with the flashing light on the pacemaker or with an ECG tracing. Repeat this procedure several times with the patient taking deep breaths. Second, test the patient's escape rate and rhythm by slowly decreasing the pacemaker rate when the pacemaker sensitivity is set on approximately 3 mv. Do not unnecessarily test for escape rate and rhythm if the pacemaker rate is decreased to 45 and the patient does not begin to override the pacemaker. Third, test the threshold by slowly decreasing the current output of the generator until capture is lost. Increase the current output until capture reoccurs. This current on the pacemaker control dial is the current threshold. If it approaches 20 mA, then no safety margin exists should pacing fail during induction. After determining the threshold, set the pacemaker to twice the threshold.

Anesthetic Drugs

All anesthetic drugs have been successfully used in patients with temporary pacemakers. Do not change your anesthetic drug management because the patient requires a pacemaker. Both narcotic and inhalational techniques are reasonable.

Monitoring

The question concerning monitoring with a pulmonary arterial (PA) catheter versus a central venous catheter assumes major importance. The incidence of dislodging a temporary ventricular electrode when floating a pulmonary arterial catheter remains unknown. It is reasonable to float a pulmonary arterial catheter in a critically ill patient who will benefit from your knowing the cardiac output. Several suggestions may help:

1. Include in your preoperative note the reasons for inserting the PA catheter.

2. Insert a PA catheter that has pacing capabilities such as a Swan-Ganz pacing catheter or the Swan-Ganz paceport catheter.

3. Insert the PA catheter to the central venous pressure (CVP): atrial position and float the catheter to the wedge position after opening the chest.

4. Consider using esophageal or transcutaneous pacing. An esophageal probe could be inserted after induction. The transcutaneous pacing electrode must be moved to the left side of the chest to clear the operative area. This could potentially increase the threshold so that transcutaneous pacing might not be possible.

Causes of Intraoperative Pacemaker Failure

There are several causes of failure of a temporary pacemaker.

Mechanical Problems
Disconnections and low battery should be ruled out by changing the generator and assuring that the pacing cable is securely connected to the generator.

Electrode Dislodgment
Electrode dislodgment also could be a likely cause of loss of pacing in this patient. This problem arises when induction of anesthesia causes preload or afterload related changes in heart size. Also, a change in ventilatory pattern can cause loss of pacing. If pacing is lost in these situations, increase the current output of the generator.

Special Problems

External sequential pacemakers are designed with two current outputs: one to the atrium and one to the ventricle. The atrial output occasionally inhibits the ventricular output if the R-wave sensitivity is set at a very low number. Simply decrease the atrial output or set the R-wave sensitivity on a higher number to eliminate this internal inhibition of ventricular output.

Potassium Shifts

Acute potassium shifts cause both a decreased and an increased pacemaker threshold. With acute hyperventilation, potassium shifts into the cells. This potassium shift creates a more negative resting membrane potential. For this reason, if the pacemaker output remains constant, it is more difficult to raise the membrane to threshold. This could be another explanation for the pacemaker failure.

Infarction

Myocardial infarction results in loss of pacing by increasing the surface area of the electrode. The metallic electrode has a specific surface area. With constant generator output, the current spreads over the electrode. When the current density on the electrode reaches a critical level, the myocardium surrounding the electrode reaches threshold. If the myocardium infarcts, that tissue no longer responds to electrical impulses; however, it continues conducting the impulses. The area of the electrode enlarges to include that of the infarcted area. Because the same current spreads over a larger surface area, the current density decreases; no area of myocardium reaches threshold, and pacing is lost. This patient requires electrode replacement if increasing the generator output does not reestablish pacing.

Electrocautery

The electrocautery inhibits pacemakers that have the R-wave sensitivity set at a very low number. Although anodal, asynchronous pacing has been associated with ventricular dysrhythmias,[7-9] it might be necessary to asynchronously pace in the intraoperative setting by setting the R-wave sensitivity to asynchronous or to a high number.

Summary

This case highlights the reason for establishing more than one pacing modality before anesthetizing a temporarily paced, critically ill patient with a temporary pacemaker. This is especially true if the patient is scheduled to have a cardiac procedure redone in which the surgeon cannot quickly open the chest. Changes in preload associated with ventilation and changes in preload and afterload associated with anesthetic drugs potentially affect the electrode position, resulting in the loss of pacing. If pacing loss occurs before the chest is prepped, the patient may require CPR and sternotomy in unsterile conditions. In this particular case, I strongly recommend inserting a pacing Swan-Ganz catheter or a Swan-Ganz paceport catheter with electrode, since a temporary electrode is already in place.

REFERENCES

1. Atkins JM, Leshin SH, Blomqvist G, et al: Ventricular conduction blocks and sudden death in acute myocardial infarction: Potential indictation for pacing. *N Engl J Med* 1973; 288:281–284.
2. Gann D, Balachandran PK, Sherif NE, et al: Prognostic significance of chronic versus acute bundle branch block in acute myocardial infarction. *Chest* 1975; 67:298–303.
3. Lowan B, Kosowsky B: Artificial cardiac pacemakers. *N Engl J Med 1970; 283:971–977.*
4. Zaidan JR, Waller JL, Lonergan JH: Hemodynamics of pacing after aortic valve replacement and coronary artery surgery. *Ann Thorac Surg* 1983; 36:69–73.
5. Hartzler GO, Maloney JD, Curtis JJ, et al: Hemodynamic benefits of atrioventricular sequential pacing after cardiac surgery. *Am J Cardiol* 1977; 40:232–236.
6. Leinbach RC, Chamberlain DA, Kaster JA, et al: A comparison of the hemodynamic effects of ventricular and sequential A-V pacing in patients with heart block. *Am Heart J* 1969; 78:502–508.
7. Zaidan JR: Pacemakers. *Anesthesiology* 1984; 60:319–334.
8. Preston TA: Anodal stimulation as a cause of pacemaker-induced ventricular fibrillation. *Am Heart J* 1973; 86:366–372.
9. Merx W, Han J, Yoon MS: Effects of unipolar cathodal and bipolar stimulation on vulnerability of ischemic ventricles to fibrillation. *Am J Cardiol* 1975; 35:37–41.

PART TWO

Congenital Heart Disease

12

Pulmonary Hypertension and Systemic Desaturation

Recommendations by Paul N. Samuelson, M.D.

A well sedated 7-year-old child with ventricular- and atrial-septal defects and pulmonary hypertension had anesthesia induced with halothane, nitrous oxide, and oxygen by mask. An intravenous catheter was placed and preparations were made for endotracheal intubation. At this time the child was noted to be dusky in color, the O_2 saturation on the pulse oximeter decreased from 75% to 53%, the blood pressure dropped to 60/30 mm Hg, and the heart rate decreased from 110 to 58 beats per minute.

ANALYSIS OF THE PROBLEM

The drop in oxygen saturation by the pulse oximeter to 53% as well as the associated drop in blood pressure to 60/30 mm Hg and the decrease in heart rate from 110 to 58 beats per minute signifies to us a problem. My initial assessment of this problem would be that, in fact, vasodilatation and/or cardiac depression had been created by the inhalation anesthetic agent; and the drop in systemic pressure thus caused an increase in the right-to-left shunting.[1-3] This creates a chain reaction of events resulting in further hypoxia, acidosis, pulmonary vasoconstriction, and decreased cardiac function leading eventually to cardiac arrest.

APPROACH TO THE PROBLEM

In most instances, the pulmonary hypertension can be easily reversed by noting and treating the problem early by increasing the systemic vascular resistance with a drug such as phenylephrine or ephedrine. Concomitantly, I would discontinue the halothane and ventilate the patient with 100% oxygen. If the heart rate did not increase, I would administer atropine 0.01 to 0.02 mg/kg. Bradycardia is a special problem in the vagotonic infant; it is probably less of a problem at this age. However, we do want the heart rate and, therefore, cardiac output to be greater, even though it is probably a reaction to the increased right-to-left shunt and systemic hypoxia.

Assuming that these measures did not improve things quickly and markedly, I would administer bicarbonate 1 mEq/kg in an attempt to alkalinize the patient and decrease any reactive and thus reversible pulmonary vasoconstriction. I would also include hyperventilation without excessive intrathoracic or end-expiratory pressure, which might add to problems with pulmonary blood flow. An arterial blood gas determination would be helpful in documenting what was going on. We have found that measuring the end-expired carbon dioxide is useful as a continuous monitor.

DISCUSSION

In our experience, this would be an unusual case, that is, the combination of an atrial- and ventricular-septal defect is not common in a child as old as 7 years. Most isolated atrial-septal defects (ASD) would be discovered by the local family physician when the patient is younger, and be referred to a cardiologist. This defect would be closed surgically if it did not close spontaneously within the first few years of life. An isolated ventricular-septal defect (VSD) is usually noted early by the patient's family physician and cardiologist; if this defect does not close spontaneously, it is closed surgically, again, within the first few years of life. Thus, the case to be discussed is somewhat out of the ordinary; however, it presents a number of interesting pathophysiologic and pharmacophysiologic points to consider.

Pathophysiology

The initial high pulmonary vascular resistance present in fetal life decreases somewhat immediately following birth with the expansion of the lungs and the breathing of room air. The pulmonary vascular resistance then further decreases over the next four months and is associated with an increased number of pulmonary artery branches and a decreased alveoli/artery ratio.[4-6]

In 1897 the Eisenmenger syndrome was reported in a 32-year-old man with exercise intolerance and cyanosis who died of heart failure and hemoptysis and at post mortem had a ventricular-septal defect.[7] This syndrome was described as an elevated pulmonary blood flow secondary to left-to-right shunt, leading to elevation in the pulmonary vascular resistance due to "endarteritis obliterans" in the peripheral arteries. Generally, as time has progressed, the conditions of patients who have this severe an increase in pulmonary vascular resistance are considered to be inoperable.

It is interesting that the elevation in pulmonary artery pressure secondary to elevations in pulmonary venous pressure (in contrast to left-to-right shunts) such as those occurring with mitral stenosis, cor triatriatum, and total anomalous pulmonary venous connection with obstruction are usually followed by a decrease in the pulmonary vascular resistance following surgery.[5, 6] The reason for being particularly concerned about the preexisting degree of pulmonary hypertension in this child is that not only are we immediately concerned with it during the anesthesia before cardiopulmonary bypass, but most likely it will affect our treatment following repair and weaning from cardiopulmonary bypass.

It is interesting that acute hypoxia results in acute vasoconstriction in normal individuals and is perhaps exaggerated in certain individuals, maybe more so in patients who already have slight elevations in pulmonary artery pressure. In animals, at least, the elevation in pulmonary artery pressure secondary to a decrease in the PaO_2 is proportional to the amount of smooth muscle existing in the pulmonary artery vasculature. It is also known that patients with preexisting pulmonary vascular disease are much more responsive to the pulmonary vasoconstrictive effects of a decrease in pH and an increase in $PaCO_2$. They probably also are more sensitive to the various endogenous vasoactive mediators such as histamine, serotonin, bradykinin, cathecholamines, and others as well as exogenous anesthetic and hemodynamically active pharmacologic agents.[5-7]

Patients with an isolated secundum ASD usually have normal pulmonary vascular resistance in childhood; however, the defect is diagnosed by their local physician because of the murmur of relative pulmonary stenosis or elevated pulmonary blood flow secondary to the left-to-right shunt through the ASD. About 20% of these patients will show a progressive increase in the pulmonary vascular resistance after the third decade in life. This increase in pulmonary vascular resistance later in life is the reason for surgically closing atrial-septal defects usually before the child begins school.[6] Patients with isolated ventricular-septal defects usually go through the normal reduction in pulmonary vascular resistance following birth. However, about 15% of the infants then have a progressive increase in the pulmonary vascular resistance in late infancy or early childhood. These patients are detected by the murmur related to either the VSD or the elevated pulmonary artery blood flow. A reasonably large percentage of these VSDs will close spontaneously; however, those that do not should be repaired within the first two years of age before elevations in pulmonary vascular resistance become potentially irreversible.[6] Frequently, the combination of an ASD and VSD is associated with a defect in the mitral valve and termed an "AV canal." Almost all of these patients have elevations in pulmonary artery pressure and somewhat irreversible increases in pulmonary vascular resistance very early in life.[6]

The patient presented in this case did not have an AV canal, but, in fact, had a separate ASD and VSD. It is possible that this patient was not detected early in life because the infantile pulmonary vascular resistance remained elevated and, therefore, the patient never had a left-to-right shunt large enough for murmurs to be noted. Then, as the patient became older and the shunt reversed, the defect was discovered because of cyanosis and exercise intolerance. It is also conceivable that the early murmur was present and either missed or ignored and then the persistent left-to-right shunt resulted in a gradual increase in the pulmonary vascular resistance secondary to altered growth and development of the pulmonary vascular musculature due to the hemodynamic state. The murmur then would become less noticeable as the pulmonary artery pressure and the pulmonary vascular resistance increased and eventually the shunt would be "balanced," or variable, at times becoming right-to-left and noticeable because of cyanosis. Nevertheless, we are presented with a 7-year-old with an atrial-septal defect and a ventricular septal defect who has "pulmonary hypertension."

Preanesthetic Evaluation

It would be particularly interesting in this case to obtain the catheterization data, which should include pulmonary artery pressure, pulmonary vascular resistance, and the ratio of pulmonary to systemic blood flow. We would want to determine under what basal anesthetic conditions and percentage of oxygen these catheterization data were obtained. We would also like to know if, in fact, exercise increased the pulmonary artery pressure and pulmonary vascular resistance and to what degree. It would be helpful to know if breathing 100% oxygen or some drug intervention such as tolazoline dropped the pulmonary artery pressure. All these data would help to delineate the severity of the "pulmonary hypertension." I think that we can assume that the cardiologist and surgeon taking care of this patient believed that, in fact, the pulmonary hypertension was in some degree related to a left-to-right shunt and that it would regress following surgical closure of the ASD and VSD. There are a couple of pieces of information that are particularly troublesome. The initial blood pressure during anesthesia is not given nor is the inspired oxygen concentration

(FIO$_2$); however, the initial oxygen saturation by pulse oximeter of 75% suggests that, in fact, the child was initially shunting, at least to some degree, right-to-left, for this would correlate with a PaO$_2$ of about 40 mm Hg at pH 7.4.

Anesthetic Management

A preoperative visit would be made to ascertain the physiologic state of the patient, the physical appearance, the laboratory data, and especially the catheterization data as noted above. In addition, the procedures and risks would be discussed with the family.

The patient would be medicated with pentobarbital, 5 mg/kg; morphine, 0.1 mg/kg; and scopolamine, 0.01 mg/kg intramuscularly, one hour prior to arrival in the operating room.

If the patient was sleepy and cooperative upon arrival in the operating room, intravenous administration of anesthesia would be started. If the patient was not sleepy and cooperative, the anesthetic induction would be carried out as in the case history; that is, light inhalation anesthesia with halothane, nitrous oxide, and oxygen would be administered until an intravenous route was obtained. At this point the inspired halothane would be decreased and the anesthetic switched over to more of a "balanced" technique, utilizing fentanyl 10 to 30 ug/kg and oxygen and nitrous oxide as tolerated per hemodynamics and pulse oximetry. The blood pressure initially would be monitored with blood pressure cuff and then with an intra-arterial catheter placed after the patient was asleep. The pulse oximeter as used in this case history is extremely useful in this setting. End-expired CO$_2$ measurement would also help to ensure sufficient ventilation and avoid respiratory acidosis.

Postbypass Management

If necessary, we have used some phenylephrine to facilitate myocardial reperfusion and washout of the cardioplegic solution after the cross clamp is removed and have frequently added small amounts of intravenous nitroglycerin for its effect on reperfusion of the myocardium as well as perhaps some theoretical decreases in pulmonary vascular resistance. We use hyperventilation and systemic alkalinization with bicarbonate as well as deep anesthesia with either fentanyl or sufentanil to assure the minimum amount of endogenous catecholamine response at the end of bypass.[8–10] When the atrial-septal defect and ventricular-septal defect are closed in this patient, we are going to be confronted with the problem of whether or not the right ventricle is going to be able to pump against the elevated pulmonary artery pressure and, in fact, how much of the initial elevation in pulmonary vascular resistance will be reversed both immediately following surgery and postoperatively. It would be very helpful to monitor—at a minimum—the right and left atrial pressures before and after cardiopulmonary bypass in this patient to follow their ratio. In addition, determination of the right ventricular and pulmonary artery pressures before and after repair of the ASD and VSD would be of particular help.

If the right-sided pressures remain markedly elevated they, in fact, may result in right ventricular failure. This problem is extremely hard to handle and, in addition to the above pharmacology, we would try a combination of dopamine and nitroglycerin or perhaps dopamine and phentolamine to aid in preserving systemic cardiac function and decreasing pulmonary vascular resistance. In fact, when the pulmonary vascular resistance is relatively fixed, it is extremely hard to manipulate pharmacologically. In some of these instances, the clinician must reinstitute cardiopulmonary bypass and perforate the ventricular-septal defect patch, thus allowing a release of the blood from the right ventricle and a "vent" leading to some right-to-left shunt. This allows the right ventricle to work at a slightly lower pressure and thus prevents severe right ventricular failure.

Summary

This patient presents the opportunity to review the factors involved in the evolution of pulmonary hypertension in patients with congenital heart disease, its evaluation preoperatively, and the management intraoperatively—both before and following the surgical repair.

REFERENCES

1. Stoelting RK, Longnecker DE: The effect of right-to-left shunt on rate of increase of arterial anesthetic concentration. *Anesthesiology* 1972; 36:352–356.
2. Rao TLK, Mathru M, Azad C, et al: Bronchoscopy and reversal of intracardiac shunt. *Anesthesiology* 1979; 51:558–560.
3. Gronert GA, Messick JM, Cucchiara RF: Paradoxical air embolism from a patent foramen ovale. *Anesthesiology* 1979; 50:548–549.
4. Heymann MA, Hoffman JIE: Persistent pulmonary hypertension syndromes in the newborn, in Weir KE, Reeves JT (eds): *Pulmonary Hypertension*. Mount Kisco, NY, Futura Publishing Co, 1984, pp 45–71.
5. Hoffman JIE, Heymann MA: Pulmonary arterial hypertension secondary to congenital heart disease, in Weir KE, Reeves JT (eds): *Pulmonary Hypertension*. Mount Kisco, NY, Futura Publishing Co, 1984, pp 73–114.
6. Rabinowitch M: Pulmonary hypertension, in Adams FH, Emmanouilides GC (eds): *Heart Disease in Infants, Children, and Adolescents*, ed 3. Baltimore, Williams & Wilkins Co, 1984, pp 669–692.

7. Alpert JS, Irwin RS, Dalen JE: Pulmonary hypertension. *Curr Probl Cardio* 1981; 5:1–39.

8. Hickey PR, Hansen DD: Fentanyl- and sufentanil-oxygen-pancuronium anesthesia for cardiac surgery in infants. *Anesth Analg* 1984; 63:117–124.

9. Hickey PR, Hansen DD, Wessel D, et al: Pulmonary and systemic hemodynamic responses to fentanyl in infants. *Anesth Analg* 1985; 64:483–486.

10. Hickey PR, Hansen DD, Wessel D, et al: Blunting of stress responses in the pulmonary circulation of infants by fentanyl. *Anesth Analg* 1985; 64:1137–1142.

13

Hemodilution, Arterial Flow Rates, and Cardiopulmonary Bypass

Recommendations by Susan Craig Nicolson, M.D., and David R. Jobes, M.D.

A 3-year-old child was scheduled to have total correction of tetralogy of Fallot. The child had a hemoglobin level of 18 gm/dl. Use of cardiopulmonary bypass was planned, with cooling to 30° C before occlusion and to 20° C after aortic occlusion. The question of appropriate bypass flow rates and hemodilution was raised by the surgeon.

ANAYLSIS OF THE PROBLEM

This 3-year-old child represents a prototype of a small pediatric patient with a complex cyanotic congenital heart defect presenting for definitive surgical repair. The presence of a ventricular-septal defect in conjunction with obstruction to right ventricular outflow in tetralogy of Fallot leads to right-to-left shunting of blood across the ventricular-septal defect, resulting in arterial desaturation. Hypoxemia stimulates hemoglobin production yielding increased red blood cell mass and decreased plasma volume. Blood viscosity increases coincidentally with the increase in hematocrit reading. If red blood cell mass is maintained with institution of hypothermia, blood viscosity will increase as temperature falls. Reduction of bypass flow further increases the likelihood of impaired flow in the capillary beds. Elevated viscosity causes poor peripheral perfusion, sludging, and embolic phenomena.

Multiple abnormal components of the coagulation mechanism have been cited to explain the coagulopathy that has long been observed in many patients with polycythemic cyanotic congenital heart disease. Some children have thrombocytopenia, others have platelet dysfunction. The diminished plasma volume in polycythemic patients results in a reduction in the amount of circulating plasma coagulation factors that may contribute to the bleeding tendency. Right ventricular failure may lead to passive hepatic congestion, with further reduction of the factors that are synthesized in the liver.

The small heart size coupled with the proportionately large bypass cannulae and instruments and the potential for pulmonary collateral flow draining into the heart can pose problems in achieving an acceptable surgical field. Reduction in pump flow rate—to the extreme of circulatory arrest, exsanguination, and cannulae removal—may be necessary to improve surgical conditions. To safely reduce pump flow, hypothermia and consequently a degree of hemodilution need to be instituted.

APPROACH TO THE PROBLEM

Standard preoperative orders regarding oral intake and premedication may be written. Anesthesia is induced and, following placement of monitoring and vascular access lines, surface cooling is begun. Ambient temperature is 22° C to 25° C; the cooling blanket under the patient is set at 20° C. Assuming the patient weighs 15 kg and has a hematocrit reading of 54%, the priming volume of the pump should be approximately 1,300 cc of clear fluid to produce a 25% hematocrit reading while on cardiopulmonary bypass (CPB). A method to calculate the amount of nonhemic priming volume necessary to hemodilute this patient to the desired hematocrit reading is shown in Table 13–1. Our nonhemic prime consists of crystalloid in the form of Plasmalyte buffered to a pH of 7.40, heparin 100 units/100 cc crystalloid, furosemide 1 mg/kg, and methylprednisolone 30 mg/kg. The patient is placed on cardiopulmonary bypass and cooled to a core temperature of 20° C with a flow rate set at 1.5 L/minute (100 cc/kg/min). This flow rate and temperature will be maintained until just before the aortic cross clamp is to be removed, at which time rewarming may begin and a higher flow rate instituted to facilitate rewarming. Following commencement of warming, 0.5 gm/kg of mannitol is added to further promote diuresis with resultant hemoconcentration. If pulmonary collateral flow is large and obstructs the operative field during bypass, the flow rate may temporarily be reduced by as much as 75% (375 cc/minute). Circulatory arrrest may be used in the extreme case for up to 45 minutes.

TABLE 13–1.

Calculations for Hemodilution in a 3-Year-Old 15-kg Child With Hematocrit Reading of 55%

PRIME VOLUME (PV)	=	TOTAL HEMODILUTED VOLUME (THV)	−	ESTIMATED BLOOD VOLUME (EBV)
I. EBV	=	patient's weight (kg) × 75 ml/kg		
EBV	=	15 kg × 75 ml/kg = 1,125 ml		
II. THV	=	$\dfrac{\text{Preperfusion Hematocrit Reading (\%)}}{\text{Desired hematocrit value during CPB (\%)}}$ × EBV (ml)		
THV	=	$\dfrac{55}{25}$ × 1,125 ml = 2,475 ml		
III. PV	=	2,475 ml − 1,125 ml = 1,350 ml		

DISCUSSION

Cardiac size, anatomy of the right ventricular outflow tract and pulmonary arteries, collateral blood flow, and skill and preference of the surgeon will influence the surgeon's decision to perform the procedure using two venous cannulas and intermittent reduced flow rates vs. using a single venous cannula and circulatory arrest. There is no upper age or weight limit to using the technique of deep hypothermia and circulatory arrest. Given that the child is to be cooled to a rectal temperature of 20° C using cardiopulmonary bypass and the ambient temperature remains at 22° C to 25° C, intermittent reduced flow rate to the extreme of 45 minutes of arrest time is compatible with preservation of vital organ function. Circulatory arrest offers the advantage of shortening repair and bypass time and minimizing damage to clotting factors and platelets in situations in which the heart is small and/or pulmonary venous return is of such a magnitude to necessitate prolonged intervals of low flow and high-volume cardiotomy suction return.

A primary goal of hypothermia and hemodilution is to produce a favorable balance between tissue oxygen supply and demand. Commonly employed flow rates at normothermia are 120 to 150 cc/kg/minute for infants under 5 kg, 100 to 120 cc/kg/minute for infants 5 to 10 kg and 100 cc/kg/minute for children 10 to 30 kg. No clearly defined limits of acceptable reduction in flow rates are established; however, clinical results have demonstrated that flow rates can be reduced with temperature reduction without compromising vital organ function. Oxygen supply is slightly improved by the enhanced tissue oxygen solubility and is minimally jeopardized by the shift to the left of the oxygen hemoglobin dissociation curve with lowering of body temperature.[1] Oxygen consumption and cerebral metabolism decrease 5% to 6% per degree centigrade. Empirically, flow rates can be reduced proportional to the degree of hypothermia achieved. Forty-five minutes of circulatory arrest at 20° C has been utilized without significant sequelae.[3] Flow rates may be reduced while monitoring mixed venous oxygen saturation. Normal acid-base status will result when 80% mixed venous saturation is maintained.[6] Hemodilution lowers viscosity and improves flow characteristics. The reduction in oxygen-carrying capacity secondary to hemodilution plus reduced flow is well tolerated provided that the metabolic demand is proportionately reduced by hypothermia. The extreme example of hemodilution dictated by nonclinical circumstances (Jehovah's Witnesses) demonstrates that hematocrit readings as low as 10% to 15% do not adversely affect outcome in similar pediatric patients.[2] The relationship of oxygen-carrying capacity and metabolic demand ultimately at normothermia at the end of bypass are important. If the hematocrit is kept at 20% or greater, only a normal cardiac output should be needed. At a 25% hematocrit value, a modest reserve in oxygen supply will be achieved. Viscosity changes between a 20% and 25% hematocrit reading are slight.[4] Therefore, a compromise is achieved at a hematocrit value of 25%.

Another indication for hemodilution in patients with cyanotic heart disease is the improvement in coagulation seen when a hematocrit reading of 30% or less is achieved during cardiopulmonary bypass. Reduction in consumption of coagulation factors with improved tissue perfusion induced by hemodilution improve hemostasis postbypass resulting in decreased blood loss and decreased use of blood and blood products.[5]

REFERENCES

1. Fisher A, Foex P, Emerson P, et al: Oxygen availability during hypothermic cardiopulmonary bypass. *Crit Care Med* 1977; 5:154–158.
2. Henling CE, Carmichael MJ, Keats AS, et al: Cardiac operation for congenital heart disease in children of Jehovah's Witnesses. *J Thorac Cardiovasc Surg* 1985; 89:914–920.
3. Messmer B: Psychomotor and intellectual development after deep hypothermia and circulatory arrest in infancy. *J Thorac Cardiovasc Surg* 1972; 72: 495.
4. Messmer B: Hemodilution. *Surg Clin North Am* 1975; 55:659.
5. Milam JD, Aushn SF, Nuhill MR, et al: Use of sufficient hemodilution to prevent coagulopathies following surgical correction of cyanotic heart disease. *J Thorac Cardiovasc Surg* 1985; 89:623–629.
6. Winkler M, Lamberti J, Rohrer C: Perfusion considerations for infants weighing ten kilograms or less. *J Extra-Corporeal Tech* 1985; 17:31–36.

14

Safe Period of Circulatory Arrest

Recommendations by Paul R. Hickey, M.D.

A 4-day-old infant with simple transposition of the great vessels was to undergo complete anatomical correction. Induction and sternotomy were uneventful. The infant was surface cooled to 32° C, placed on cardiopulmonary bypass, and core-cooled to 18° C. At this point the arterial and venous cannulas were removed and total circulatory arrest was instituted. After 60 minutes of circulatory arrest, the corrective procedure was still incomplete and the surgeon stated he needed more time.

ANALYSIS OF THE PROBLEM

This case illustrates a commonly asked question in hospitals where circulatory arrest is used during cardiac surgery. The question is: what is the safe period of circulatory arrest?

APPROACH TO THE PROBLEM

If the surgeon in the present case needs significantly more time to finish the essential parts of the complex anatomical repair of transposition of the great arteries before rewarming can take place, cardiopulmonary bypass could be resumed for a brief period of time, approximately 10 to 15 minutes, while the infant is kept profoundly hypothermic. During this brief period of reperfusion, reoxygenation of tissues, washout of acidotic metabolic products, and perhaps recooling can take place. After this period of reperfusion, another period of circulatory arrest can be utilized by the surgeon to finish the repair.

A number of centers have employed a second approach: using two shorter periods of circulatory arrest with an intervening period of perfusion at normal flow rates during deep hypothermia so that longer *total* periods of deep hypothermic circulatory arrest (DHCA) will be tolerated without permanent neurologic damage. The period of reperfusion between separate periods of DHCA allows reoxygenation, recooling if necessary, and washout of metabolic wastes. This technique is being used clinically in a number of centers (including our own) without notable problems in the limited number of cases in which surgeons cannot complete the repair within the "safe period" of circulatory arrest. Although it is being used clinically, this technique of adding another period of circulatory arrest to the initial period of arrest following a brief period of reperfusion has not been formally studied. It would seem preferable for the surgeon to plan on two shorter periods of circulatory arrest if he suspects that it will take him more than 60 minutes of total arrest time to accomplish the critical parts of the repair.

Although no safe time limit for the second period of hypothermic circulatory arrest has been established, there are anecdotal reports of unusual cases in which two consecutive periods of circulatory arrest as long as 50 or 60 minutes in length were used for a cumulative circulatory arrest period of over 100 minutes without gross neurologic damage. Whether reversible or subtle irreversible neurologic damage is cumulative with this technique is unknown.

DISCUSSION

Background

Despite extensive use of deep hypothermic circulatory arrest (DHCA) in cardiac surgery since the initial reports of its use appeared in the late 1960s,[1-3] significant controversy continues over the "safe period" of DHCA. The safe period at any given temperature is defined as the maximum continuous arrest time tolerated by the central nervous system without permanent neurologic damage. There are still no clearly defined safe time limits for circulatory arrest even after almost 20 years of clinical use of DHCA. Many cardiac surgical centers employ prolonged DHCA extensively, while other centers have minimized or avoided use of DHCA entirely because of concerns about the safety of prolonged circulatory arrest techniques. Instead the centers where its use is largely avoided employ low-flow cardiopulmonary bypass at deep levels of hypothermia or brief periods of circulatory arrest.

Use of DHCA provides ideal operating conditions for the surgeon, shortens cardiopulmonary bypass time, and maximizes myocardial protection by preventing rewarming of the myocardium from adjacent organs and from washout of cardioplegic solutions by the noncoronary collateral circulation to the heart. In addition to these advantages, some operations, such as aortic arch reconstruction, simply cannot readily be done without the use of circulatory arrest.

Pathophysiology of Neonatal Transposition of the Great Arteries

In simple transposition of the great vessels, the pulmonary artery originates from the left ventricle and the aorta originates from the right ventricle. Viability of the neonate depends on adequate mixing of the pulmonary and systemic circulations at some point in the central circulation. Neonates who require surgery usually have an intact ventricular septum. They are dependent on a patent ductus arteriosus or a patent foramen ovale for mixing of the two otherwise separate circulations. By infusing prostaglandin E$_1$, the ductus arteriosus can be kept open for many weeks,[4] or alternatively, the foramen ovale can be enlarged into an atrial-septal defect using a Raskind balloon septostomy. Neonates with transposition and a ventricular-septal defect usually have adequate mixing at the ventricular level and surgery in these neonates can be safely deferred until they are 3 to 6 months of age.

Anatomical correction of transposition involves division of both the aorta and the pulmonary artery above the semilunar valves and reanastomosis of these great vessels to the left and right ventricles, respectively. The coronary arteries must be transplanted along with the aorta over to the outlet of the left ventricle from their original position at the right ventricular outlet in order to provide an oxygenated, high pressure coronary circulation. Since the coronary arteries of the neonate are only 1 or 2 mm in diameter, the operation is technically very demanding. A slight malalignment or rotation in the reanastomosis of the coronary arteries to the aortic root can result in coronary ischemia, myocardial infarction, and death. Offsetting these risks is the advantage that anatomical repair of transposition establishes continuity of the left ventricle with the systemic circulation. In contrast, Mustard or Senning intraatrial repair of transposition leaves the right ventricle in continuity with the systemic circulation. Late systemic (right) ventricular dysfunction has been reported after these latter two types of repair of transposition in infants.

The size of these structures in the neonate and the complexity of the anatomical repair make accurate operative repair in the neonate difficult during perfusion of the systemic circulation on cardiopulmonary bypass. The bulk of perfusion cannulae, atrial cannulae, and suction cannulae, along with blood return from the coronary sinus and thebesian veins, all make visualization and precise surgical repair difficult in the tiny neonatal heart. During complete anatomical correction, mobilization, division, and reanastomosis of the aorta, coronaries, and pulmonary artery make continued perfusion from the aortic root problematic during much of the operation. These considerations make DHCA the technique of choice for this operation in some institutions. However, the technical problems cited above make it difficult to complete the essential parts of the procedure during the time limit imposed by the "safe" period of circulatory arrest.

Pathophysiology of Deep Hypothermic Circulatory Arrest

Protection of the central nervous system by deep hypothermia during prolonged periods of circulatory arrest is poorly understood, leading to the confusion over the safe period in DHCA. Although hypothermia depresses metabolic rate and oxygen consumption in the brain for a Q_{10}* of about 2.2 to 2.7[5, 6], this depression is not sufficient by itself to account for the brain's prolonged tolerance to ischemia below 20° C. It is now becoming clear that hypothermia acts in a number of other ways to protect the integrity of the brain not only during ischemia, but also upon reperfusion *after* ischemia.

Upon reperfusion after normothermic ischemia, large areas of the microcirculation in the brain shut down, leading to the "no reflow" lesion and subsequent infarction of the affected areas of the brain. These "no reflow" lesions are prevented by hypothermia, which preserves the integrity of the microcirculation,[7] possibly by preventing damage to the endothelial cells lining the arterioles and capillaries. Hypothermia preserves intracellular pH at higher levels during ischemia in the brain because of the elevation of the neutral pH of water with lower temperatures.[8] This higher intracellular pH level appears to maintain membrane integrity, probably by allowing continued enzyme activity and maintenance of substrate stores during ischemia. Hypothermia has been shown to maintain levels of adenosine triphosphate (ATP) in rat brain during ischemia and to allow preischemic levels of creatine phosphate to be readily regenerated upon reperfusion.[8] In contrast, during similar periods of normothermic ischemia, severe decreases in high energy phosphate levels occur in the brain and appreciable regeneration of the levels of high energy phosphates does not take place upon reperfusion.[8]

Another mechanism of cellular damage after ischemia at normal temperatures is massive calcium influx during initial reperfusion of previously ischemic areas.[9] This calcium influx is probably due to the opening of calcium channels during ischemia and is prevented by hypothermia.[10] Once large amounts of calcium gain access to the cell, activation of lipolytic enzymes and severe damage to membranes occurs. Although these and other mechanisms of cellu-

---

*Q_{10} = factor of change in metabolic rate for 10° C change in body temperature.

lar damage with ischemia and reperfusion are incompletely understood, it is clear that deep hypothermia is effective in protecting against much of the damage that takes place during and immediately after ischemia.

Experience with Deep Hypothermic Circulatory Arrest

The safe period of deep hypothermic circulatory arrest originally was thought to be approximately 45 minutes. This value stems from experimental evidence in animals that suggested that 45 to 60 minutes of circulatory arrest was well tolerated at brain temperatures below 20° C[6, 11, 12] as well as from initial clinical experience.[1–3] Subsequent extensive clinical experience in many centers has shown empirically that up to 60 minutes and sometimes longer periods of circulatory arrest at temperatures of less than 20° C are tolerated by the central nervous system of virtually all infants without demonstrable long-term neurologic deficit.[13–16] Although many studies do report a significant incidence of transient seizures (4%to10%) occurring in the immediate postoperative period, the seizures have been shown not to be a sign of permanent brain damage.[17] While a few reports have appeared of isolated severe neurologic deficits occurring at periods of DHCA as short as 45 minutes,[18, 19] centers with a large DHCA experience report remarkably few neurologic problems after prolonged periods (approximately 60 minutes) of DHCA in infants.

There is some clinical and experimental evidence that the central nervous system of infants may better tolerate prolonged periods of circulatory arrest than that of older children and adults, but this has not been well studied.[20, 21] When the period of circulatory arrest appreciably exceeds 60 minutes at temperatures of 15° C to 20° C, the incidence of postoperative neurologic problems increases significantly. While some experimental evidence suggests that temperatures lower than those currently used (down to 10° C) may substantially extend the safe period of circulatory arrest to as long as 90 minutes, the use of temperatures of around 10° C is strictly experimental.[22]

In contrast to the excellent clinical experience with DHCA in many centers, the approach of some pediatric cardiac centers is that the safe period may be substantially less than 45 minutes and DHCA is often avoided. This view is based partly on experimental studies in animals by Kirklin's group at Alabama showing decreases in neurologic function and in the proportions of normal neurons remaining after more than 45 minutes of circulatory arrest in gerbils.[23] A study from another group of investigators has shown microscopic cellular damage in brains of all dogs cooled to 18° C with cardiopulmonary bypass, whether or not circulatory arrest was used, so that deep hypothermia by itself may be responsible for some of the damage seen experimentally with DHCA.[24]

This conservative view of DHCA is further supported by recent clinical evidence showing that long periods of deep hypothermic circulatory arrest cause subclinical but reversible damage to the central nervous system that is not readily apparent. Mild decreases in brain mass by computed tomography were found postoperatively in two infants who had undergone periods of circulatory arrest longer than 60 minutes.[25] Neither of these two children had abnormal neurologic findings postoperatively and the abnormalities in the brains subsequently returned to normal by 6 to 12 months after the operation. Ten other infants in this study with shorter periods of circulatory arrest showed no postoperative changes in the brain by computed tomography.[25]

Additional support for this approach comes from functional evidence that the central nervous system does sustain a considerable, but apparently reversible, insult during prolonged periods of circulatory arrest. Coles et al.[19] showed that although cortical-evoked potentials do disappear during profound hypothermia, they take a variable amount of time to recover normal latency after rewarming subsequent to prolonged periods of DHCA in infants. The recovery time of these cortical-evoked potentials has been shown to be linearly related to the product of the time of circulatory arrest and the temperature during the arrest. This demonstrated that recovery of cortical functions is delayed for a considerable period after DHCA despite normal brain temperature and presumably normal brain blood flow. The latency to recovery of continuous EEG activity (another cortical function) after rewarming also was related to the duration of circulatory arrest in another study of infants undergoing DHCA.[26] In contrast, brain stem auditory-evoked potentials recover much more quickly upon rewarming after comparable periods of DHCA, as might be expected from the well-documented better tolerance of the brain stem to ischemia.[27]

This evidence of subclinical but apparently reversible neurologic dysfunction following DHCA supports the concern that subtle, irreversible neurologic damage may occur with prolonged DHCA times ($>$ 40 minutes). The contention is that this results in a more frequent occurrence of decreased intellectual capacity and development in children after DHCA than the gross neurologic deficits that are rarely seen after DHCA. A number of studies of intellectual development performed years after DHCA have provided some evidence to support this position,[28–30] but other studies have found no relationship between DHCA times up to 60 to 70 minutes and subsequent intellectual function.[31, 32] While the most recent clinical report suggested that arrest periods as long as 70 to 75 minutes may be tolerated at temperatures of 15° C to 16° C without gross neurologic damage, routine postoperative assessment of intellectual development was not carried out in this study.[13] Since differences in techniques of DHCA make it hazardous to extrapolate clinical practices and results from one institutional setting to another, these results may not be applicable in other institutions.

The contradictions apparent in studies cited above make it clear that understanding of DHCA is inadequate at present. The empirically developed techniques of DHCA used in some centers have been documented to be reasonably safe for 60 minutes of DHCA, but the precise aspects of the DHCA technique responsible for this success have not been defined. In centers that have extensive experience with this technique, approximately 60 consecutive minutes of circulatory arrest at brain temperatures between 15° C to 20° C is probably the *maximum* safe limit, but in all centers and especially in those using DHCA only occasionally, shorter periods of circulatory arrest clearly are preferable.

Management Options

When the period of circulatory arrest is prolonged to more than 70 minutes, it is clear that the incidence of major neurologic sequelae, such as cortical blindness, goes up dramatically.[19] The approach suggested for our problem case has been effective in preventing major neurologic complications after prolonged total periods of circulatory arrest, substantially beyond 70 minutes, but this technique is an empiric one and has not been formally studied. In the usual case in which this problem arises, the surgeon has not planned on exceeding the ''safe period,'' but as the end of this period nears, realizes that more time is needed. Thus, the initial period of circulatory arrest is generally long and the subsequent period is generally shorter.

An alternative to this approach is to reinstitute bypass with low flows, while maintaining deep hypothermia. Studies by Fox et al.[33] and by Govier et al.[34] suggest that cerebral blood flow and metabolic rate are well maintained during deep hypothermic hemodiluted cardiopulmonary bypass at very low levels of pump flow, as low as 0.5 L/minute/m^2 regardless of the perfusion pressures achieved. Since the brain appears to be able to preferentially divert flow to itself at low levels of flow and temperature, these low flows may protect the viability of the brain while providing the surgeon with acceptable, if not optimal, operating conditions.

The effect of different methods of anesthetic management on the outcome in DHCA has not been well studied. There is no single recognized optimal approach to anesthesia for DHCA, nor are there any published clinical studies of the effect of different anesthetic techniques on outcome after DHCA. A few limited experimental studies of different anesthetic techniques for circulatory arrest using surface cooling and surface rewarming have shown that the use of the potent inhalation agents (halothane and isoflurane) resulted in significant neurologic dysfunction after only 30 minutes of DHCA in dogs, whereas use of ether anesthesia in the same studies was not associated with any neurologic disturbances upon recovery after 30 minutes of circulatory arrest.[35–37] The investigators doing these studies have recommended use of a halothane-diethyl ether azeotrope for anesthesia in these cases of surface-induced hypothermic circulatory arrest.[38] Unfortunately, these studies have limited clinical applicability since few institutions currently use the surface cooling and surface rewarming techniques studied in these investigations. Surface cooling and rewarming techniques without use of cardiopulmonary bypass considerably complicate the use of deep hypothermic circulatory arrest.

Some clinicians have advocated use of barbiturates or other agents just before the initiation of circulatory arrest to help provide cerebral protection. The available evidence suggests that the protective effect of barbiturates in cerebral ischemia is additive to that of moderate hypothermia.[39] However, when cerebral electrical activity ceases at deep hypothermic levels, barbiturates no longer provide additive protection to that of deep hypothermia because barbiturates reduce only the portion of cerebral metabolic oxygen consumption that is related to neuronal electrical activity.[40,41] No clinical studies of these pharmacologic means of cerebral protection and their influence on the safe period have been carried out in the setting of DHCA.

Experimental work and theoretical considerations suggest that an alternative approach to cerebral protection after prolonged periods of DHCA may be the prevention of reperfusion injury in the brain. Use of calcium channel blockers such as nimodipine,[42] calcium antagonists such as magnesium or cobalt,[43, 44] free radical scavengers such as superoxide dismutase and catalase,[45] reduction of prearrest glucose levels,[46] or infusions of adenosine or inosine[47] upon reperfusion may do much to prevent or ameliorate reperfusion injuries and help extend the safe period. This work is, however, entirely experimental at present and extensive laboratory and clinical studies must be done before these approaches to cerebral protection after prolonged periods of DHCA can be recommended.

REFERENCES

1. Hikasa Y, et al: Open heart surgery in infants with an aid of hypothermic anesthesia, I. *Arch Jap Chir* 1967; 36:495.
2. Hikasa Y, et al: Open heart surgery in infants with an aid of hypothermic anesthesia, II. *Arch Jap Chir* 1968; 37:399.
3. Mohri H, Dillard DH, Crawford EW, et al: Method of surface-induced deep hypothermia for open heart surgery in infants. *J Thorac Cardiovasc Surg* 1969; 58:262–270.
4. Yokota M. Muraoka R, Aoshima M, et al: Modified Blalock-Taussig shunt following long-term administration of prostaglandin E_1 for ductus-dependent neonates with cyanotic congenital heart disease. *J Thorac Cardiovasc Surg* 1985; 90:399–403.
5. Michenfelder JD, Theye RA: Hypothermia: Effect on canine brain and whole body metabolism. *Anesthesiology* 1968; 29:1107–1112.

6. Perna AM, Gardner TJ, Tabaddor K, et al: Cerebral metabolism and blood flow after circulatory arrest during deep hypothermia. *Ann Surg* 1973; 178:95–101.

7. Norwood WI, Norwood CR, Castaneda AR: Cerebral anoxia: Effect of deep hypothermia and pH. *Surgery* 1979; 86:203–209.

8. Norwood WI, Norwood CR, Ingwall JS, et al: Hypothermic circulatory arrest: 31-Phosphorus nuclear magnetic resonance of isolated perfused neonatal rat brain. *J Thorac Cardiovasc Surg* 1979; 78:823–830.

9. Kass IS: Blocking Ca^{++} entry protects against anoxic brain damage in vitro. *Anesthesiology* 1984; 61:A367.

10. Rich TL, Langer GA: Calcium depletion in rabbit myocardium: Calcium paradox protection by hypothermia and cation substitution. *Circ Res* 1982; 51:131–141.

11. Connolly JE, Boyd RJ: The effects of hypothermia on the brain. *Ann Chir Thorac Cardiovasc* 1962; 1:677.

12. Sade RN, Fisher EG, Castaneda AR: Hypothermic circulatory arrest: Cerebral circulation and metabolism, abstracted. *Eur Surg Res* 1975; 8(suppl 2):35–36.

13. Tharion J, Johnsol DC, Celermajer JM, et al: Profound hypothermia with circulatory arrest. *J Thorac Cardiovasc Surg* 1982; 84:66–72.

14. Lamberti JJ, Lin CY, Cutiletta A, et al: Surface cooling and circulatory arrest in infants undergoing cardiac surgery. *Arch Surg* 1978; 113:822–826.

15. Venugopal P, Olszowka J, Wagner H, et al. Early correction of congenital heart disease with surface induced deep hypothermia and circulatory arrest. *J Thorac Cardiovasc Surg* 1973; 66:375–385.

16. Bender HW, Fisher DR, Walker WE, et al: Reparative cardiac surgery in infants and small children: Five years experience with profound hypothermia and circulatory arrest. *Ann Surg* 1979; 190:437–443.

17. Ehyai A, Fenichel GM, Bender HW: Incidence and prognosis of seizures in infants after cardiac surgery with profound hypothermia and circulatory arrest. *JAMA* 1984; 252:3165–3167.

18. Brunberg JA, Doty DB, Reilly EL: Choreoathetosis in infants following cardiac surgery with deep hypothermia and circulatory arrest. *J Pediatr* 1974; 84:232.

19. Coles JG, Taylor MJ, Pearce JM, et al: Cerebral monitoring of somatosensory evoked potentials during profoundly hypothermic circulatory arrest. *Circulation* 1984; 70:96–102.

20. Messmer BJ, Schallberger U, Galliker R, et al: Psychomotor and intellectual development after deep hypothermia and circulatory arrest in early infancy. *J Thorac Cardiovasc Surg* 1976; 72:495–502.

21. Mohri H, Barnes H, Wintersheid LC, et al: Challenge of prolonged suspended animation: A method of surface induced hypothermia. *Ann Surg* 1968; 168:779.

22. Haneda K, Sands MP, Thomas R, et al: Prolongation of the safe interval of hypothermic circulatory arrest: 90 minutes. *J Cardiovasc Surg* 1983; 24:15–21.

23. Treasure T, Naftel DC, Conger KA, et al: The effect of hypothermic circulatory arrest time on cerebral function, morphology, and biochemistry. *J Thorac Cardiovasc Surg* 1983; 86:761–770.

24. Molina JE, Einzig S, Mastri AR, et al: Brain damage in profound hypothermia: Perfusion versus circulatory arrest. *J Thorac Cardiovasc Surg* 1984; 87:596–604.

25. Muraoka R, Yokota M, Aoshima M, et al: Subclinical changes in brain morpholo-

gy following cardiac operations as reflected by computed tomographic scans of the brain. *J Thorac Cardiovasc Surg* 1981; 81:364–369.

26. Weiss M, Weiss CJ, Nocolas F, et al: A study of the electroencephalogram during surgery with deep hypothermia and circulatory arrest. *J Thorac Cardiovasc Surg* 1975; 70:316.

27. Kaaga K, Takiguchi T, Myokai K, et al: Effects of deep hypothermia and circulatory arrest on the auditory brain stem responses. *Arch Otorhinolaryngol* 1979; 225:199–205.

28. Wells FC, Coghill S, Caplan HL, et al: Duration of circulatory arrest does influence the psychological development of children after cardiac operation in early life. *J Thorac Cardiovasc Surg* 1983; 86:823–831.

29. Wright JS, Hicks RG, Newman DC, et al: Deep hypothermic arrest: Observation on later development in children. *J Thorac Cardiovasc Surg* 1979; 77:466–468.

30. Settergren G, Ohqvist G, Lundberg S, et al: Cerebral blood flow and cerebral metabolism in children following cardiac surgery with deep hypothermia and circulatory arrest: Clinical course and follow-up of psychomotor development. *Scand J Thor Cardiovasc Surg* 1982; 16:209–215.

31. Dickinson DF, Sambrooks JE: Intellectual performance in children after circulatory arrest with profound hypothermia in infancy. *Arch Dis Child* 1979; 54:1–6.

32. Clarkson PM, MacArthur BA, Barratt-Boyes BG, et al: Developmental progress after cardiac surgery in infancy using hypothermia and circulatory arrest. *Circulation* 1980; 62:855–861.

33. Fox LS, Blackstone EH, Kirklin JW, et al: Relationship of brain blood flow and oxygen consumption to perfusion flow rate during profoundly hypothermic cardiopulmonary bypass. *J Thorac Cardiovasc Surg* 1984; 87:658–664.

34. Govier AV, Reves JG, McKay RD, et al: Factors and their influence on regional cerebral blood flow during nonpulsatile cardiopulmonary bypass. *Ann Thorac Surg* 1984; 38:592–600.

35. Mohri H, Dillard DH, Merendino KA: Hypothermia: Halothane anesthesia and the safe period of total circulatory arrest. *Surgery* 1972; 72:345–351.

36. Sato S, Vanini V, Mohri H, et al: A comparative study of the effects of carbon dioxide and perfusion rewarming on limited circulatory occlusion during surface hypothermia, under halothane and ether anesthesia. *Ann Surg* 1974; 180:192.

37. Sato S, Vanini V, Sands MP, et al: The use of Forane anesthesia for surface-induced deep hypothermia. *Ann Thorac Surg* 1975; 20:299.

38. Sands MP, Dillard DH, Hessel EA, et al: Improved anesthesia for deep surface-induced hypothermia: The halothane-diethyl ether azeotrope. *Ann Thorac Surg* 1978; 29:123–129.

39. Quasha AL, Tinker JH, Sharbrough FW: Hypothermia plus thiopental: Prolonged electroencephalographic supression. *Anesthesiology* 1981; 55:636–640.

40. Steen PA, Newberg L, Milde JH, et al: Hypothermia and barbiturates: Individual and combined effects on canine cerebral oxygen consumption. *Anesthesiology* 1983; 58:527–532.

41. Artru AA, Michenfelder JD: Influence of hypothermia or hyperthermia alone or in combination with pentobarbital or phenytoin on survival time in hypoxic mice. *Anesth Analg* 1981; 60:867–870.

42. Steen PA, Gisvold SE, Milde JH, et al: Nimodipine improves outcome when given after complete cerebral ischemia in primates. *Anesthesiology* 1985; 62:406–414.
43. Vacanti FX, Ames A III: Mild hypothermia and Mg^{++} protect against irreversible damage during CNS ischemia. *Stroke* 1984; 15:695–698.
44. Kass IS: Blocking Ca^{++} entry protects against anoxic brain damage in vitro. *Anesthesiology* 1984; 61:A367.
45. Werns SW, Shea MJ, Driscoll EM, et al: The independent effects of oxygen radical scavengers on canine infarct size: Reduction by superoxide dismutase but not catalase. *Circ Res 1985; 56:895–898.*
46. Myers RE, Yamaguchi S: Nervous system effects of cardiac arrest in monkeys. *Arch Neurol* 1977; 34:65–74.
47. Goldhaber SZ, Pohost GM, Kloner RA, et al: Inosine: A protective agent in an organ culture model of myocardial ischemia. *Circ Res* 1982; 51:181–188.

15

Pulmonary Artery Hypertension and Right Ventricular Failure

An 8-month-old child with truncus arteriosus with reactive pulmonary hypertension underwent total anatomic correction. Immediately after cardiopulmonary bypass, the pulmonary artery pressure was systemic; right atrial pressure was 20 mm Hg and cardiac index was 1.6 L/min/m^2.

Recommendations by M. Jerome Strong, M.D.

ANALYSIS OF THE PROBLEM

The case presentation at the beginning of this chapter contains problems common during surgical repair of pulmonary truncus arteriosus. The 8-month-old infant is older than the average patient presenting for correction of pulmonary truncus arteriosus at the University of California, San Francisco Medical Center. It is likely that, by the age of 8 months, the degree of pulmonary hypertension might be more severe. Although clinical evidence suggests that pulmonary hypertension appears earlier and in a more malignant form in a truncus than in other congental cardiac defects having identical right-to-left shunts, the degree of pulmonary hypertension is highly variable and does not necessarily correlate with age. Occasionally, palliative pulmonary-artery banding is performed to protect the pulmonary bed from high systemic pressures. Definitive repair follows when the infant is 2 to 3 months of age.

APPROACH TO THE PROBLEM

Among the postoperative surgical complications following repair of the truncus defect (e.g., bleeding), reactive pulmonary hypertension is consistently the most serious threat to the patient's survival. Acute pulmonary hypertension results in right ventricular strain, hypotension, bradycardia, and, finally, ventricular fibrillation. Apart from the influences of hypoxia and hypercarbia, it is not understood what factors trigger the postoperative reactivity of the pulmonary vascular bed. Pain or discomfort from any source and suctioning of the endotracheal tube have been identified as factors, but there is no consistent pattern.

One study[6] suggests that fentanyl might blunt stress responses causing reactive pulmonary hypertension. However, this study involved a series of patients having ventricular-septal defects, atrial-ventricular canals, and tetralogy of Fallot, not all of which tend to develop the severe degrees of reactive pulmonary hypertension that characterize pulmonary truncus arteriosus. It would appear that fentanyl facilitated ventilation by maintenance of high PO_2 and low CO_2, rather than by any specific pharmacologic action.

No specific therapy is currently available to treat pulmonary hypertension. In our experience, treatment using a combination of drugs that sedate and paralyze the patient and ensure sufficient ventilatory patterns to sustain high PO_2, PCO_2 less than 40, and pH above 7.4 is most successful.

There are also no prognostic guides to indicate the length of time the pulmonary vascular bed will remain reactive, nor is there sufficient data to recommend any particular anesthetic agent, technique, or postoperative regimen that will ultimately influence outcome.

DISCUSSION

Persistent truncus arteriosus is a rare congenital cardiac defect that results from failure of the embryologic trunk to separate into a discrete pulmonary artery (PA) and aorta. The consequence of this failure is a condition in which all of the three circulations (systemic, pulmonary, and coronary) arise from a single arterial trunk. If left untreated, all patients die. The median age at death varies from a few weeks to six months. Symptoms include failure to thrive, dyspnea, and congestive failure. Varying degrees of cyanosis may also be present.

Functional Anatomy

The embryologic dysfunction in persistent truncus arteriosus involves the sixth pair of aortic arches. Normally, these separate from the aorta to form the pulmonary trunk from which the pulmonary arteries arise. However, in pulmonary truncus arteriosus, a single trunk becomes the outflow vessel connecting with the arteries and continuing as the aorta. The points at which the pulmonary arteries emerge from the trunk vary. Their location determines the classification of pulmonary truncus arteriosus into types I, II, III, and IV (Fig. 15–1).

Type I is distinguished by a T-shaped branching of the truncus that forms the right and left pulmonary arteries. Type II is characterized by right and left pulmonary arteries emerging from separate posterior sites on the truncus; type III, by right and left pulmonary arteries emerging from separate lateral sites. Each of these classifications conforms to the anatomic definition of truncus arteriosus because the three circulations share a common outflow tract.

In type IV, however, the pulmonary circulation is derived from the bronchial arteries that connect to the descending thoracic aorta. This configuration should not be considered a true truncus but, rather, a pulmonary atresia with a ventricular-septal defect. Functionally, it is similar to tetralogy of Fallot in that it is characterized by a large right-to-left shunt accompanied by severe cyanosis.

The direction of blood flow in pulmonary truncus arteriosus is illustrated in Figure 15–2. Unoxygenated blood enters the right atrium (RA) from the venae cavae, flows through the tricuspid valve into the right ventricle (RV), then exits through an obligatory ventricular-septal defect (VSD) into the left

FIG 15–1.
Types of pulmonary truncus arteriosus. *A,* type I is identified by T-shaped branching of the right and left pulmonary arteries; *B,* type II, by separate posterior right and left pulmonary arteries; *C,* type III, by separate lateral right and left pulmonary arteries; and *D,* type IV, by bronchial arteries connected to the descending thoracic aorta.

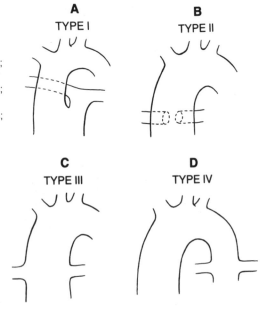

A
TYPE I

B
TYPE II

C
TYPE III

D
TYPE IV

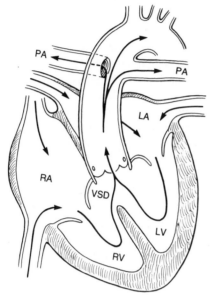

FIG 15–2.
Blood flow in pulmonary truncus
arteriosus.

ventricle (LV), where it mixes with oxygenated blood returning normally to the heart from the pulmonary circulation. The result is an enormous volume of blood entering the left ventricle and causing left ventricular failure, increases in pressures in the left atrium (LA), and consequent congestive heart failure.

Hemodynamic Consequences of Truncus

The blood flow through the pulmonary and systemic circulations is determined by the ratio of the resistances offered by each circulation. Normally, the systemic circulation functions at pressures and resistances higher than that of the pulmonary circulation. At birth, systemic vascular resistance usually increases in response to the loss of the low resistance of the placental circulation. The PO_2 also increases, fetal hypoxic pulmonary constriction is abolished, and there is an increase in pulmonary blood flow resulting from decreased pulmonary vascular resistance.

Infants born with pulmonary truncus arteriosus have a pulmonary circulation subjected to high systemic pressures and, consequently, an abnormally high pulmonary blood flow returning to the left side of the heart. Because the left ventricle does not have time to adapt to the increases in pressure and volume, left ventricular failure rapidly follows. Additional stress occurs because the pulmonary vascular circulation is exposed to high pressure and flow during both diastole and systole. The high diastolic run-off secondary to pulmonary truncus arteriosus decreases diastolic pressure, which, in turn, decreases the diastole-dependent coronary blood flow. This results in compromised myocardial function.

Exposure of the vasculature to high pulmonary pressure appears to delay normal dissolution of the muscular layer in the pulmonary arterioles.[1-3] Simultaneously, the walls of the pulmonary vessels begin to thicken to accommodate the higher pressures and flow, leading to progressive, obliterative structural changes. The natural course of the truncus defect is therefore determined by increases in pulmonary vascular resistances and subsequent decreases in pulmonary blood flow. Treatment may include pharmacologic therapy and surgical repair.

Clinical Features

Pulmonary hypertension occurs in three broad but overlapping clinical stages dependent on the structural changes in the pulmonary arterioles.[3]

In the initial stage, pulmonary blood flow is extremely high and alterations in vascular resistance may be low but quite labile. Clinical symptoms include a large left-to-right shunt, prominent dyspnea, and failure to thrive. Because of mixing of blood between the right and left ventricles below the truncal valve, clinical cyanosis is minimal. These symptoms typically appear in the second and third months of life, but they may also become evident during the newborn's first few hours. Treatment during this first stage is directed primarily at symptoms of congestive heart failure, utilizing digitalis and diuretics.

During the second stage, increases in pulmonary vascular resistance are accompanied by decreases in pulmonary flow. The symptoms of heart failure disappear because of the decrease in pulmonary flow and the infant appears to thrive. There may be some slight cyanosis accompanying crying. The apparently improved clinical picture is misleading, because infants at this stage are at high risk during surgical repair due to the changes in pulmonary vascular resistance.

In the third and final stage, pulmonary vascular resistance is high and fixed. Cyanosis is marked. The reversal of the left-to-right shunt may indicate that the condition of the patient is inoperable.

In first-stage and second-stage patients, reactive pulmonary hypertension is aggravated by hypoxia and hypercarbia. However, pulmonary hypertension is known to decrease in the presence of hyperoxia, hypocarbia, and an alkaline pH level, conditions that decrease pulmonary vascular resistance. Postoperative treatment of these patients with hyperoxia and hypocarbia will be discussed later in this chapter. Although the drug tolazoline has been used to reduce pulmonary hypertension, because of concomittant systemic hypotension, it is not extensively used for treatment of reactive pulmonary hypertension.

Surgical Correction

Mair et al.[4] have demonstrated that prognosis following surgery is good when patients having pulmonary truncus arteriosus have a preoperative resting systemic O_2 saturation of 85% or higher. A preoperative systemic O_2 saturation lower than 85% suggests a poor outcome. The preoperative presence of lowered O_2 saturation in these patients is due to an increase in right-to-left shunt, resulting from an increase in pulmonary vascular resistance.

Total surgical correction of the truncus defect is illustrated in Fig. 15–3. The pulmonary arteries are excised from the trunk and the opening on the trunk oversewn. An incision is made in the right ventricle and the ventricular-septal defect is closed. A valved Dacron conduit is then used to join the right ventricle to the free distal portion of the pulmonary arteries. Various surgical techniques are applied to the distal pulmonary arteries, depending on the type of defect. Blood flow following correction is illustrated in Fig. 15–4.

Several concerns persist following total correction. First, most total corrections are now done in infancy.[5] As the child grows, the conduit to the pulmonary artery will become too small relative to body size, resulting in inadequate pulmonary blood flow. The conduit must therefore be replaced one or more times.

A second concern is compromised myocardial function. Because the

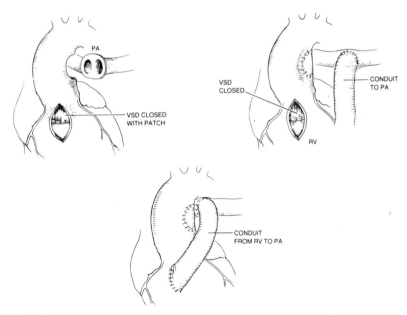

FIG 15–3.
Steps in total surgical correction of pulmonary truncus arteriosus.

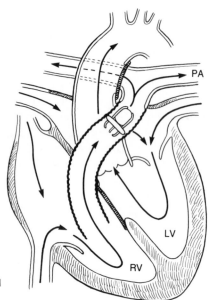

FIG 15–4.
Blood flow following correction of
pulmonary truncus arteriosus. Valved
conduit in place from RV to PA.

coronary circulation is inadequate during uncorrected truncus arteriosus, myocardial function may become impaired and may remain so even after correction. The final and most important concern is the postsurgical ability of the right ventricle to pump blood into the pulmonary vascular bed. This ability depends almost entirely on the degree of pulmonary hypertension and is independent of whether it is reactive or fixed.

REFERENCES

1. Heath D, Edwards JE: The pathology of hypertensive pulmonary vascular disease: A description of six grades of structural changes in the pulmonary arteries with special reference to congenital cardiac septal defects. *Circulation* 1958; 18:533–547.
2. Marcelleti C, McGoon DC, Mair DD: The natural history of truncus arteriosus. *Circulation* 1976; 54:108–111.
3. Kidd BSL: Persistent truncus arteriosus, in Keith JD, Rowe RD, Vlad P (ed): *Heart Disease in Infancy and Childhood*. New York, Macmillan Publishing Co, Inc, 1978, pp 457–469.
4. Mair DD, Ritter DC, Davis GD, et al: Selection of patients with truncus arteriosus for surgical correction. *Circulation* 1974; 49:144–151.
5. Ebert PA, Turley K, Stanger P, et al: Surgical treatment of truncus arteriosus in the first six months of life. *Ann Surg* 1984; 39:451–456.
6. Hickey PR, Hansen DD, Wessel DL, et al: Pulmonary and systemic hemodynamic responses to fentanyl in infants. *Anesth Analg* 1985; 64:483–486.

16

Tachyarrhythmias After Cardiopulmonary Bypass

A 1-year-old child was scheduled for correction of a complete atrioventricular (AV) canal defect. After successful closure of the defect and weaning from cardiopulmonary bypass, the patient developed a rapid tachycardia of 220 to 250 beats per minute. The arrhythmia was associated with hypotension and marked hemodynamic instability.

Recommendations by William J. Greeley, M.D.

ANALYSIS OF THE PROBLEM

Arrhythmias occur frequently during cardiac surgery. This is especially true during pediatric cardiovascular surgery in which intracardiac repair is associated with a higher incidence of arrhythmogenesis when compared to that of adults.[1] As significant hemodynamic compromise can result from these arrhythmias, such as is seen in this patient, rapid and accurate detection is important. Additionally, the correct diagnosis of arrhythmias in the period immediately following cardiopulmonary bypass has important therapeutic and prognostic significance.[2]

A fundamental knowledge of the various etiologies of arrhythmias is necessary for the management of rhythm disturbances that occur during anesthesia and surgery. Generally speaking, the occurrences of intraoperative arrhythmias may be due to either intrinsic or extrinsic mechanisms. *Intrinsic* causes of arrhythmias are due to underlying disease states. The potential for arrhythmogenesis exists prior to surgery and the various exogenous stimuli that occur during anesthesia and surgery provoke the occurrence of specific rhythm disturbances. The most common intrinsic cause of arrhythmias in pediatric patients occurs with Wolff-Parkinson-White (WPW) syndrome and related conduction disorders.[3] Pediatric patients who are symptomatic from this syndrome usually have a history of symptomatic atrial arrhythmias, in which the specific electrophysiologic diagnosis of the disorder and effective antiarrhythmic therapy are known. Other intrinsic causes of arrhythmias occur in association with congenital heart disease; for example, Ebstein's anomaly of the tricuspid valve is associated with supraventricular tachycardias.[4] Another example is L-transposition of the great vessels, which is associated with supraventricular tachycardias as well as complete heart block. Other congenital heart defects associated with tachyarrhythmias are ventricular-septal defect (VSD), double-outlet right ventricle, and univentricular hearts. Reentrant tachycardias and ventricular arrhythmias such as those that occur with myocarditis, cardiomyopathy, valvular heart disease, and coronary artery disease are rare causes of intrinsic arrhythmias that may become manifested during surgery. Finally, a large group of patients with intrinsic arrhythmias are those children in whom prior cardiac surgery has created persistent arrhythmias.

The importance of identifying those patients with intrinsic or preexisting arrhythmias is that anesthesia and surgery may provoke the occurrence of these arrhythmias intraoperatively. Therefore, a fundamental knowledge of the history of a patient's specific rhythm disturbance and effective therapy is essential to management of their arrhythmias in the operating room. Arrhythmias that occur in children on an intrinsic basis outside the operating room will most likely reappear, given the right set of conditions, within the operating room.

Extrinsic causes of intraoperative arrhythmias arise de novo without preexisting arrhythmogenic potential and are usually related to anesthesia or surgery. Extrinsic causes of arrhythmias in pediatric patients can be due to autonomic imbalance of either the sympathetic or parasympathetic nervous system, anesthetic agents, certain vasoactive drugs especially the sympathomimetics, metabolic derangements, hypothermia, and conduction injury due to surgical intervention.

The occurrence of sympathetic overstimulation during pediatric cardiovascular surgery is a common extrinsic cause for arrhythmogenesis. Light anesthesia, endotracheal intubation, hypercarbia, acidosis, and/or hypoxemia increase circulating levels of catecholamines, which increase automaticity in cardiac tissue and may shift pacemaker activity producing various arrhythmias. Hemodynamic changes, such as elevated blood pressure, also alter automaticity and increase the risk of ectopy. The effect of various anesthetic agents on cardiac conduction tissue has been well described.[5] For example, halothane directly decreases the rate of depolarization and increases nonuniform repolarization in cardiac conduction tissue, thereby potentiating reentrant arrhythmias. Indirectly, it is well known that halothane sensitizes the myocardium to the arrhythmogenic action of catecholamines via β-receptor stimulation. Succinyl-choline, when administered to young infants and neonates who possess an autonomic imbalance favoring the parasympathetic system, often can produce significant sinus bradycardia, sinus arrest, or ventricular arrhythmias. Pancuronium, as another example, often produces a sinus tachycardia due to muscarinic blockade.

Metabolic causes of arrhythmogenesis during pediatric cardiac surgery usually are due to potassium metabolism. Hyperkalemia depresses depolarization as well as atrioventricular (AV) conduction leading to progressive heart block. Hypokalemia, on the other hand, increases the rate of depolarization and increases the rate of automaticity potentiating arrhythmogenesis. Another extrinsic cause of arrhythmias occurs after cardiopulmonary bypass in those children who are not sufficiently rewarmed. Hypothermia will depress AV node conduction and heart rate, potentiating ectopy, especially of ventricular pacemakers. Finally, one of the most common causes for arrhythmias occurs in those patients undergoing surgical repair of congenital heart defects in which intracardiac repair is associated with a greater incidence of specific arrhythmias. Intra-atrial repair such as a Mustard or Senning procedure for transposition of the great vessels may disrupt normal atrial conduction, placing the patient at risk for both tachyarrhythmias and bradyarrhythmias, which occur both in the immediate period following cardiopulmonary bypass and later on a long-term basis. During other surgical procedures such as a VSD closure or an AV-canal defect repair, in which the conduction system runs along the rim of the ventricular defect, the conduction tissue is at risk for injury due to the proximity of repair. After surgical procedures in which ventriculotomies are performed such as in tetralogy of Fallot repair or a Rastelli procedure, the risk of ventricular arrhythmias on a reentrant or ectopic basis is significant. Additionally, indirect precipitants of arrhythmias during surgery may be due to ischemia secondary to insufficient myocardial protection during aortic cross-clamping or due to reperfusion injury after unclamping and rewarming.

In general, then, causes of intraoperative arrhythmias during pediatric cardiovascular surgery are extensive and in the final analysis the exacting etiology is often multifactorial. For example, direct surgical stimulation of the heart in a patient with intrinsic arrhythmogenic potential and with residual myocardial ischemia due to reperfusion injury after bypass is often sufficient to produce a sustained tachyarrhythmia.

APPROACH TO THE PROBLEM

The specific management of this 1-year-old child with a tachyarrhythmia after surgical repair is predicated upon the principles of general management out-

lined below. The first step in management is to diagnose the rhythm disturbance accurately. Presumably, this tachyarrhythmia at a rate of 220 to 250
beats per minute would be very difficult to diagnose using the surface ECG
alone and additional information will be necessary in order to accurately diagnose the rhythm disturbance. This can be done by utilizing an esophageal lead
for ECG monitoring and is best accomplished during anesthesia by utilizing a
pediatric esophageal stethoscope modified with an esophageal lead (Portex,
Inc.) in which electrode wires can be attached to any ECG surface recording
system, establishing a bipolar esophageal lead. Another approach is to utilize
atrial epicardial pacing wires, establishing a bipolar circuit to produce well-
defined atrial activity. Either of these techniques will further characterize the
rhythm disturbance in this child in order to diagnose the arrhythmia correctly.

While the specific diagnosis of the rhythm disturbance is being made, an
assessment of potential etiologic factors should be performed. Specifically, an
arterial blood gas and a serum potassium level should be determined in order to
assess ventilation and metabolic status, respectively. The level of anesthesia
should be assessed, as inadequate levels may lead to elevated circulating
catecholamines, initiating and perpetuating this arrhythmia. Preoperative and
intraoperative anesthetic and vasoactive drug therapy should be assessed for its
arrhythmogenic potential. Also, surgical manipulations of the heart should be
stopped during this arrhythmia.

The most likely cause of rhythm disturbance in this patient is probably related to injury to the conduction system due to surgical technique, inadequate
myocardial protection, or reperfusion injury. In infants with AV-canal defects,
the conduction tissue is abnormal in that the AV node and penetrating bundles
are posteriorly oriented near the crux of the heart and are intimately involved
with the rim of the ventricular septal defect. Because the surgical repair necessitates valve reconstruction at the crux of the heart as well as closure of atrial
and ventricular septal defects, conduction tissue is at high risk for injury and
resultant arrhythmogenesis.

Although AV dissociation or complete heart block would be the most
common rhythm disturbance to occur secondary to this particular surgical procedure, tachyarrhythmias, especially those atrial in origin, are not infrequent.
These tachyarrhythmias can occur due to inadequate myocardial protection or
residual reperfusion injury. Despite the fact that these causes may lead to temporary arrhythmogenesis, the nature of these injuries is such that the rhythm
disturbance will be self-perpetuating, probably reciprocating, and antiarrhythmic therapy will be necessary.

Based on the occurrence of this arrhythmia immediately after cardiopulmonary bypass, the intrinsic prognosis should be considered poor for a self-
limiting disorder. Furthermore, the rate of the arrhythmia as well as the hypotension suggests that immediate antiarrhythmic therapy is warranted. Such

rhythm disturbances, if left untreated, will often degenerate into ventricular tachycardia and ventricular fibrillation.

Having decided to utilize antiarrhythmic therapy after correctly diagnosing the rhythm disturbance and treating underlying secondary factors, the clinician should employ simple maneuvers and medications first. The objective in treating a rhythm disturbance of this magnitude is to control and protect the ventricular rate and to convert the arrhythmia to a normal sinus rhythm. In approaching antiarrhythmic therapy, the clinician should know a few drugs very well, avoid combinations of drug therapy, and only use antiarrhythmic agents and/or defibrillation when precipitating factors cannot be identified and the situation warrants therapy, such as in this case. As noted above, the need for immediate therapy in this patient is based on a rhythm disturbance with a poor prognosis as well as hemodynamic compromise.

With the clinician utilizing an esophageal lead or an atrial epicardial lead for diagnosis, if the rhythm disturbance is noted to be a wide QRS tachycardia, the presumptive diagnosis would be ventricular tachycardia. Knowing that a small percentage of wide QRS tachycardias in children can be atrial in origin, the clinician must assume the worst and treat for ventricular arrhythmias. The preferred approach would be synchronous defibrillation using low-voltage therapy. Prophylaxis against recurrent ventricular tachycardia can be accomplished by a continuous lidocaine infusion as a first choice; procainamide (Pronestyl) infusion as a second choice; or phenytoin (Dilantin) therapy if digitalis intoxication is suspected.

In this patient the most likely origin of the tachyarrhythmia is an atrial site. The potential atrial arrhythmias in order of frequency are: nonreciprocating junctional ectopic tachycardia (NRJET), paroxysmal atrial tachycardia (PAT), or atrial fibrillation (AF) with a rapid ventricular response. The first, NRJET is characterized by identifiable atrial activity dissociated from chaotic QRS ventricular activity on the esophageal or atrial epicardial lead (Fig 16–1). This rhythm disturbance is best treated with immediate digitalization and atrial pacing.[2] Defibrillation is usually unsuccessful due to the ectopic nature of the arrhythmia. Hemodynamic stability is achieved by inotropic support while awaiting conversion of this rhythm disturbance. The second line of drug therapy for this rhythm is either phenytoin or propafenone.[8]

Paroxysmal atrial tachycardia is characterized by a narrow QRS tachycardia with identifiable atrial activity and a consistent PR interval on the esophageal lead. The preferred treatment for this arrhythmia is atrial overdrive pacing, utilizing either the atrial epicardial leads or the esophageal lead. Second-line therapy for this arrhythmia would be either propranolol, verapamil, or digoxin. Vagal maneuvers may be employed; however, their success rate is low. Atrial fibrillation with a rapid ventricular response will be characterized by chaotic atrial activity and an irregularly occurring QRS complex when

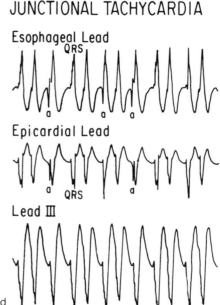

JUNCTIONAL TACHYCARDIA

Esophageal Lead

Epicardial Lead

Lead III

FIG 16–1.
Nonreciprocating junctional ectopic tachycardia (NRJET), best diagnosed by the esophageal or atrial epicardial electrograms, is characterized by identifiable atrial activity (A) dissociated from chaotic ventricular (QRS) activity.

viewed either from the surface or esophageal lead. Antiarrhythmic therapy initially should be directed at slowing the ventricular response since this is the single most important factor in controlling hemodynamic compromise.[9] The preferred approach would be synchronous defibrillation, initially using a low dose of voltage. Digoxin may also be used to convert the rhythm. However, in a setting of acidosis and fluctuating potassium levels, as well as in the presence of hemodynamic compromise, this therapy is generally not recommended immediately. The ventricular response may be slowed to an acceptable level with either propranolol or verapamil.

DISCUSSION

The successful management of arrhythmias during pediatric cardiovascular surgery depends upon several general principles:

1. Correct diagnosis and characterization of the arrhythmia must be obtained.

2. Etiologic factor or factors for arrhythmogenesis should be sought.

3. Intrinsic prognosis of the rhythm disturbance should be known.

4. Associated hemodynamic changes should be noted.

5. Recognition of the time of onset during anesthesia should be observed.

6. The type of cardiac congenital heart disease and the operative procedure should be intimately known.

The intraoperative diagnosis of arrhythmias can be made by reviewing the surface electrocardiogram, especially in leads II and AVF where P-wave depolarization is maximized.[6] In general, the surface electrocardiogram is useful only in identifying sinus rhythms in children. When the surface ECG is viewed intraoperatively, diagnostic errors are frequent in children whose heart rates are faster during surgery when compared to those of adults.[7] This is especially true during tachyarrhythmias in which P-wave identification, essential for diagnosis, is not always possible.

Esophageal electrocardiography has recently been reported to be a valuable tool for arrhythmia analysis during pediatric cardiac surgery and can overcome the inaccuracies of the surface ECG monitoring.[7] This is primarily due to the proximity of the esophageal lead to atrial tissue, resulting in large distinct A waves representing atrial depolarization. The esophageal lead has been shown to be superior in identifying rhythm disturbances, when compared to the surface ECG leads, especially during tachyarrhythmias. Atrial epicardial pacing wires placed during surgery also have proved to be helpful in the immediate postoperative period for diagnosing rhythm disturbances. For example, Figure 16–2 shows a narrow QRS tachycardia that occurred after cardiopulmonary bypass. Of note is the lack of identifiable P-wave activity on the surface leads II and AVF during the tachycardia. The esophageal electrogram and the atrial epicardial electrogram both produce well defined A-wave deflections, where the temporal relationship between the atrial and ventricular activation is obvious, indicating a diagnosis of sinus tachycardia. Therefore, to diagnose rhythm disturbances during pediatric cardiovascular surgery correctly, a combination of the surface electrocardiogram and an esophageal or epicardial lead is essential.

At the time of recognition of the arrhythmia, an understanding should be sought as to the etiologic factors causing the rhythm disturbance. Treating the rhythm disturbance with drug therapy without correcting the underlying etiologic factors may result in only a temporary solution to the problem. Therefore, during the occurrence of an arrhythmia, an assessment should be made of hemodynamic changes, ventilation, surgical manipulation, ongoing drug therapy, level of anesthesia, and metabolic status. Correction of any abnormalities in these factors may result in the resumption of sinus rhythm.

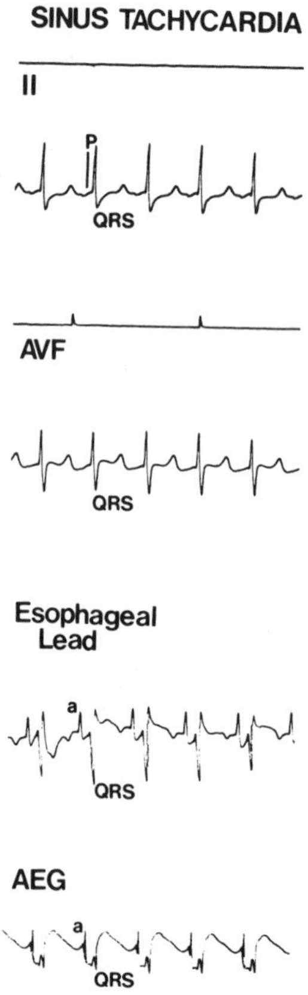

SINUS TACHYCARDIA

II

AVF

Esophageal
Lead

AEG

FIG 16–2.
Clear identification of A waves from the esophageal and
atrial epicardial electrograms allowed precise
confirmation of sinus tachycardia. Lack of distinct P
waves in leads II and AVF made definitive diagnosis
from these leads impossible.

Next, the intrinsic prognosis of the rhythm disturbance diagnosed should
be assessed. Simply stated, rhythm disturbances such as ventricular tachycardia, multifocal premature ventricular contractions, atrial fibrillation with a rapid ventricular response, and sinus bradycardia all have a poor prognosis in that
they may precipitously lead to immediate hemodynamic compromise and/or a
worsening of the rhythm disturbance. Rapid detection and therapy are essential
in their management. Other rhythm disturbance such as premature atrial contractions and sinus tachycardia are often well tolerated initially; in such cases
immediate therapy is not often necessary. Paroxysmal atrial tachycardia and
junctional tachycardia may or may not be well tolerated in the period immediately following cardiopulmonary bypass, depending on the presence or absence
of myocardial dysfunction and because their reciprocating nature would suggest refractoriness to conventional therapy. Since these rhythm disturbances
can cause hemodynamic compromise over a short period of time, therapy

should not be unduly delayed. Figure 16–3 demonstrates the intraoperative diagnosis of paroxysmal atrial tachycardia at a heart rate of 240 beats per minute in a 7-month-old infant who underwent intra-atrial repair of transposition of the great vessels. As can be seen, the surface leads II and AVF are not sufficiently accurate to diagnose the rhythm disturbance. However, the esophageal lead accurately diagnoses the rhythm as PAT. Since the arrhythmia was associated with significant hypotension, the patient was immediately treated with propranolol. This treatment led to the disruption of the reentrant or ectopic tachycardia converting the rhythm disturbance to a sinus mechanism, with a resultant increase in blood pressure.

Hemodynamic changes should be sought during the episodes of arrhythmogenesis. Most hemodynamic changes such as hypotension are usually secondary changes due to the rhythm disturbances. The degree of hemodynamic compromise associated with any primary rhythm disturbance is usually influenced by two factors: the state of the myocardium (whether it is diseased or normal) and the rate of ventricular response to the arrhythmia. For example, in pediatric patients with a cardiomyopathy or immediately after cardiopulmonary bypass (at which time the myocardium may be considered diseased due to the effects of extracorporeal circulation), arrhythmias are often associated with hypotension when compared to normal functioning hearts during the same arrhythmias. The faster the rate of ventricular response, the more likely the

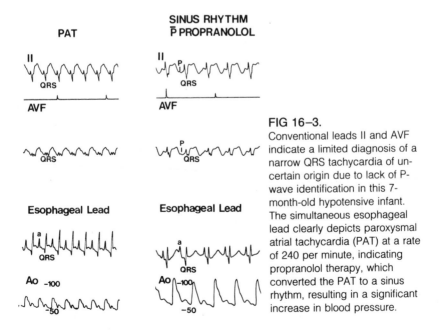

FIG 16–3.
Conventional leads II and AVF indicate a limited diagnosis of a narrow QRS tachycardia of uncertain origin due to lack of P-wave identification in this 7-month-old hypotensive infant. The simultaneous esophageal lead clearly depicts paroxysmal atrial tachycardia (PAT) at a rate of 240 per minute, indicating propranolol therapy, which converted the PAT to a sinus rhythm, resulting in a significant increase in blood pressure.

rhythm disturbance is to produce hemodynamic compromise. Infrequently, primary hemodynamic changes such as hypertension and hypotension in pediatric patients can lead to a secondary rhythm disturbance. Under these circumstances, the hemodynamic changes should be corrected.

When considering management for arrhythmias, the particular time of onset during the anesthesia has important prognostic implications. In general, arrhythmias that have been precipitated during the induction of anesthesia or during intubation are self-limiting arrhythmias and require no further management. Arrhythmias due to intrinsic heart disease or conduction defects or due to metabolic disturbances such as hypokalemia usually are self-perpetuating arrhythmias that will require therapeutic intervention. Arrhythmias due to anesthetic or vasoactive drugs or to autonomic imbalance may be self-perpetuating and their resolution depends upon the speed of recognition of the disturbance and the correction of the etiologic factors.

The final principle in managing arrhythmias during pediatric cardiovascular surgery is a detailed, intimate knowledge of the patient's congenital heart defect and the specific operation. As mentioned previously, there are certain congenital heart defects that produce specific arrhythmias. Furthermore, specific operations place certain parts of the conduction tissue at risk for direct injury during repair, precipitating certain arrhythmias.

Summary

In this patient the causes of intraoperative arrhythmias after cardiopulmonary bypass are multiple. The correct diagnosis of the tachyarrhythmia and identification of the etiologic factors have important therapeutic and diagnostic significance. The important factors that influence the management of tachyarrhythmias in this setting are the correct diagnosis of the rhythm disturbance and its etiologic factors, the intrinsic prognosis of the rhythm disturbance, associated hemodynamic changes, the time of onset during surgery, and the intrinsic heart disease of the patient and the nature of the corrective repair. Since pediatric patients are at risk for arrhythmias due to intracardiac repair and the overall immediate and long-term success of the repair depends upon management of the arrhythmias, tachyarrhythmias such as the one presented here represent a challenge to anesthesiologists; their management provides rewarding and satisfying results.

REFERENCES

1. Mardini MK, Varghese PJ, Nugent EW, et al: A comparative study of the natural history of post-surgical (acquired) and spontaneous (congenital) junctional rhythm. *Pediatr Res* 1974; 8:352.

2. Grant JW, Serwer GA, Armstrong BE, et al: Treatment of post-operative nonparoxysmal junctional tachycardia (NJT). *J Am Coll Cardiol* 1985; 5:428.
3. Gillette PC, Garson A Jr, Kugler JD: Wolff-Parkinson-White syndrome in children: Electrophysiologic and pharmacologic characteristics. *Circulation* 1979; 60:1487.
4. Guntheroth WG: Arrhythmias in children. *Circulation* 1981; 64:647.
5. Pratila MG, Vasilios P: Anesthetic agents and cardiac electromechanical activity. *Anesthesiology* 1978; 49:338–360.
6. Prodhomme G, Dinh CD, Scheydeker JL, et al: Pediatric ECG monitoring: 2,500 pediatric patients under anaesthesia. *Anesth Analg* (Paris) 1979; 36.
7. Greeley WJ, Kates RA, Bushman GA, et al: Intraoperative esophageal electrocardiography for arrhythmia analysis and therapy in pediatric cardiac surgical patients. *Anesthesiology* 1986; 65:669–672.
8. Garson A, Gillette PC: Juntional ectopic tachycardia in children: Electrocardiography, electrophysiology and pharmacologic response. *Am J Cardiol* 1979; 44:298.
9. Radford DJ, Izukawa T: Atrial fibrillation in children. *Pediatrics* 1977; 59:250.

17

Coarctation and Systemic Hypertension

An 8-year-old child underwent a successful resection of coarctation of the aorta. Upon emergence from anesthesia and after extubation, the child developed systemic hypertension with blood pressures ranging from 160/90 mm Hg to 200/110 mm Hg.

Recommendations by Michael F. Sweeney, M.D., Jorge A. Estrin, M.D., Ph. D. and Thomas E. Stanley III, M.D.

ANALYSIS OF THE PROBLEM

This is a classic case of paradoxical hypertension following coarctation repair.

APPROACH TO THE PROBLEM

Aggressive antihypertensive therapy has been successful in decreasing the incidence and severity of paradoxical hypertension and the postcoarctectomy syndrome.[6,4] This pharmacologic management can be applied in a rational way based on the pathophysiology of the disease.

Prior to surgery, no attempt is usually made to control the hypertension proximal to the coarctation. Preoperative loading with orally administered β-adrenergic blocking drugs over a two-week period has been shown to decrease the incidence and severity of paradoxical hypertension without lowering preoperative blood pressure.[8] Whether this regimen has any advantage over shorter term oral blockade or perioperative intravenous therapy is unknown.

Successful management of postcoarctectomy hypertension depends primarily on accurate blood pressure measurement. The most reliable method available is an intra-arterial cannula in the right upper extremity. The left arm is avoided in case the subclavian flap procedure is used for the coarctectomy. The lower extremities can also be used for blood pressure monitoring postoperatively, provided no residual coarctation exists. Occasionally, a patient has an anomalous right subclavian artery take off from the descending aorta below the coarctation. In this case, blood pressure can be followed intraoperatively with a temporal arterial catheter. At the end of the procedure, this should be changed to another site. Central venous access is advisable, not only to allow assessment of intravascular volume, but also to reliably administer infused antihypertensives such as nitroprusside. A bladder catheter is also recommended.

Typically, the coarctectomy is performed via a left lateral thoracotomy. General endotracheal anesthesia with a potent inhalation agent carried by air and oxygen mixtures is utilized and supplemented as needed with narcotics and muscle relaxants.

The decision to treat perioperative hypertension should be based upon reasonable guidelines of acceptable blood pressures. Maximum blood pressure measurements for different age groups are presented in Table 17–1. If unacceptable hypertension exists, all other causes for this condition must be excluded prior to treatment. Intraoperatively, an adequate level of anesthesia must be maintained. Sufficient analgesia and sedation must be provided in the postoperative period, especially if the endotracheal tube is still in place. Intercostal nerve blocks can be very useful for this purpose. Hypercarbia, hypoxemia, and hypothermia must be ruled out. The patient's neurologic status should be followed closely. Finally, an assessment of the patient's intravascular volume status should be made and diuretic therapy started if hypervolemia is present. If examining these variables does not yield a cause for the hypertension, pharmacologic intervention is undertaken.

Since the primary cause of early paradoxical hypertension is sympathetic hyperactivity, adrenergic blocking drugs form the first line of therapy. Of these agents, propranolol is the most widely used. Its nonspecific β-adrenergic

TABLE 17–1.

Maximum Blood Pressure Measurements for Different Age Groups

AGE	SYSTOLIC	DIASTOLIC
Young infant	100	70
Older infant	110	75
Toddler	120	80
School-aged	130	85
Adolescent	140	90

blocking effect decreases cardiac output by decreasing stroke index and heart rate. It does this by direct negative inotropic action as well as by a milder indirect inhibition of central adrenergic outflow. It also directly suppresses renin release, and is therefore useful for treating the delayed phase of paradoxical hypertension as well. Blood pressure and heart rate measurements are used to monitor the efficacy of therapy. The initial dose of propranolol is 0.02 mg/kg intravenously. This dose is repeated or doubled until: (1) the blood pressure is normal or (2) the heart rate is in the middle of the normal range for age. Usually no more than 0.2 mg/kg over 30 minutes is needed to attain either of these goals. The total dose required is then repeated as needed, usually every 4 to 12 hours. If the desired heart rate is attained but the blood pressure remains elevated, inappropriate vasoconstriction is present. Therefore, sodium nitroprusside is begun at 1 μg/kg/minute and quickly increased until the blood pressure is normal. Usually no more than 8 μg/kg/minute is needed. This infusion is then weaned as tolerated.

Using this drug regimen,[24] all of the coarctectomy patients at our hospital have been maintained normotensive, and the incidence of clinically significant mesenteric arteritis has been reduced to a very low level. When oral intake is resumed, propranolol is begun at 1 to 2 mg/kg orally every 8 to 12 hours. Also, if sodium nitroprusside cannot be weaned in 48 to 72 hours, captopril is begun orally to limit renin-angiotensin II mediated vasoconstriction. The dose used is 1 to 2 mg/kg/day in three divided doses. Oral medications are later withdrawn as tolerated.

The safety of the aforementioned therapy is excellent. Metoprolol can be substituted for propranolol in patients with reactive small airways disease. Propranolol should also be used cautiously in patients with myocardial conduction defects or severely impaired contractility. Sodium nitroprusside gives rapidly titratable direct smooth muscle relaxation. Its effect is gone less than five minutes after discontinuing infusion, a feature that makes sodium nitroprusside very useful in the immediate postoperative period, when cardiovascular lability

TABLE 17–2.

Management of Paradoxical Hypertension

Rule out	Metabolic, neurologic causes
	Discomfort/anxiety, hypervolemia
Treatment	
Early hypertension	β-adrenergic blockade, vasodilator if needed
Delayed hypertension	Vasodilator, especially captopril

or bleeding can occur. At the infusion levels and duration of therapy needed for these cases, cyanide and thiocyanate toxicity are rare. Captopril is also safe, though its effect is less controllable due to its requirement for oral administration and long elimination half-life. Rarely, neutropenia necessitates its discontinuance. The management of paradoxical hypertension is summarized in Table 17–2.

Alternative approaches to therapy include the use of methyldopa, clonidine, reserpine, trimethaphan, α-adrenergic blockers, calcium channel blockers, prazosin, hydralazine, and diazoxide. All of these drugs have been used with good efficacy. Their main disadvantage relates to difficulty of rapid titratability. In addition, some of these drugs such as methyldopa, clonidine, reserpine, and trimethaphan have other central nervous system effects that make them less advantageous.

DISCUSSION

Coarctation of the aorta is a well-recognized congenital cardiovascular defect, representing approximately 10% of all diagnosed congenital cardiovascular anomalies. The coarctation is a high-grade stenosis of the aortic isthmus that usually occurs at the ductus or ligamentum arteriosum, just distal to the origin of the left subclavian artery. This lesion tends to be associated with numerous other congenital cardiac defects, most commonly patent ductus arteriosus, atrial- and ventricular-septal defects, and anomalies of the aortic valve. In combination with these defects, coarctation can present with symptoms of severe congestive heart failure. Depending on the number and severity of the associated anomalies, infants with coarctation and cardiac failure face a significant mortality despite aggressive medical and surgical therapy.

Fortunately, the more common mode of presentation of coarctation is asymptomatic hypertension with decreased pulses in the lower extremities. Under these circumstances, the diagnosis may not be made until the child is several years of age. There are usually no other defects save a 40% incidence of bicuspid aortic valve. Surgery at an early age has become popular in these cases, and perioperative mortality is less than 5%.[9,10,15]

Hypertension occurs in the arterial distribution proximal to the coarctation. Obviously, the mechanical stenosis caused by the lesion is the primary etiologic factor for this blood pressure elevation. However, an additional cause of sustained hypertension in these patients can be a secondary hyperreninemia and subsequent hypervolemia, stimulated by the relative hypotension in the arterial tree distal to the coarctation. This hypertension plays a dominant role in the natural history of the disease. In a review of 104 patients with coarctation,

Reifenstein et al. reported that three fourths of deaths in these patients were the result of complications of the hypertensive state, such as dissecting aortic aneurysm, cardiac failure, and intracranial hemorrhage.[16]

Attempts to treat this hypertension medically have failed. Definitive treatment of coarctation of the aorta is surgical and is currently performed in many patients shortly after the diagnosis is made, regardless of the mode of presentation. Although several operative techniques have been developed, the two most popular are complete resection of the coarcted segment with end-to-end anastomosis, and the subclavian flap procedure, which is a partial resection that incorporates the proximal left subclavian artery into the anastomosis. In a large series published in 1957, it was reported that coarctectomy successfully normalized resting blood pressure in 95% of patients.[18] However, the postoperative course of these patients is rarely as benign as these figures suggest.[7,11]

The phenomenon of paradoxical hypertension following coarctectomy affects 15% to 60% of these patients and occurs most frequently in older patients who have severe long standing hypertension preoperatively. Disastrous complications may then ensue. The term paradoxical is used to emphasize that often a greater degree of hypertension occurs after the repair. This puzzling observation was reviewed in 1967 by Sealy,[20] who described two components of postcoarctectomy hypertension. The first is an acute phase, occurring 12 to 24 hours postoperatively, marked by a predominant systolic blood pressure elevation. This is followed within two to three days by the delayed phase, characterized by a predominant diastolic pressure rise. The latter component can be transient or can last for prolonged periods of time.[14]

The acute phase usually lasts no more than a week, and its occurrence coincides with an elevation of plasma norepinephrine to levels as high as 750% of normal postoperative values.[3, 20] Rocchini et al.[17] demonstrated a damped cold pressor response in these patients, indicating an elevation of resting sympathetic tone. Fox et al.[6] postulated that this enhanced sympathetic activity is the result of the triggering of a spinal reflex originating at the aortic isthmus. Mechanical stimulation of afferent nerve fibers in the isthmus has been shown to cause increases in blood pressure, heart rate, and maximum rate of rise of left ventricular systolic pressure via a reflex mechanism localized at the spinal cord level. These effects on hemodynamic parameters tend to augment the original stimulation at the isthmus, thus constituting a positive feedback mechanism for the reflex.[12] Support for this spinal reflex theory comes from reports that a similar hypertension may be seen after other types of procedures in the aortic isthmus area.[6] Interestingly, paradoxical hypertension did not occur in patients who had nonsurgical repair of their coarctations by balloon dilatation.[5]

Classic carotid and aortic baroreceptor reflexes will tend to normalize paradoxical hypertension, but this effect may be attenuated. Long-standing proximal hypertension preoperatively may cause a resetting of these baroreceptors to a level of diminished sensitivity.[2, 7, 19] Sehested et al.[22] demonstrated greater mechanical rigidity of the precoarctation aortic wall as compared to that of the distal aorta and theorized that this biomechanical change might have an effect on the pressure transducing ability of the baroreceptors.

If the norepinephrine level falls to normal within a few days, the hypertension usually resolves. Otherwise, the patient may pass into the delayed phase of paradoxical hypertension. This component of the hypertensive phenomenon is associated with elevated plasma renin levels. The cause of hyperreninemia is probably a stimulation of renin release by the persistent elevation of sympathetic nervous system activity in these patients.[17, 25]

A serious complication of coarctectomy that is almost always accompanied by paradoxical hypertension is the postcoarctectomy syndrome. First described in 1953,[21] this syndrome is characterized by nonlocalized abdominal pain and distention, decreased bowel sounds, fever, and leukocytosis. In some patients, there is a progression to bloody diarrhea, bowel perforation, or infarction. Exploratory laparotomy is sometimes required. The syndrome occurs in 2% to 28% of all coarctectomies, and nearly all of these have paradoxical hypertension.[17, 23] This potentially fatal complication is thought to be the result of an acute superior mesenteric arteritis, and much work has been done to characterize and predict its appearance. Mays and Sergeant[13] have theorized that after coarctectomy, the superior mesenteric artery suffers intimal damage and throm-

TABLE 17–3.

Pathophysiology of Paradoxical Hypertension

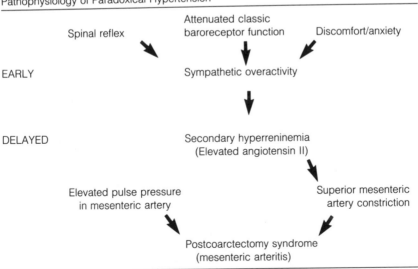

bosis because of the acute increase in pulsatile blood flow to this arterial bed. The mesenteric vessels are particularly prone to this damage since they lack significant supportive tissue. In addition, experimental work has shown that the superior mesenteric artery possesses a marked sensitivity to circulating angiotensin II, which can result in a disproportionate decrease in bowel perfusion if angiotensin II levels are elevated.[1]

The pathophysiology of paradoxical hypertension is summarized in Table 17–3.

Summary

We have discussed the pathophysiology of paradoxical hypertension following repair of coarctation of the aorta and have seen that it is characterized by sympathetic nervous system overactivity and a secondary high plasma renin state. Management is initially directed along the lines of reliable detection of hypertension with an arterial catheter, followed by the rapid exclusion of possible metabolic, pain/anxiety, or central nervous system explanations for the blood pressure elevation. Intravascular volume status is then assessed, and diuretic given as needed. Propranolol is relied upon as the first-line medication, with sodium nitroprusside and captopril used to relieve inappropriate vasoconstriction in the presence of adequate β-adrenergic blockade. With this aggressive regimen, paradoxical hypertension and its potentially fatal complications are readily controlled.

REFERENCES

1. Adar R, Franklin A, Salzman EW: Disproportionate reduction in superior mesenteric artery flow during dehydration and cardiac tamponade. *Surg Forum* 1975; 26:295.
2. Beekman RH, Katz BP, Moorehead-Steffens C, et al: Altered baroreceptor function in children with systolic hypertension after coarctation repair. *Am J Cardiol* 1983; 52:112–117.
3. Benedict CR, Grahame-Smith DG, Fisher A: Changes in plasma catecholamines and dopamine β-hydroxylase after corrective surgery for coarctation of the aorta. *Circulation* 1978; 57:598–602.
4. Casta A, Wolf WJ, Conti VR, et al: Captopril for management of paradoxical hypertension after coarctation repair. *Pediatr Res* 1983; 17:110A.
5. Choy M, Rocchini AP, Beekman RH, et al: No paradoxical hypertension after balloon angioplasty of coarctation of the aorta. *Circulation* 1985; 72:1038A.
6. Fox S, Pierce WS, Waldhausen JA: Pathogenesis of paradoxical hypertension after coarctation repair. *Ann Thorac Surg* 1980; 29:135–141.
7. Freed MD, Rocchini A. Rosenthal A, et al: Exercise-induced hypertension after surgical repair of coarctation of the aorta. *Am J Cardiol* 1979; 43:253–258.

8. Gidding SS, Rocchini AP, Beekman R, et al: Therapeutic effect of propranolol on paradoxical hypertension after repair of coarctation of the aorta. *N Engl J Med* 1985; 312:1224–1228.
9. Glass IH, Mustard WT, Keith JD: Coarctation of the aorta in infants: A review of twelve years experience. *Pediatrics* 1960; 26:109–121.
10. Hartmann AF, Goldring D, Strauss AW, et al: Coarctation of the aorta, in Moss AJ, Adams FH, Emmanouilides GC (eds): *Heart Disease in Infants, Children and Adolescents,* ed 2. Baltimore, Williams & Wilkins Co, 1977, pp 199–209.
11. Liberthson RR, Pennington DG, Jacobs ML, et al: Coarctation of the aorta: Review of 234 patients and clarification of management problems. *Am J Cardiol* 1979; 43:835–840.
12. Lioy F, Malliani A, Pagani M, et al: Reflex hemodynamic responses initiated from the thoracic aorta. *Circ Res* 1974; 34:78–84.
13. Mays ET, Sergeant CK: Postcoarctectomy syndrome. *Arch Surg* 1965; 91:58–66.
14. Nanton MA, Olley PM: Residual hypertension after coarctectomy in children. *Am J Cardiol* 1976; 37:769–772.
15. Pennington DG, Liberthson RR, Marshall J, et al: Critical review of experience with surgical repair of coarctation of the aorta. *J Thorac Cardiovasc Surg* 1979; 77:217–229.
16. Reifenstein GH, Levine SA, Gross RE: Coarctation of the aorta. *Am Heart J* 1947; 33:146–168.
17. Rocchini AP, Rosenthal A, Barger AC, et al: Pathogenesis of paradoxical hypertension after coarctation resection. *Circulation* 1976; 54:382–387.
18. Rumel WR, Bailey CP, Samson PC, et al: Surgical treatment of coarctation of the aorta. Report of the Section on Cardiovascular Surgery, American College of Chest Physicians. *JAMA* 1957; 164:5–7.
19. Samanek M, Goetzova J, Fiserova J, et al: Differences in muscle blood flow in upper and lower extremities of patients after correction of coarctation of the aorta. *Circulation* 1976; 54:377–381.
20. Sealy WC: Coarctation of the aorta and hypertension. *Ann Thorac Surg* 1967; 3:15–28.
21. Sealy WC: Indications for surgical treatment of coarctation of the aorta. *Surg Gynecol Obstet* 1953; 97:301–306.
22. Sehested J, Baandrup U, Mikkelsen E: Different reactivity and structure of the prestenotic and poststenotic aorta in human coarctation: Implications for baroreceptor function. *Circulation* 1982; 65:1060–1065.
23. Verska JJ, De Quattro V, Woolley MM: Coarctation of the aorta. *J Thorac Cardiovasc Surg* 1969; 58:746–753.
24. Will RJ, Walker OM, Traugott RC, et al: Sodium nitroprusside and propranolol therapy for management of postcoarctectomy hypertension. *J Thorac Cardiovasc Surg* 1978; 75:722–724.
25. Zanchetti A, Stella A: Neural control of renin release. *Clin Sci Mol Med* 1975; 48:215S.

18

Early Postoperative Ventilation

A 5-year-old child with Down's syndrome and moderate mental retardation underwent successful closure of an atrial-septal defect (ASD), and ventricular-septal defect (VSD). One hour postoperatively, the patient began to awaken from general anesthesia, became very agitated and restless, and was difficult to ventilate mechanically.

Recommendations by Susan C. Nicolson, M.D.
and Russell C. Raphaely, M.D.

ANALYSIS OF THE PROBLEM

Improper or incomplete fusion of the major endocardial cushions results in abnormalities in development of the atrioventricular canal and manifests as one or more defects of the atrioventricular (AV) septum and/or AV valve(s). This 5-year-old child with trisomy 21 has two such lesions, an atrial-septal defect (ASD) and a ventricular-septal defect (VSD), which constitute a partial AV canal.

The congenital lesion commonly referred to as an AV canal consists of a spectrum of defects.[1] A complete canal refers to a defect consisting of an intra-atrial communication, a large intraventricular communication, and a single common AV orifice. An intra-atrial communication, a small intraventricular communication and a divided or nearly divided AV orifice constitutes an intermediate or transitional AV canal. A partial defect is associated with four abnormalities that may occur alone or in combination: primum atrial-septal defect, para-tricuspid inlet ventricular-septal defect, widened medial tricuspid commissure, and cleft mitral valve.

The entire spectrum of endocardial cushion defects, from partial to complete, occur in 0.137 patients per 1000 live births.[2] This lesion ranks sixth in frequency among lesions and accounts for 5.3% of congenital defects in infants. Of the endocardial defects 35% to 40% occur in children with Down's syndrome.[2] The site and size of the left-to-right shunt, the magnitude of the AV valve regurgitation, and the amount of pulmonary artery hypertension influence the clinical findings in patients with this abnormality. In patients with partial canal with no evidence of mitral insufficiency, symptoms develop late in life, often as a result of pulmonary hypertension secondary to pulmonary vascular occlusive disease which occurs in 25% to 40%[3] of untreated cases. Usually a large amount of blood is shunted from left to right across the septal defects, resulting in biventricular volume overload and increased pulmonary blood flow. The ventilation-perfusion mismatch and increased bronchial secretions that result secondary to increased pulmonary flow make preoperative atelectasis and lower respiratory tract infections more likely in these patients. Long-term increased pulmonary blood flow results in increased pulmonary artery pressure. The pulmonary arterioles respond to the increased flow under an increased pressure head with hypertrophy of the muscular layer followed by thickening of the intimal layer resulting in increased pulmonary vascular resistance late in the patient's course.

The surgical repair in the patient described above consisted of patch closure of the ASD and VSD, usually done through a right atriotomy, using cardiopulmonary bypass and cooling to 28° C to 30° C. A 5% overall mortality is associated with surgical correction of the partial and uncomplicated intermediate types and increases to 10% to 35% for repair of a complete AV canal defect.[3]

Because this child awakened from general anesthesia one hour following arrival in the intensive care unit, we assume that the anesthetic consisted of a combination of potent inhalational agent and neuromuscular blocker with or without low-dose narcotic.

APPROACH TO THE PROBLEM

The agitated and restless child who becomes difficult to ventilate mechanically in the early postoperative period is a problem frequently encountered by those who care for pediatric patients following open heart surgery. Successful outcome demands prompt systematic evaluation to determine etiology (Table 18–1) and immediate intervention to assure adequate oxygenation and ventilation.

As a first step, we advocate transferring the child from the mechanical ventilator to a system permitting manual ventilation using a modified T-piece

TABLE 18–1.

Differential Diagnosis of Agitation in the Child Following Congenital Heart Surgery

Respiratory
  Artificial airway
    Displacement
    Obstruction
  Barotrauma
  Natural airway
    Bronchospasm
  Breathing system malfunction
Hemodynamic
  Low cardiac output
    Preload
    Afterload
    Contractility
      Structural problems
      Operative trauma
    Rate/rhythm
Pain and fear

attached to a compliant reservoir bag receiving a high flow of 100% oxygen. The partially inflated reservoir bag should be inspected visually and tactilely for deflation synchronous with the child's inspiratory effort and inflation during exhalation. When dry gas is administered from a compressed gas source that is not humidified, droplets appear on the inner wall of the tracheal tube as the water vapor contained in the exhaled gas condenses as the gas cools during its passage over the tracheal tube. If these maneuvers fail to establish the tube's position in the trachea, laryngoscopy is immediately performed to confirm proper tube placement.

Next, we determine the magnitude of impedence to gas flow into the lungs during manual inflation, using the experienced anesthetist's hand to judge the tidal volume and sense impediment to flow. Synchronizing the clinician's manual inflation with the child's spontaneous inspiratory effort differentiates asynchrony of the child and ventilator from other causes of impedence to gas flow into the lungs. If a block in the circuit was suspected, it must now lie between the endotracheal tube and the lung, as the remainder of the circuit that had been in question when the child was on the ventilator was removed when the child was transferred to the manual system. Passing a large suction catheter down the tracheal tube lumen serves to identify a kink in the tube or blockage by inspissated secretions or blood. If secretions or blood are found, vigorous flushing of the tube with saline and repeat suctioning may remove the obstruction. Failing to satisfy ourselves that the tube is patent demands the removal of the suspect artificial airway and replacement with another tracheal tube.

Bronchomotor hyperreactivity that causes impedence to gas flow may respond to β2-agonists, like metaproterenol sulfate (Alupent), administered by inhalation. This bronchodilator possesses minimal hemodynamic effect.

Pneumothorax may be detected by physical examination revealing diminished breath sounds and increased tympany in the involved hemithorax. Chest roentgenogram confirms the presence of pleural air. In the presence of hypoxemia, hypercarbia, acidemia, or hemodynamic instability, immediate decompression by thoracostomy of the involved hemithorax should occur with physical examination evidence only.

Low cardiac output may lead to the child's restlessness and agitated state. Physical signs indicating low output include hypotension, diminished peripheral pulses, cool extremities, and pallor or grey color of the skin. Examination of the contour of the systemic arterial pressure wave form, determination of the AV oxygen content difference, and analysis of arterial blood to look for nonrespiratory acidemia helps us decide if cardiac output is meeting the metabolic needs. Cardiac output determinations by dye or thermal dilution prove useful in patients with congenital defects if no intracardiac or pulmonary to systemic connections exist.

Once low cardiac output is identified, the clinician determines which of the four determinants (preload, afterload, contractility, or rate/rhythm) is the culprit.

In our experience, hemorrhage or tamponade commonly alters preload. Replacement of losses titrated against filling pressures and systemic blood pressure constitutes the best remedy for hemorrhagic preload depletion. Compression of the chest on either side of the sternal incision, irregular tidal volumes and frequency by manual inflation, and movement and vigorous suctioning of the mediastinal tube usually evacuate the accumulated blood in the mediastinum and relieve tamponade, thus avoiding surgical reexploration.

If cardiac output is decreased, we immediately seek structural etiologies as the cause. The myocardium following cardiopulmonary bypass copes poorly with extra pressure or volume burdens. In this child, AV valve regurgitation or septal patch dehiscence occupy the highest positions in our differential. Echocardiography is useful in identifying these problems. Pressures measured through catheters whose orifices are located in the left atrium, right atrium, and pulmonary artery, as well as the oxygen saturation of hemoglobin in the blood sampled from those structures help to determine and locate a shunt. Once structural causes have been eliminated, the impaired myocardial performance attributable to disturbed biochemistry and other trauma of cardiopulmonary bypass requires pharmacologic treatment. Inotropic support with or without an afterload reducing agent is begun.

Finally, low output could result from a primary rate/rhythm disturbance. The nature of the disturbance is identified and appropriate therapy begun.

Once cardiorespiratory function has been eliminated as the cause of the child's agitation and restlessness, we turn our attention to pain and fear. Incisional pain, discomfort from the tracheal, nasogastric, vascular, mediastinal, pleural, and urinary catheters all cause noxious input to the central nervous system. Fear can result from the child's inability to comprehend his/her plight and unfamiliar surroundings and his/her inability to express the same. Formulating a plan to treat pain or fear as the etiology of agitation requires consideration of the two postoperative ventilation management options, i.e., spontaneous ventilation with a natural airway versus mechanical ventilation via an artificial airway and deciding on the optimal time for extubation.

Table 18–2 outlines the eight parameters to be evaluated in determining the ideal time to remove the tracheal tube following cardiac surgery. At the time of extubation, the patient's cardiac output should be acceptable on minimal, if any, pharmacologic support; the rhythm stable; and no active bleeding should exist. Body temperature should be normal. The surgeon should be confident that the repair is optimal and no evidence should exist for a residual shunt or mitral insufficiency. The child's pulmonary status is assessed to be certain that following tracheal tube removal, adequate oxygenation and ventilation can be sustained with an inspired oxygen fraction (FIO_2) of less than 0.5 and minimal work.

Our experience indicates that patients with left-to-right shunting have increased pulmonary vascular resistance are at increased risk for developing low cardiac output, arrhythmias, or respiratory insufficiency within the first 24 hours following surgery. For these reasons, we advocate mechanical ventilation until the morning of the first postoperative day. Maintaining a secure airway and ensuring adequate oxygenation and ventilation with minimal patient work through this period eliminates these variables as contributors to the child's impaired cardiac performance should it arise.

Since we favor continued mechanical ventilation via an artificial airway,

TABLE 18–2.

Parameters to Assess in Considering a Child a Candidate for Extubation Following Cardiac Surgery

Cardiac output
Rhythm
Hemostasis
Temperature
Anatomy
Pulmonary function
Neuromuscular function
State of consciousness

we would treat the agitation and restlessness arising from pain and fear initially with narcotic administration. We believe that fentanyl disturbs hemodynamic function least. Our initial dose is 1 to 5 µg/kg. We have observed on occasion, that fentanyl, even with higher doses, was ineffective in achieving tranquility and produced dysphoria in a few patients. When narcotic alone fails to eliminate agitation induced by pain and fear, we have added diazepam, droperidol, or chloral hydrate with success. We prefer, when possible, to avoid the use of neuromuscular blocking agents in controlling postoperative agitation. Preserving the patient's ability to breathe spontaneously minimizes the impact of a mechanical ventilation system failure. We continuously measure end tidal CO_2 and utilize the pulse oximeter to alert us to inadequate gas exchange.

DISCUSSION

An alternative approach to managing treatment of a child with acceptable cardiopulmonary function and satisfactory hemostasis who becomes agitated and restless secondary to pain and fear in the early postoperative period is to proceed with extubation of the trachea. Proponents of early extubation of the trachea cite the risks inherent to artificial airways, mechanical ventilation, and the potentially adverse hemodynamic consequences of administering drugs to control agitation as reasons to remove the artificial airway sooner.[4]

We liberate patients from the ventilator by reducing mechanical breath frequency in decrements of 2 breaths per minute, stopping if tachypnea, retractions, and respiratory acidemia occur, or until we reach 6 ventilatory breaths per minute. We believe a patient's spontaneous breathing effort augmented by a mechanical ventilator delivering tidal volumes that are judged to move the chest wall at this low frequency produces conditions equivalent to the child breathing on his own without an artificial airway. If the alveolar-arterial oxygen gradient (Aa DO_2) remains less than 240 mm Hg on 3 to 5 cm of end expiratory pressure, spontaneous breathing effort is acceptable and no respiratory acidemia exists. With the child breathing under these conditions for one to two hours, if the Aa DO_2 remains less than 240 mm Hg on 3 to 5 cm of end-expiratory pressure, spontaneous breathing effort is acceptable and no respiratory acidemia exists, we measure the maximum inspiratory force and vital capacity,[4] seeking further evidence of the child's ability to sustain adequate gas exchange with his/her own breathing effort.

We then administer 100% oxygen for three to five minutes with a reservoir bag, mask, tracheal tube, laryngoscope, and drugs available. We clear the mouth and pharynx of secretions and remove the tracheal tube while applying positive pressure to the manual breathing system attached to the patient's tracheal tube. Following early extubation, the patient remains in the intensive care unit until the next morning to certify cardiopulmonary stability.

No data exist demonstrating that patient outcome is influenced by the timing of tracheal extubation, provided that the patient meets criteria for extubation and that skilled personnel observe the child following extubation in an intensive care setting.

Finally, communication between caregivers ensures that all members of the team involved in the care of children with critical illness share in the judgments related to therapeutic intervention.

REFERENCES

1. Feldt RH, Edwards WD, et al: Atrial septal defects and atrioventricular canal, in Adams FH, Emmanouilides GC (eds): *Heart Disease in Infants, Children, and Adolescents,* ed 3. Baltimore, Williams & Wilkins Co, 1983, pp 118–134.
2. Fyler DC: Report of the New England Regional Infant Cardiac Program. *Pediatrics* 1980; 65:377.
3. Norwood WI, Castaneda AR: Atrio-ventricular canal defects: Partial, intermediate, and complete, in Glenn WWL, Baue AE, et al (eds): *Thoracic and Cardiovascular Surgery,* ed 4. Norwalk, Conn, Appleton-Century-Crofts, 1983, pp 757–769.
4. Barash PG, Lescovich F, Katz JD, et al: Early extubation following pediatric cardiothoracic operation: A viable alternative. *Ann. Thorac Surg* 1980; 29:228.

PART THREE

Acquired Valvular Heart Disease

19

Hypotension and Severe Aortic Stenosis

Aortic valve replacement was scheduled for a 55-year-old man with severe aortic stenosis. The patient had a history of chest pain and results of his ECG and chest roentgenogram were compatible with a diagnosis of left ventricular hypertrophy. Anesthesia was induced with pancuronium 2 mg, followed by 50 μ/kg of fentanyl intravenously over five minutes while the patient was breathing O_2. At this time, prior to the adminstration of the remaining pancuronium (0.1 mg/kg), the blood pressure dropped from 120/80 mm Hg to 70/50 mm Hg and the rhythm was sinus at a rate of 50 beats per minute.

Recommendations by **William A. Lell, M.D., and Michael Scarbrough, M.D.**

ANALYSIS OF THE PROBLEM

In the case presented, induction of anesthesia with fentanyl results in bradycardia and hypotension. Fentanyl-induced stimulation of the central vagal nucleus causes the bradycardia. Rapid administration of high doses of the drug to patients breathing 100% oxygen potentiates the response. [1]

Could the observed hypotension result from fentanyl-induced changes in systemic vascular resistance (SVR) or stroke volume as well as bradycardia? High-dose fentanyl induction in patients with coronary artery disease usually produces a small decrease or no change in SVR. [1] Insufficient data are available to predict with certainty the response in patients with aortic stenosis. Profound hypotension associated with fentanyl induction has been reported in patients with valvular disease and/or severe left ventricular dysfunction. [2] Although unsubstantiated, fentanyl-induced central vagal stimulation in association with decreased central sympathetic outflow could cause vagal dominance resulting in bradycardia, vasodilatation, impaired contractility, and, ultimately, profound hypotension. Interventions to prevent or control these factors are particularly important in patients with aortic stenosis.

APPROACH TO THE PROBLEM

Pharmacologic interventions cannot correct anatomical obstructions. The goal of drug therapy is to restore a hemodynamic state compatible with survival until cardiopulmonary bypass and valve replacement can be completed. Because pharmacodynamics are unpredictable, careful titration of drugs to effect is preferred over bolus administration. Data derived from invasive monitoring are extremely useful in guiding drug therapy. However, supraventricular or ventricular arrhythmias induced by pulmonary artery catheterization can be life threatening. Appropriate equipment for electrical cardioversion must be immediately available.

Bradycardia.—It is unlikely that the vagolytic effects of 2 mg of pancuronium alone would be sufficient to prevent fentanyl-induced bradycardia. Larger doses of pancuronium (0.05 to 0.1 mg/kg) or pancuronium (2mg) and glycopyrrolate (0.2 mg intravenously at induction)[3] are more likely to be effective. Fentanyl-induced bradycardia can be treated with atropine alone. β-Adrenergic agonists may also be used to normalize the autonomic imbalance that results in vagal dominance and bradycardia. When used together, vagolytic and β-adrenergic agents must be carefully titrated to avoid uncontrolled tachycardia. A heart rate in the range of 70 to 90 beats per minute is appropriate.

Vasodilatation.— α-Adrenergic agonists and volume expansion correct vasodilatation-induced decreases in myocardial perfusion pressure and ventricular filling. Overcorrection must be avoided to prevent undesirable increases in afterload and preload. Although phenylephrine-induced increases in impedance to aortic ejection are relatively small compared to the resistance imposed by mechanical obstruction, even a minimal increase in SVR may severely compromise stroke volume.[4] Thus, the margin for error in maintaining adequate coronary perfusion pressure without depressing cardiac output is small.

Inotropic Agents.—Positive inotropic agents augment ventricular ejection across the stenotic valve and may correct any reductions in contractility resulting from fentanyl-induced autonomic imbalance. However, prolonged administration of high doses is likely to precipitate or potentiate myocardial ischemia and its sequelae.

In summary, careful titration of drugs guided by invasive monitoring should achieve the following goals:

1. Provide sufficient chronotropic action to reverse fentanyl-induced bradycardia without producing tachycardia.

2. Increase SVR sufficiently to maintain coronary perfusion pressure without depressing stroke volume.

3. Provide positive inotropic support without potentiating ischemia.

A sympathomimetic agent with combined α- and β-agonist activity is the drug of choice. The use of these agents combined with fluid administration when indicated to correct volume deficits resulting from vasodilatation or preexisting diuretic therapy is the preferred method of treatment.

DISCUSSION

The symptomatic patient with critical aortic stenosis frequently presents for aortic valve replacement in a precariously compensated condition, with limited capability for augmenting a fixed low cardiac output. Uneventful induction of anesthesia in these patients necessitates minimal disruption of the delicately balanced hemodynamic state. Avoidance of hypotension associated with myocardial ischemia, dysrhythmias, vasodilatation, or other causes is particularly important in preventing rapid and irreversible myocardial damage. Why is hypotension such a life-treatening event to the patient with aortic stenosis? The answer to this question is based on a thorough understanding of the pathophysiologic consequences of chronic left ventricular outflow obstruction.

The physiologic response to chronic aortic stenosis, regardless of etiology, is an increase in systolic and diastolic ventricular pressure. The compensatory morphological response to ventricular hypertension is concentric hypertrophy, characterized by a marked increase in wall thickness and left ventricular mass. As long as the ventricle hypertrophies in proportion to the increased intraventricular pressure, ventricular volumes, ejection fraction, and wall stress are all normalized. Late but rapid deterioration occurs when ventricular hypertrophy can no longer compensate for ventricular hypertension.[5] At this point, perhaps in association with intrinsic depression of myocardial contractility or rarely myocardial fibrosis, ejection fraction decreases and ventricular end diastolic pressure increases, resulting in clinical signs and symptoms of low cardiac output and pulmonary venous hypertension. Long-term survival now depends not on ventricular hypertrophy but surgical relief of the outflow obstruction.

Ventricular hypertrophy, although essential as a morphological compensatory mechanism, enhances susceptibility to ischemic myocardial damage. Vulnerability is further potentiated by the physiologic changes associated with chronic left ventricular outflow obstruction that alter myocardial oxygen demand and delivery. When decompensation occurs, uncompensated increases in wall tension increase myocardial oxygen consumption. Increased left ventricular systolic and diastolic pressure and prolongation of the systolic ejection period can also adversely affect a tenuous oxygen delivery. Systolic coronary blood flow is virtually eliminated by extravascular compression of penetrating vessels. Differential distribution of intramural forces results in blood being directed away from the subendocardium toward the epicardium,[6, 7] (Fig 19–1). Diastolic coronary blood flow is compromised by the decrease in coronary perfusion pressure resulting from the increased ventricular diastolic pressure and a shortened diastolic interval due to prolonged systolic ejection. Other factors potentiating myocardial ischemia include a pressure-dependent reduction in coronary vasodilator reserve[8] and the frequent occurrence of obstructive

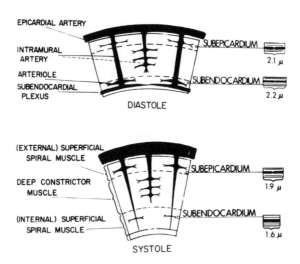

FIG 19–1.

Schematic cross section of a normal left ventricular wall during end-diastole and end-systole; relative sarcomere lengths are depicted at the right. Note: (1) greater subendocardial contraction and therefore energy requirements and (2) extravascular compression of the intramural arteries during systole with an intramyocardial pressure gradient from subendocardium to subepicardium. In the hypertrophied ventricle of aortic stenosis, a much larger mass of myocardium is rendered vulnerable to ischemia. (From Bell JR, Fox AC: Pathogenesis of subendocardial ischemia. *Am J Med Sci* 1974; 268:2. Used by permission.)

coronary atherosclerosis.[9] In view of the increased vulnerability to ischemia, it is not surprising that angina occurs in approximately two thirds of symptomatic patients with aortic stenosis. Persistent ischemia impairs contractility and results in a further reduction of the already compromised cardiac output. The subsequent fall in coronary blood flow promotes further ischemia. A vicious cycle ensues, rapidly culminating in bradyarrhythmias and ventricular fibrillation. Closed chest cardiac compressions are relatively ineffective in maintaining cardiac output because of the mechanical obstruction to ventricular ejection and poor filling of the noncompliant left ventricle. The end result is extensive myocardial infarction and death. Because the determinants of myocardial oxygen consumption are relatively fixed in patients with aortic stenosis and difficult to manipulate, prevention of myocardial ischemia and its sequelae depends on the maintenance of adequate oxygen delivery. Even a small reduction in pressure-dependent coronary blood flow to the hypertrophied left ventricle can trigger rapid and irreversible ischemic damage. Thus, hypotension is a life-threatening event for the patient with aortic stenosis.

Prevention of hypotension depends on the recognition and control of causative factors. Hypotension can result from a decrease in peripheral vascular resistance and/or cardiac output. Vasodilatation is difficult to control and in general poorly tolerated by patients with aortic stenosis. In clinical practice, the adverse effects of decreasing pressure-dependent coronary blood flow usually prevail over the theoretical advantages of decreasing afterload and increasing stroke volume. Thus, decreases in peripheral vascular resistance are best controlled by avoiding agents and techniques known to cause excessive vasodilatation.

Hypotension due to decreased cardiac output results from decreases in stroke volume and/or heart rate. Hypotension resulting from a decrease in stroke volume most likely occurs secondary to impaired contractility and/or inadequate "preloading." The adverse effects of ischemic-induced depression of contractility are discussed above. Maintenance of adequate stroke volume also depends on effective filling of the noncompliant hypertrophied left ventricle. As ventricular diastolic pressure increases with failure, passive diastolic filling is reduced and the active atrial contribution to ventricular filling becomes progressively more important. Arrhythmias, resulting in a loss of a coordinated atrial contraction, are likely to cause dramatic decreases in stroke volume and profound hypotension. Late in the natural history of patients with aortic stenosis, compensatory mechanisms become ineffective in maintaining normal flow across the stenotic valve. Stroke volume can no longer increase and cardiac output becomes rate dependent. At this point, control of heart rate is essential to the prevention of ischemic myocardial damage. Bradycardia results in decreased cardiac output, hypotension, and inadequate pressure-dependent coronary perfusion. Tachycardia increases cardiac output but potentiates ischemia by increasing oxygen demands and decreasing the duration of diastolic coronary blood flow.

Summary

The hypertrophied left ventricle resulting from chronic outflow obstruction is extremely vulnerable to hypotensive-induced ischemic damage. Successful management depends on the control of factors known to cause hypotension. Although pharmacologic intervention may temporarily maintain hemodynamic stability, every effort should be directed toward expediting the surgical repair.

REFERENCES

1. Bovill JG, Sebel PS, Stanley TH: Opioid analgesics in anesthesia: With special reference to their use in cardiovascular anesthesia. *Anesthesiology* 1984; 61:731–755.
2. Hug CC: Anesthetic agents and the patient with cardiovascular disease, in Ream AK, Fogdall RP, (eds): *Acute Cardiovascular Management: Anesthesia and Intensive Care*. New York, JB, Lippincott Co, 1982, pp 272–273.
3. Bailey PL, Pace NL, Stanely TH: Rigidity and hemodynamics during fentanyl induction: Pretreatment with diazepam and pancuronium. *Anesthesiology* 1983; 59:A316.
4. Perloff JK, Binnion PF, Caulfield WH, et al: The use of angiotensin in the assessment of left ventricular function in fixed orifice aortic stenosis. *Circulation* 1967; 35:347.
5. Ross J: Afterload mismatch in aortic and mitral valve disease: Implications for surgical therapy. *J Am Coll Cardiol* 1985; 5:811–826.
6. Rembert JC, Kleinman LH, Fedor JM: Myocardial blood flow distribution in concentric left ventricular hypertrophy. *J Clin Invest* 1978; 62:379–386.
7. Bertrand EM, Lasianoppe JM, Tilmant PY, et al: Coronary sinus blood flow at rest and during exercise in patients with aortic valve disease. *Am J Cardiol* 1981; 47:199–205.
8. Marcus ML, Doty DB, Hiratzka LF, et al: Decreased coronary reserve: A mechanism for angina pectoris in patients with aortic stenosis and normal coronary arteries. *N Engl J Med* 1982; 307:1362–1366.
9. Hancock EW: Aortic stenosis, angina pectoris, and coronary artery disease. *Am Heart J* 1977; 93:382–393.

BIBLIOGRAPHY

1. Braunwald E: Valvular heart disease, in Braunwald E (ed): *Heart Disease: A Textbook of Cardiovascular Medicine*. Philadelphia, WB Saunders Co, 1984, pp 1095–1105.

2. Chambers DA: Anesthesia for the patient with acquired valvular heart disease, in Kaplan JA (ed): *Cardiac Anesthesia*. New York, Grune & Stratton, 1979, pp 220–226.

3. Rapaport E: Natural history of aortic and mitral valve disease. *Am J Cardiol* 1975; 35:221–225.

4. Trenmouth RS, Phelps NC, Neill WA: Determinants of left ventricular hypertrophy and oxygen supply in chronic aortic valve disease. *Circulation* 1976; 53:644–650

20

Atrial Fibrillation With Severe Aortic Stenosis

Aortic valve replacement was scheduled for a 55-year-old man with severe aortic stenosis and ischemic heart disease. He had a past history of atrial fibrillation for which he took digoxin, but at the time of induction he had a normal sinus rhythm. He had an uneventful induction with fentanyl, vecuronium, and oxygen. Filling pressures were: right atrial, 5 mm Hg; and pulmonary artery wedge, 8 mm Hg.

With surgical manipulation of the atrium (placement of atrial purse strings), atrial fibrillation occurred with a ventricular response of 110 beats per minute, a decrease in cardiac index to 1.6 L/minute/m^2, a blood pressure of 80/60 mm Hg, and a pulmonary artery wedge pressure of 22 mm Hg.

Recommendations by John F. Viljoen, M.D., and John F. Fragola, Jr., M.D.

ANALYSIS OF PROBLEM

Anesthesia was induced and maintained with fentanyl, vecuronium, and oxygen. The patient had a normal sinus rhythm prior to manipulation of the atrium, at which point atrial fibrillation occured. The ventricular rate was 110 beats per minute; the arterial pressure fell to 80/60 mm Hg; the cardiac index was 1.6 L/minute/m^2, and the pulmonary artery wedge pressure 22 mm Hg. Clearly, cardiac output fell after the rhythm change.

APPROACH TO THE PROBLEM

Management can be classified as either aggressive or conservative as shown in the algorithm (Fig 20–1).

154

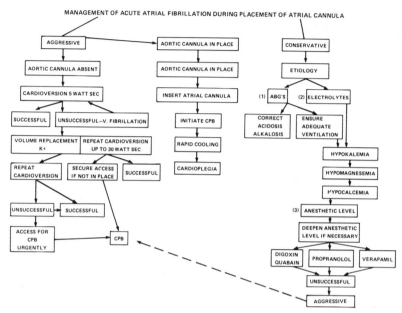

MANAGEMENT OF ACUTE ATRIAL FIBRILLATION DURING PLACEMENT OF ATRIAL CANNULA

FIG 20–1.
Management plan in patient with aortic stenosis who develops atrial fibrillation.

1. Aggressive Approach
   a. If the aorta is already cannulated, venous access can be rapidly established, bypass initiated, rapid cooling performed, the aorta cross clamped and opened, and the cardioplegic solution introduced.
   b. If the aortic cannula is not in place, as it should have been, or venous access not available, internal cardioversion should be attempted. Direct current (DC) cardioversion should begin with 5 watts-second and if unsuccessful should be gradually increased to 30 watts-second. It is of course advisable to correct conditions predisposing to arrhythmias (for example, hypokalemia, hypovolemia) as soon as possible, but the clinician may elect to proceed with cardioversion without delay.

      It should be remembered that DC cardioversion can precipitate intractable ventricular arrhythmias or asystole. This is more likely to occur in the presence of a high digoxin level, or abnormal acid-base status. Cardioversion causes transmembrane electrolyte shifts as well as local catecholamine release. These may actually potentiate digoxin toxicity.
2. Conservative Approach
   a. Correct conditions predisposing to arrhythmias: The presence of hy-

pokalemia, acidosis, hypoxia, or hypercarbia should be determined and, if present, remedial measures should be pursued.

b. Because atrial fibrillation may be due to increased sympathetic discharge secondary to an inadequate depth of anesthesia, deepening the level should be considered (a low concentration of an inhalation agent can be introduced).

c. If a and b above do not control the rhythm and vital signs remain unstable, additional pharmacologic interventions can be attempted as follows:

   (1) Digoxin is given in doses of 0.25 to 0.5 mg intravenously (IV) or ouabain 0.1 to 0.2 mg IV. It should be remembered that blood levels necessary for control of arrhythmias are often in the toxic range. Moreover, after cardiopulmonary bypass, changes in electrolytes and/or acid base status can potentiate digitalis toxicity.

   (2) Propranolol (Inderal) can be added in doses of 0.2 to 0.5 mg IV every 2 minutes up to 2 mg. Some authorities would question the use of a β-blocker in a patient with aortic stenosis and a low cardiac output.

   (3) Verapamil 2.5 to 5.0 mg IV (up to 10 mg) can be given over 1 to 3 minutes. Verapamil can precipitate hypotension, sinus node arrest, atrioventricular (AV) block, and/or decreased myocardial function. Lidocaine would not be advisable just prior to cardioverson as it can increase AV conduction leading to an accelerated ventricular response.

DISCUSSION

Background

Aortic stenosis is the most common valvular disorder in the older age group. Patients may present after a long asymptomatic period, sometimes as long as 50 years. The most common symptoms are angina, syncope, and congestive heart failure (CHF), all of which represent an advanced stage of the pathologic process. If surgery is not performed, the average life span is less than five years after the appearance of the above symptoms (sudden death can occur in 0.4% to 0.5% of patients).

Pathophysiology

Aortic stenosis is caused by calcification of the valve, which is either congenitally deformed (bicuspid) or simply affected by the aging process. The aortic valve area (AVA) is decreased in size (normally 2.6 to 4.0 sq cm). The major problem is one of systolic pressure overload due to obstruction of left ventricular ejection. As the aortic valve orifice gets smaller, the left ventricle must overcome a higher than normal gradient. The initial compensatory mechanism is to increase the duration of the ejection period. When this is no longer effective, the stroke volume will fall. In the process the left ventricle increases its mass by concentric hypertrophy. The increase in wall thickness leads to a reduction in ventricular compliance during diastole. This necessitates a higher left ventricular filling pressure to maintain stroke volume. Synchronized left atrial contraction is thus of crucial importance because passive left ventricular diastolic filling is less effective. Cardiac output is often maintained by increasing the heart rate, thereby reducing diastolic time. This in turn deleteriously affects subendocardial left ventricular perfusion. Onset of rhythms other than sinus, i.e., atrial tachycardia or atrial fibrillation, cause higher left atrial pressure. This will lead to pulmonary congestion, dyspnea, and eventually cardiac failure.

Other problems associated with aortic stenosis are: (1) an increased baseline oxygen demand secondary to increased left ventricular mass; (2) an increase in myocardial oxygen consumption due to elevated wall tension; and (3) decreased oxygen supply due to diminished coronary perfusion (effective coronary perfusion pressure = aortic diastolic pressure minus left ventricular end-diastolic pressure). The presence of coronary artery disease will further limit oxygen supply.

As the disease progresses, decreased contractility will occur on the basis of subendocardial ischemia. Cardiac dilatation will ensue, leading to a decreased stroke volume. Cardiac output can only be sustained by increasing the heart rate. This will in turn increase oxygen consumption and decrease supply by shortening diastolic filling time. A vicious cycle is thereby established.

Preoperative Considerations

Before embarking on therapeutic strategies, the anesthesiologist should have the following information available:

1. Whether the patient had been treated for symptoms of CHF or if it was solely the presence of arrhythmias that necessitated the use of medications.

2. Whether the electrocardiogram showed ischemic changes, a prior infarction, or signs of electrolyte or drug-induced changes.

3. The catheterization findings (specifically, left ventricular function, i.e., ejection fraction) and results of coronary angiography demonstrating the degree and location of myocardial perfusion deficits.

Prophylactic digitalization is controversial. Some believe it helps avoid unexpected postoperative arrhythmias or cardiac decompression; others feel the margin of safety is so small that arrhythmias can be produced. If patients show signs of congestive cardiac failure (apparently not the case in our patient), digoxin should be administered for one to three days prior to surgery. If atrial fibrillation exists, digoxin is given to: (1) slow the rapid ventricular rate by decreasing conduction; and (2) possibly convert the patient's heart rate to a sinus rhythm. This is more likely to occur if the atrial fibrillation is not chronic.

Since the patient had been receiving digoxin, it is appropriate to closely examine the ECG and check findings of serum electrolyte studies (since hypokalemia, hypocalcemia, or hypomagnesemia can all unmask digitalis toxicity). Arterial blood gas analysis will reveal the presence of hypoxia and/or hypercarbia or acid-base abnormalities, which increase the likelihood of digitalis toxicity. The digoxin level should be within the normal range of 1.5 to 3.0 ng/ml. This latter information has an important bearing on the decision whether or not to use cardioversion in the case.

General Comments

Premedication.—This must be generous enough to sedate the patient, but not sufficient to cause respiratory depression with accompanying hypoxia or hypercarbia. Hypotension due to venodilation will cause a drop in preload that is particularly deleterious in this situation.

Monitoring.—In patients with aortic stenosis, ischemic heart disease, and atrial fibrillation, electrocardiographic monitoring of V_5 and lead II are essential. Monitoring of V_5 will detect left ventricular ischemia in approximately 85% to 87% of cases, and lead II provides valuable information with regard to arrhythmias.

The placement of a pulmonary-artery catheter to measure filling pressures, cardiac output, and systemic vascular resistance is helpful as the clinician is better able to assess volume status and the efficacy of pharmacologic interventions. The use of a pulmonary artery catheter is not without risk, however, and the possibility of precipitating refractory ventricular arrhythmias is always present. Placement of a left atrial pressure catheter introduced once the chest is open is an alternative approach.

Anesthesia.—A narcotic-based technique is a good choice and, when judiciously used, can achieve excellent hemodynamic stability. Some clinicians regard an inhalation agent as a poor choice for the following reasons:

1. Myocardial depression can be produced.

2. Patients with aortic stenosis cannot compensate for a fall in peripheral resistance, as this causes a reduction in diastolic pressure with the potential for significant myocardial ischemia. Other clinicians argue that a low concentration of an inhalation anesthetic can cause a reduction in myocardial oxygen demand without significantly affecting contractility. Furthermore, a slower heart rate is beneficial in patients with valvular stenosis. The establishment of an adequate depth of anesthesia will also reduce sympathetic response to surgical stimulation.

Volume Replacement.—Maintenance of intravascular volume is of crucial importance as the relationship of left ventricular end diastolic volume to pressure is delicately balanced in patients with this disease. Monitoring filling pressure is thus mandatory. It is a strong clinical impression that hypovolemic patients are particularly liable to develop atrial fibrillation during cannulation of the great vessels. The patient in the case described above had a wedge pressure of 8 mm Hg. Under normal circumstances this value would not suggest the presence of hypovolemia. In patients with aortic stenosis, however, left ventricular compliance is greatly reduced, so that a pressure of 8 mm Hg is compatible with a diagnosis of volume depletion.

Summary

Multiple concerns are evident in considering patients with aortic stenosis. Acute atrial fibrillation in the circumstances described above can cause rapid deterioration of the patient's condition. Treatment involves sound medical judgment based on a thorough understanding of the pathophysiology of this condition. For the reasons given in this discussion, it is recommended that aortic cannulation should always be performed before venous access is attempted.

BIBLIOGRAPHY

1. Braunwald E: *Heart Disease: A Textbook of Cardiovascular Medicine*. Philadelphia, WB Saunders Co, 1984.
2. Chambers DA: Acquired valvular disease in Kaplan JA (ed): *Cardiac Anesthesia*. New York, Grune & Stratton, 1979, vol. 1, pp 197–240.
3. Frank S, Johnson A, Ross J Jr: Natural history of valvular aortic stenosis. *Br Heart J* 1979; 35:41.
4. Merin RG: Calcium channel blockers. 34th Annual ASA Refresher Course Lectures, No. 404. American Society of Anesthesiologists, 1983.
5. Reves JG: Anesthesia for acquired cardiac disease. 35th Annual ASA Refresher Course Lectures, No. 123. American Society of Anesthesiologists, 1984.
6. Rogers MC: Recognition of cardiac dysthythmias. 35th Annual ASA Refresher Course Lectures, No. 201. American Society of Anesthesiologists, 1984.

7. Thomas SJ (ed): *Manual of Cardiac Anesthesia.* New York, Churchill Livingstone Inc, 1984.
8. Thomas SJ, Lowenstein E: Anesthetic management of patients with valvular heart disease. *Int Anesthesiol Clin* 1979; 17:67.
9. Waller JL: Inotropes and vasopressors, in Kaplan JA (ed): *Cardiac Anesthesia.* New York, Grune & Stratton, 1983, vol 2, pp. 283–287.

21

Stuck Mitral Prosthesis

A 45-year-old woman had a Starr-Edwards mitral prosthesis inserted five years previously, correcting a rheumatic mitral stenosis. Over the last few weeks, she had noted several occasions of lightheadedness and once "nearly passed out." Echocardiography revealed an improperly functioning ball in the Starr-Edwards prosthesis. After sternotomy for emergency surgery, the pulmonary artery pressure would rise and suddenly fall with reciprocal changes in systemic pressures.

Recommendations by Roberta Hines, M.D.

ANALYSIS OF THE PROBLEM

In the patient described above all appears well until the time of sternotomy when a sudden rise in pulmonary capillary wedge pressure is associated with a sudden fall in systemic blood pressure. Differential diagnoses here will include: (1) arrhythmia (predominantly tachycardia); (2) manipulation of the heart; or (3) malfunction of the prosthetic mitral valve mechanism. In this case the patient's rhythm remained unchanged at a normal sinus rate of 80 beats per minute. The second hypothesis is easily eliminated by noting that no surgical manipulation is occurring at this point in the procedure. We must assume it is indeed a mechanical malfunction of mitral valve prosthesis that is responsible for this patient's deterioration. By palpation of the left atrium, the surgeon would be able to confirm the diagnosis.

APPROACH TO THE PROBLEM

Having identified the etiology of the patient's myocardial dysfunction, steps to resolve the mechanical obstruction should be instituted rapidly. The most effective method to relieve the obstruction is manual manipulation by the surgical staff until definitive valve replacement may be accomplished. This will result in only temporary resolution of the obstruction and all efforts must be directed to placing this patient on cardiopulmonary bypass as soon as possible to accomplish definitive valve replacement.

DISCUSSION

Mitral Stenosis

Rheumatic fever is the most frequent cause of mitral stenosis. However, only 50% of patients will relate a history compatible with prior rheumatic fever. Although most patients remained asymptomatic for up to 20 years, onset of stenosis begins approximately 2 years after the primary bout of rheumatic fever. Incidence of mitral stenosis peaks in the fourth decade of life, with a high female-to-male prevalence (4:1).

Initially, surgical treatment of mitral stenosis consisted of a closed digital commissurotomy.[1] This technique was replaced with open valvulotomy and by the mid 1960s prosthetic replacement of deformed valves had become the standard of surgical care.[2] A recent review of valve replacement performed at our institution over a ten-year period reveals an incidence of mechanical valve failure of approximately 0.1% to 0.2% per patient year. The highest failure rate was seen with Björk-Shiley prostheses, with a decreasing incidence of dysfunction occurring with St.Jude's and Starr-Edwards prostheses.

Pathophysiology

Regardless of the etiology, mitral stenosis results in a progressive thickening of valve leaflets and in shortening and fusion of the chordae tendineae, with a resultant decrease in the cross sectional area of the mitral valve. At a given rate of flow, pressure at the mitral orifice varies inversely with a square of its diameter.[3] Normal left ventricular function is maintained until the mitral orifice is reduced to approximately 1.5 to 2.5 sq cm (normal 4 to 6 sq cm), at which point the stenosis becomes hemodynamically significant. In the early stages of the disease, the left ventricle suffers from volume underloading, while the left atrium is subjected to increases in both volume and pressure.[4] Ejection fraction, defined as stroke volume divided by end diastolic volume, will remain normal as both components are decreased proportionately with the progression of the disease.

With long-standing mitral stenosis the increased pressure of the left atrium is reflected by elevations of pressure in the pulmonary artery, veins, and capillaries. These elevations in pulmonary pressures result in ventilation-perfusion abnormalities, a decrease in lung compliance, and an increased work of breathing.[5] Clinically this becomes manifest as dyspnea, which is often the earliest presenting complaint of this disease. At first the shortness of breath occurs only after vigorous exercise, but as the valve narrows and pulmonary vascular resistance increases, dyspnea occurs at rest. Cardiac rhythm is usually normal until the age of 40 when atrial fibrillation commonly develops. By the age of 60, atrial fibrillation is present in 80% of patients with mitral stenosis.[6]

Preanesthetic evaluation

When evaluating the patient with mitral stenosis, a detailed history and careful physical examination will aid in assessing the physiologic progression of the disease process. In this patient, the specific details of the "lightheadedness" should be carefully addressed. It is important to know what events may have precipitated these attacks and what physical sequelae accompany these (i.e. shortness of breath, palpitations, etc.).

On physical examination a murmur consistent with mitral stenosis will be present. This murmur will be a low-pitched rumbling diastolic murmur heard best at the apex. The murmur is more pronounced following exercise and heard best with the patient tilted slightly to the left.

A preoperative electrocardiographic examination is vital to determine cardiac rhythm, especially the presence or absence of atrial fibrillation. Other associated electrocardiographic findings may include P mitrale and a pattern of right ventricular hypertrophy in cases associated with pulmonary artery hypertension.

Anesthetic Management

The optimum premedication dosage in patients with mitral stenosis will be guided by the severity of the valvular lesion. As the mitral valve area decreases, a concomitant decrease in premedication requirement should be anticipated. Under most circumstances morphine, 0.05-0.08 mg/kg, in combination with scopolamine, 0.3 to 0.4 mg intramuscularly (IM), given to the patient 90 minutes prior to arrival in the operating room will provide adequate sedation without cardiovascular or respiratory compromise. All patients and especially those with any evidence of pulmonary artery hypertension should be receiving supplemental oxygen while in transport to the operating room.

Monitoring should be designed to provide a maximum physiologic data base. Electrocardiographic monitoring is essential, with an optimal combination consisting of a Lead II and V_5.[7] Arterial pressure monitoring is valuable in providing a continuous determination of systemic blood pressure as well as a means for obtaining arterial blood gas samples. Pulmonary artery catheters allow for measurement of pulmonary capillary wedge pressure (PCWP) as well as determination of cardiac output by thermodilution. In the absence of significant mitral valve disease, the pulmonary capillary wedge pressure will reflect left atrial pressure (LAP), which is in turn a reflection of left ventricular end diastolic pressure (LVEDP). However, in the case of mitral stenosis, PCWP (LAP) will be higher than the LVEDP by the amount of the gradient across the valve. Therefore, the left ventricular filling pressure will be consistently lower than the pressure reflected by the PCWP (LAP) measurements.

The induction and maintenance of anesthesia should be aimed at maintaining optimal intravascular volume and avoiding tachycardia. Tachycardia is especially detrimental as it produces a profound increase in PCWP with a resultant decrease in left ventricular volume and cardiac output.[8] Prior to induction, a full hemodynamic patient profile should be obtained. This should include heart rate, mean blood pressure, right atrial pressure (RAP), pulmonary artery pressure (systolic, diastolic, mean), pulmonary capillary wedge pressure (PCWP), and cardiac output (CO). These measurements will allow for calculation of systemic vascular resistance and the left ventricular stroke work index.

Induction with a narcotic-oxygen base will provide hemodynamic stability, even in those patients with evidence of pulmonary artery hypertension. The choice of narcotic is an individual one based upon the anesthesiologist's experience. In this patient, I would choose fentanyl, 50 μg/kg as a loading dose, followed by a continuous infusion of fentanyl at 0.5 μg/kg/minute. This dosage regimen will result in a plasma concentration of fentanyl of approximately 15 to 18 ng/ml.[9]

Patients with mitral stenosis have a relatively fixed stroke volume and therefore are highly dependent on heart rate for the maintenance of their cardiac output. A relatively stable heart rate should be the aim when choosing a muscle relaxant for intubation and use throughout the procedure. Metocurine or vecuronium would be an excellent choice for muscle relaxation, as both produce minimal change in heart rate. Pancuronium and gallamine should be avoided for their propensity to generate a tachycardia. Similarly, the bradycardia often seen following the administration of succinylcholine produces a reduction in cardiac output as well.

Summary

We are presented with a patient with mitral stenosis who is hemodynamically unstable and has a documented (by echocardiography) malfunctioning mitral valve prosthesis. The pathophysiologic basis for these hemodynamic events result from failure of the valve to open, resulting in a rise in left atrial pressure. Consequently, the left ventricle receives progressively less and less

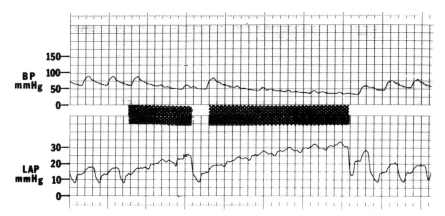

FIG 21–1.

A continuous tracing during normal sinus rhythm of systemic blood pressure (BP) and left atrial pressure (LAP) after placement of a mitral valve prosthesis. *Crosshatched* areas indicate time that the valve occluder malfunctioned, inhibiting blood flow from the left atrium to the left ventricle. Note the decreased systemic BP associated with markedly elevated LAP during obstruction and the increase in BP with proper mitral prosthesis performance indicated by the reduced LAP. Paper speed is 25 mm/second. (From Reves J, Schonlau E: Use of a left atrial pressure monitor to diagnose a malfunctioning mitral valve prosthesis. *Anesthesiology* 1979; 50:248. Used by permission.)

volume during diastole, causing a decreased stroke volume and resulting systemic hypotension.

The importance of continuous pulmonary capillary wedge pressure and left atrial pressure monitoring in patients undergoing mitral valve replacement was shown by Reves and Schonlau.[10] They report a case in which a precipitous rise in left atrial pressure with concomitant systemic arterial hypotension was observed in the patient undergoing a prosthetic mitral valve replacement. They confirmed the diagnosis of mechanical malfunction based upon the arterial pulse contour and the left atrial pressure tracing (Fig 21–1). Treatment, as in this case, was prompt surgical correction.

REFERENCES

1. Bower BD, Gerard JW, Abram AL, et al: Two cases of congenital mitral stenosis treated by valvotomy. *Arch Dis Child* 1953; 28:91.
2. Young D, Robinson A: Successful valve replacement in an infant with congenital mitral stenosis. *N Engl J Med* 1964; 270:660.
3. Gorlin R, Gorlin SG: Hydraulic formula for calculation of the area of the stenotic mitral valve, other cardiac valves and central circulatory shunts. *Am Heart J* 1951; 41:1.

4. Grossman W, McLaurin LP: Diastolic properties of the left ventricle. *Ann Intern Med* 1976; 84:316.

5. Laver M, Hallowell P. Goldblat A: Pulmonary dysfunction secondary to heart disease: Aspects relevant to anethesia and surgery. *Anesthesiology* 1970; 33:161–192.

6. Glenn W, Liebow A, Lindskog G: *Thoracic and Cardiovascular Surgery With Related Pathology,* ed 3. New York, Appleton-Century-Crofts, 1975.

7. Blackburn H: The exercise electrocardiogram: Technological, procedural and conceptual development, in *Measurements in Exercise Electrocardiography: The Ernst Simonson Conference.* Springfield, Ill, Charles C Thomas Publisher 1967.

8. Stott D, Marpole M, Kolslin F, et al: The role of left atrial transport in aortic and mitral stenosis. *Circulation* 1970; 41:1031–1041.

9. Lunn J, Stanley T, Eisele J, et al: High dose fentanyl anesthesia for coronary artery surgery: Plasma fentanyl concentrations and influence of nitrous oxide on cardiovascular responses. *Anesth Analg* 1979; 58:390–395.

10. Reves J, Schonlau E: Use of a left atrial pressure monitor to diagnose a malfunctioning mitral valve prostheses. *Anesthesiology* 1979; 50:247–249.

22

Unrecognized Idiopathic Hypertrophic Subaortic Stenosis (IHSS)

A 46-year-old man with a history of chest pain underwent cardiac catheterization. He had an "innocent" systolic ejection murmur. He was well sedated and relaxed during the catheterization, which revealed subtotal occlusion of the LAD and right coronary artery. No aortic ventricular pressure gradient was noted. Coronary artery bypass surgery was scheduled for him. Induction and sternotomy were unremarkable except on one occasion when the cardiac output had declined and a bolus of 5 mg of ephedrine was administered. The blood pressure failed to improve and the cardiac output declined even further, but cardiopulmonary bypass was successfully instituted. After saphenous vein aortocoronary bypass grafting, discontinuation of CPB was complicated by hypotension, low cardiac output, and an elevated pulmonary artery wedge pressure (PAWP). Administration of nitroglycerine and dopamine failed to improve the hemodynamic status.

Recommendations by David J. Torpey, Jr., M.D.

ANALYSIS OF THE PROBLEM

An anesthesiologist when approached by the Devil on the Last Judgment Day asked, "Why?"

The Devil exclaimed, "I didn't say you've been bad, you've just made some bad choices."

The anesthesiologist's treatment of the hypotension and low cardiac output that occurred during the period before and after bypass may have been considered a "bad choice" if all the facts were available, which indeed they were *not*. The anesthesiologist was a victim of circumstances and insufficient data.

167

APPROACH TO THE PROBLEM

Low cardiac output and elevated PAWP that does not respond to positive inotropic and vasodilator therapy in a patient with a murmur must raise suspicion
of idiopathic hypertrophic subaortic stenosis (IHSS). Appropriate therapy is
use of phenylephrine and return to cardiopulmonary bypass so myectomy may
be performed. Diagnosis may be confirmed by demonstration of a gradient
between the left ventricle (LV) and aorta and/or with transesophageal echocardiography.

DISCUSSION

Background

Idiopathic hypertrophic subaortic stenosis (IHSS) is a relatively common
disorder that has an autosomal dominant pattern of inheritance, with a high degree of penetration when it occurs in families. The inherited form is frequently
associated with specific human leukocyte antigen phenotypes. A sporadic form
of the disease has also been described that predominantly (82%) affects females in the age range of 50 to 81 years. The disease may affect any age; cases
have been reported in newborns and patients 87 years of age. Idiopathic hypertrophic subaortic stenosis is more common in the elderly than heretofore
suspected. In a series of 26 patients over the age of 60 years reported by
Berger et al.,[1] the diagnosis of IHSS was only made in seven patients (27%)
prior to echocardiography. This has led most authors to recommend echocardiography in all elderly patients who have an unexplained systolic murmur,
especially when it is associated with angina, syncope, dyspnea, and left ventricular hypertrophy. Two-dimensional echo complements the M-mode technique because the distribution of left ventricular hypertrophy can be more easily discerned (Fig 22–1).

The hearts of patients with the autosomal dominant form have a greater
degree (up to 50%) of septal myofiber disorganization when compared to patients with the acquired disease. Autopsy studies have shown bizarrely shaped
and abnormally arranged bundles of myocardial fibers running in diverse directions and separated by connective tissue clefts within the hypertrophied septum.

Approximately 80% of the patients with IHSS have left ventricular outflow
tract obstruction at rest or when provoked hemodynamically. In the 20%
without obstruction, portions of the ventricular free wall may be hypertrophied
and possess bizarre, disorganized myocardial fibers, similar to those found in
the interventricular septum.

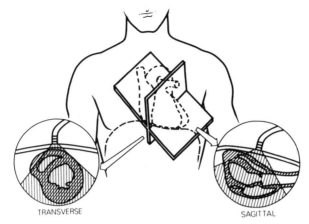

FIG 22–1.
Diagram illustrating the transverse and sagittal views obtained with two-dimensional echocardiography. (From Silverman K, et al: *Am J Cardiol* 1982; 49:27. Used by permission.)

Natural History

Reports from the United States and Great Britain approximate the annual mortality at 4% (range 3.5% to 5.5% per year). In most large series more than 50% of the deaths were sudden, probably due to arrhythmias (Johnson et al.[2]).

No reliable data are currently available that define the natural history of patients with IHSS and coexisting ischemic (atherosclerotic) coronary artery disease. Significant occlusive atherosclerotic coronary artery disease has been reported to occur in 25% of the patients who have IHSS over the age of 45 years.

Cumulative data up to 1982 have shown greater longevity for patients treated surgically (septal myectomy) when compared to medical therapy. Annual mortality for surgically treated patients approximates 2% per year. The validity of these data may be questioned today (1985) with the availability of newer β-blockers and calcium entry blockers.

A recent study by Starnes et al.[3] looked at preoperative predictors of favorable outcome in 94 patients with IHSS, refractory to medical therapy, who underwent transaortic septal myectomy. Of the patients, 97% improved postoperatively independent of presenting symptoms, functional classification, echocardiographic findings, or resting systolic gradient. They recommended myomectomy for all symptomatic patients refractory to medical therapy.

Duda et al.[4] reported the cases of 18 patients who had combined IHSS and significant atherosclerotic coronary artery disease with luminal stenosis in excess of 50%, with an operative mortality of 3%, thus demonstrating the relative safety of combined coronary artery bypass grafting and myectomy in experienced hands.

Pathophysiology

Pathologic findings of IHHS are listed in Table 22–1.

Silverman et al.[5] using two-dimensional echocardiography confirmed a "catenoidal* septal configuration" in patients with IHSS. They suggested that the catenoidal properties of the prenatal interventricular septum may result in isometric contraction of the septum with resultant local excess proliferation of cardiac muscle cells and fiber disarray leading to asymmetrical septal hypertrophy.

The catenoidal shape of the septum with a net zero curvature would develop internal tension by isometric contraction but would not contribute to the generation of pressure in the surrounding ventricle(s). The asymmetrically hypertrophied interventricular septum acts as a suspender during systolic contraction of the hyperdynamic left ventricular free wall, thereby accounting for the rapid stroke volume ejection and above normal ejection fraction, even in the presence of a reduced ventricular volume.

End diastolic volumes are smaller than normal, while end diastolic pressure is elevated; thus there is reduced left ventricular compliance. Global function of the left ventricle may be supernormal as demonstrated by increased ejection fraction and peak velocity of circumferential shortening.

TABLE 22–1.

Pathophysiology of IHHS*

PATHOLOGIC FINDINGS	FREQUENCY OF OCCURRENCE(%)
Asymmetric septal hypertrophy	80–95
Systolic anterior motion mitral valve	75–80
Midsystolic closure aortic valve	75
Outflow tract gradient, rest or provoked	80
Myofiber disarray interventricular septum	80
Ventricular cavities small to normal size	95
Dilated atria	85
Abnormal intramural coronaries	50
Cardiac output normal—elevated at rest	80–90
Pulmonary hypertension	25
Infundibular hypertrophy right ventricle	40

*Comprehensive list of the pathophysiology found in patients with IHSS and the relative frequency of occurrence as reported in the current literature.

*Catenoid has the property that every point has mutually perpendicular curvatures that are equal and opposite, thus their net curvature is zero.

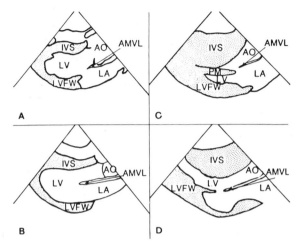

FIG 22–2.
Diagrammatic representation of echocardiographic sagittal views of heart. Normal patient, **A** and **B,** and from a patient with IHSS, **C** and **D.** End systolic views, **A** and **C.** End diastolic views, **B** and **D.** *AMVL* = anterior leaflet of mitral valve; *PM* = papillary muscle; *Ao* = aorta; *LA* = left atrium. (From Silverman K, et al: *Am J Cardiol* 1982; 49:27. Used by permission.)

The atria are dilated and often hypertrophied secondary to the increased resistance to filling of the noncompliant ventricles and mitral and/or tricuspid valve regurgitation.

Obstruction of the left ventricular outflow tract produces a gradient *inside* the ventricle that is separated from the subaortic segment by the hypertrophied septum and the anterior leaflet of the mitral valve that coapts with the septum. Obstruction may thus be viewed as both anatomical and dynamic. There is minimal correlation between heart size and the severity of outflow tract obstruction.

Figure 22–2 is a diagrammatic representation of selected echocardiograms, sagittal view, from end systole and end diastole in a normal patient and in a patient with IHSS. The diagram depicts that the hyperdynamic free wall has carried the attached mitral apparatus toward the interventricular septum. This accentuated excursion contributes to the systolic anterior motion of the mitral valve and resultant obstruction of the outflow tract.

The left ventricular free wall, which may be of normal thickness or hypertrophied during systole, encroaches upon the hypertrophied septum and results in greater obliteration of the left ventricular cavity than normal, with almost complete ejection of its contents (above normal ejection fraction).

In patients with IHSS, the septum is relatively immobile and the left ventricular free wall exhibits greatly increased excursion (Figure 22–3). The left ventricular free wall varies in its degree of hypertrophy. There is general agreement that the hypertrophied, noncompliant left ventricle constitutes the primary morphological and functional expression of the cardiomyopathic process in most patients with IHSS. Uncertainty exists as to whether left ventricular *diastolic* dysfunction, present in patients with IHSS, is the consequence of hypertrophy per se or is also present in ventricles with only mild hypertrophy or with normal thickness.

A recent report by Spirito et al.[6] employing digitized echocardiography and radionuclide angiography showed that the primary cardiomyopathic process is not limited to areas of gross wall thickening. Nonhypertrophied regions of the left ventricle were also shown to contribute to the impairment of diastolic function but to a lesser degree in most patients.

The impaired left ventricular filling (diastolic function) was shown to be secondary to prolonged isovolumetric relaxation and diminished rapid diastolic filling.

The decreased compliance of the left ventricle results in a higher left ventricular end diastolic pressure (LVEDP) for any given end diastolic volume. However, the clinician should be aware that the left ventricle is seldom dilated

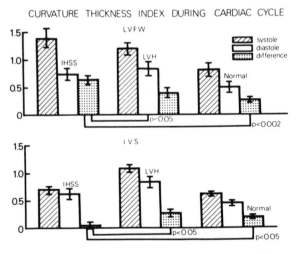

FIG 22–3.
Curvature thickness index during cardiac cycle (as calculated for the left ventricular free wall (LVFW) and interventricular septum (IVS) during systole and diastole). The significantly greater difference in the LVFW curvature thickness index between systole and diastole in IHSS correlates with its hyperdynamic state. The septum in IHSS shows significantly less change, correlating with its reduced dynamics. *LVH* = left ventricular hypertrophy. (From Silverman K, et al: *Am J Cardiol* 1982; 49:27. Used by permission.)

in patients with IHSS, even in the presence of a markedly elevated LVEDP and left atrial pressure (LAP).

In IHSS patients with associated occlusive (ischemic) coronary artery disease who have sustained an infarction, the resultant myocardial fibrosis may accentuate the varying degrees of dyssynergy during both systole and diastole. Ventricular dilatation may occur in this subset of patients.

Transmural myocardial infarctions in the absence of significant atherosclerosis of the extramural coronary arteries has been reported to occur in up to 15% of patients with IHSS (Maron et al.[7]).

Although the exact cause of transmural infarct in these patients is not known, several theories have been postulated (Maron, et al.[7]):

1. Cardiac muscle mass in excess of blood supply.

2. Medial thickening and cellular intimal proliferation resulting in narrowing of the lumens of the intracoronary arteries (small vessel disease).

3. Coronary artery spasm.

4. Frequent episodes of hypotension and tissue hypoxia with or without associated arrhythmias.

The incidence of significant occlusive coronary artery disease in patients with IHSS over the age of 45 years has been reported by numerous authors to approximate 25%. The two diseases have similar symptoms and physical findings; therefore, the clinical diagnosis of coexisting disease may be difficult. Angina may occur in up to 80% of patients with IHSS who have minimal to no atherosclerotic disease.

The murmur that occurs in IHSS may be thought to be due to papillary muscle dysfunction in patients with ischemic coronary artery disease.

Syncope is of frequent occurrence in patients with IHSS secondary to the decreased cardiac output and reduced cerebral blood flow that may accompany outflow tract obstruction and/or arrhythmias. Patients with coronary artery disease may likewise have syncopal episodes due to sinus node dysfunction or significant ventricular arrhythmias that reduce cardiac output.

Patients with combined disease may not respond to treatment with nitrates or may even have an increase in the severity of the angina. The pharmacologic effects of nitrates, namely, venous vasodilation, reduced preload, and compensatory tachycardia (treppe phenomenon), may increase the outflow tract obstruction, reduce cardiac output and systemic blood pressure, which may further reduce coronary blood flow in patients with high-grade stenotic lesions of the coronary arteries. If the presence of IHSS is not suspected in patients with known ischemic coronary artery disease, failure to respond to nitrates may lead the clinician to make the mistaken diagnosis of unstable angina.

Stewart et al.[8] recommend that "patients with angina and suspected coronary artery disease should have an echocardiogram if they demonstrate atypical signs or symptoms such as syncope, systolic murmur, and an unfavorable response to nitrate therapy." Patients over the age of 45 years with IHSS who are considered candidates for surgical correction should undergo selective coronary angiography in addition to catheterization of the right and left side of the heart to determine the presence and extent of the coronary artery disease and the ability of coronary artery bypass graft to improve myocardial blood flow.

Undiagnosed IHSS

One may ask, "Why was the diagnosis of IHSS not made preoperatively in this patient?" The diagnosis of IHSS based on results of the catheterization depends upon demonstration of an outflow tract obstruction in the left ventricle. This obstruction is dynamic and depends upon the overall size of the left ventricular outflow tract as well as the vigor of left ventricular contractility (Kerin et al.[9]).

The resting left ventricular outflow tract obstruction may be latent, labile, or persistent. In some patients no gradient may exist at rest, therefore, without provocative tests an angiographer performing selective coronary angiography without associated catheterization of the right and left sides of the heart may not observe an outflow tract gradient in a well-sedated, normovolemic patient lying in the supine position during catheterization.

Most patients with suspected ischemic coronary artery disease are receiving propranolol or some other β-blocker. Propranolol therapy may prevent the increase in outflow tract gradient even during periods of mild stress, anxiety, or exercise. It may also prevent or markedly decrease the enhancement of obstruction normally seen in these patients with provocative mechanical measures or drugs.

Angiographers may use either a multiple-hole pigtail catheter (Judkin's technique) or an end-hole catheter (Sones technique) to accomplish coronary angiography. The use of a multiple-hole pigtail catheter may neither demonstrate the obliteration of the left ventricular apex during systole nor record the systolic left ventricular outflow tract and aortic pressure gradient (Fig 22–4).

Even angiographers who use the end-hole catheters (Sones technique) for selective coronary angiography may not push the catheter tip into the left ventricular apex to avoid producing ventricular arrhythmias. Since the catheter would only be inserted, in a retrograde manner, a short distance beyond the aortic valve, the diagnosis of an outflow tract obstruction and gradient may be missed. Several patients in a reported series of 21 patients with combined IHSS and ischemic coronary artery disease who underwent surgical correction

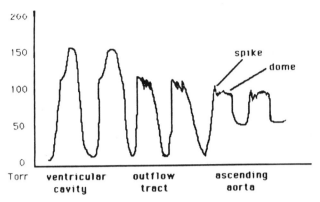

FIG 22–4.

Diagrammatic representation of changes in pressure and pressure wave forms between the cavity of the left ventricle, ventricular outflow tract, and aorta. Note the pressure gradient within the aorta and the spike-dome configuration of the aortic pulse pressure wave.

of IHSS combined with coronary artery bypass graft (CABG), or CABG alone, did not demonstrate a peak subvalvular gradient during cardiac catheterization with or without stimulation (Grill et al.[10]).

Left ventricular angiography needs to be performed with the patient in both oblique positions to determine:

1. Extent of impingement of the thickened upper end of the septum on the left ventricular outflow tract.

2. Presence and degree of mitral regurgitation and associated membranous subaortic stenosis.

Today, with emphasis on cost effectiveness, many patients may undergo coronary angiography as an outpatient in a satellite laboratory. Provocative tests may not be used unless the referring physician has alerted the invasive cardiologist of the possibility of IHSS or suspicion is aroused by an abnormal ventriculogram or hemodynamic response.

Transient hemodynamic changes may not be noted on the oscilloscope, especially if the angiographer experiences technical difficulty or concentrates exclusively on the coronary anatomy. Indeed the catheterization itself may provoke angina and outflow tract obstruction with resultant hypotension, syncope, and arrhythmias that may be attributed solely to myocardial ischemia. Treatment with sublingual nitroglycerin may further exacerbate the symptoms and cause the angiographer to terminate the procedure in the best interest of the pa-

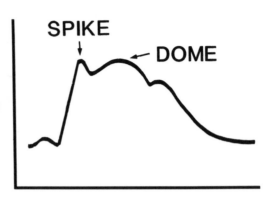

FIG 22–5.
Diagrammatic representation of an arterial pressure wave form (spike-dome pulse wave) recorded from carotid artery in patient with IHSS. Early rapid ejection phase produces a rapid ascending limb of the pulse wave. The sharp upstroke is followed by a downward dip as obstruction to outflow occurs. A second slowly rising pulse wave is produced by the continued slow ejection of ventricular contents and by reflected waves from the periphery and monitoring system (plumbing).

tient, or worse, schedule the patient for emergency coronary artery bypass surgery because of unstable angina or peri-infarction syndrome.

Therefore, neither the outflow tract obstruction nor the characteristic arterial pressure wave contour seen with IHSS, namely, "spike-dome" configuration (Fig 22–5), may be noticed unless a real time continuous paper trace is recorded and reviewed at the end of the catheterization.

The Mitral Valve in IHSS

Jeffery et al.[11] have shown that the mechanism responsible for the mitral insufficiency is the marked septal hypertrophy that causes abnormal angulation of the papillary muscles relative to the commissures of the mitral valve. During systole, contraction of the distorted papillary muscles and attached chordae tendineae holds the anterior leaflet of the mitral valve in the outflow tract with resultant obstruction. There is concomitant restriction of the posterior movement of the mitral leaflets that prevents coaptation of the leaflets and results in mitral insufficiency. Marked systolic anterior movement of the anterior mitral valve leaflet may be present in the absence of a resting potential. The anterior leaflet that opposes the septum during systole may become thickened and fibrosed secondary to the continued contact with the endocardium of the septum.

Mitral valve annular calcification is seen most frequently in the elderly patient (mean age, 61 years) and is probably the result of degenerative changes from aging and increased stress on the mitral apparatus. Mitral valve annular calcification may increase the incidence or risk of stroke in patients with IHSS. Since annular calcification occurs in the older patients who are also at greater risk for neurologic complications/sequelae from cardiopulmonary bypass, especially when combined with ventriculotomy, great care needs to be exercised by the surgeon during dissection. The increased risk for neurologic complications should be explained to the patient during the preoperative/preanesthesia visit (informed consent). In patients with hemodynamically significant mitral insufficiency and in patients for whom septal myectomy has been ineffective in relieving the mitral insufficiency, mitral valve replacement must be considered.

The combined surgical procedure of septal myectomy, coronary artery bypass graft, and mitral valve replacement carries a substantial operative and perioperative mortality. This is not unexpected, since placement of a mechanical or tissue valve in a small hypertrophied ventricular cavity as exists in IHSS may result in injury to the ventricle, the atrioventricular groove, and a significant gradient across the valve.

Arrhythmias in IHSS

Postmortem studies of patients with IHSS who experienced sudden death have shown the following (Frank et al.[12]):

1. Abnormal fibrosis of the sinus node alone or associated with narrowing of the sinus node artery in 55% of the patients.

2. Disruption or fragmentation of the AV node or His bundle in 50% of the patients.

3. Nonatherosclerotic narrowing of small coronary arteries in the ventricular septum.

These abnormalities of the conduction system predispose patients to the development of bradyarrhythmias or tachyarrhythmias that may cause sudden death.

The role of increased sympathetic neural activity as the basis for recurring ventricular fibrillation in the absence of coronary artery disease has been pointed out by Lown et al.[13] There is also increasing evidence that accessory atrioventricular connections may be present in a significant number of patients with IHSS (Sobel et al.[14]).

The subset of patients who are at increased risk for sudden death may be identified preoperatively by the following characteristics:

1. Excessively thick ventricular septum.

2. Grossly abnormal basal electrocardiogram.

3. Familial incidence of sudden death.

Electrophysiologic identification of patients suspected of having accessory atrioventricular pathways may become an important measure in the prevention of sudden death in this high risk subset of patients (Bharati et al.[15]).

Anesthetic Considerations

In formulating a plan of management for a patient with IHSS and associated ischemic coronary artery disease, the clinician must take into consideration the pathophysiology involved and the interaction of those pharmacologic agents to be used in the prescription for anesthesia.

Three factors are of prime importance:

1. Maintain normal sinus rhythm,

2. Optimize filling pressures (preload),

3. Minimize outflow tract obstruction.

Global ventricular function may be normal to supernormal, maintained by enhanced free wall dynamics, unless previous myocardial infarction has led to fibrosis and hypokinesis.

Anesthetic agents that produce global ventricular depression may reduce outflow tract obstruction in the hyperdynamic heart. Such agents, however, may reduce cardiac output and coronary blood flow in patients with impaired ventricular function especially those with dilated hypokinetic ventricles.

To choose both the correct and indicated drugs for induction and maintenance of anesthesia, the clinician must know the hemodynamic status prior to the induction of anesthesia and during the entire perioperative period.

Measurement of cardiac function, preload, and calculation of systemic and pulmonary vascular resistance are necessary for the anesthesiologist to assess the effect of his/her anesthetic technique and pharmacologic interventions. This can best be accomplished by means of a pulmonary artery thermodilution flow directed catheter with or without fiberoptics to measure continuous mixed venous oxygen saturations.

Anxiety and pain may result in the secretion of significant amounts of epinephrine. Thus, placement of invasive monitors should be accomplished in a well-sedated patient and by experienced personnel. Sedation that causes hypoventilation with resultant hypercarbia and hypoxemia due to low lung volumes in the supine geriatric patient must be avoided.

Those hospitals fortunate enough to have transesophageal echocardiographic monitors may use them to great advantage in this setting for evaluation of outflow tract obstruction, ejection fraction (left ventricular end diastolic and end systolic dimensions) and correlation of volume pressure relationships in the atria and ventricles. Decreased compliance of the stiff atria and ventricles and varying degrees of mitral insufficiency preclude reliance upon normal filling pressures to assess LVED volume. A series of ventricular function curves needs to be constructed for each patient, so that filling pressures may be established that provide optimal cardiac output, $M\dot{V}O_2$, and minimal outflow tract obstruction. The appearance of new "V" waves in the PCWP trace may signify mitral regurgitation secondary to papillary muscle distortion from increased contractility and outflow tract obstruction or may indicate myocardial ischemia. Correlation with the ECG will help in differentiating the etiology.

Direct arterial monitoring is a must for the following reasons:

1. Increases and/or decreases in outflow tract obstruction may be signified by changes in the pulse wave contour (exaggerated spike dome patterns).

2. Hypotension may be detected earlier.

3. Continuous readout of mean aortic pressure necessary to calculate systemic vascular resistance is provided.

The clinician must be certain that the "plumbing," i.e., transducers, stopcocks, and high pressure tubing, is of satisfactory quality to meet the changing hemodynamics without excess "ringing." Ringing in a pressure system may produce artifactual spikes on the arterial pressure pulse wave form and overestimate true systolic arterial pressure or lead to a mistaken diagnosis of a spike and dome configuration produced by outflow obstruction. Damping may likewise result in underestimation of the true systolic and diastolic blood pressure as well as mean aortic pressure, which will introduce error in the calculation of systemic vascular resistance (SVR)/systemic vascular resistance index (SVRI).

Multiple-lead ECG monitoring is optimal. Leads V_5 and II may be monitored to detect ischemic changes in the left and right coronary artery distribution. Esophageal ECG is ideal for determining the presence or absence of "P" waves and in making the differential diagnosis of supraventricular vs. ventricular arrhythmias and varying degrees of heart block.

The disease of IHSS is characterized by impaired left ventricular filling due to the hypertrophied septum and functional impairment of the ventricular free wall. The presence of ischemia may further decrease ventricular compliance. Ventricular filling depends greatly upon vigorous and coordinated atrial contractions. Hemodynamic deterioration resulting in acute congestive failure, decreased coronary and cerebral blood flow, ventricular arrhythmias, and sudden death may result from loss of normal sinus rhythm. Continued display of the esophageal ECG may provide the earliest indication of loss of normal sinus rhythm. If mixed venous oxygen saturations are being displayed, the hemodynamic effect of any particular arrhythmia may be readily noted.

Induction of anesthesia and endotracheal intubation should be accomplished in a well hydrated patient. Venodilatation produced by intravenous narcotics needs to be countered by fluid administration, guided by the response in filling pressures to volume administration rather than by a specific value. Transient drops in blood pressure not responding to volume infusion may be treated by titrated doses of phenylephrine given through a central line to avoid dead space sequestration.

A sufficient depth of anesthesia should be attained prior to endotracheal intubation to prevent or minimize catecholamine stimulation and outflow tract obstruction. The ability of fentanyl and the dose needed to prevent the increases in heart rate and blood pressure (sympathetic cardiovascular reflexes) resulting from endotracheal intubation and sternotomy has been questioned. Most clinicians will agree that fentanyl in doses of 60 to 100 μg/kg will attenuate any significant increase in heart rate due to endotracheal intubation and sternotomy. In patients with hyperdynamic circulation and high preinduction levels of catecholamines, the addition of diazepam and small doses of β-blockers prior to intubation and sternotomy may be helpful. Esmolol, a β₁-selective adrenergic blocker with no peripheral adrenergic-blocking effect may be used to treat tachycardia should it occur. Esmolol blunts the increase in heart rate and in the systolic and mean arterial blood pressure response due to endotracheal intubation and/or sternotomy without causing any significant decrease in diastolic blood pressure. Esmolol is currently not available except for research in the United States; thus the clinician must rely upon carefully titrated doses of propranolol to counteract catecholamine-induced tachycardia.

Care must be taken not to produce profound myocardial depression with propranolol since attempts to counteract its effect with β-agonists or calcium chloride may result in greater outflow tract obstruction and hemodynamic impairment than existed prior to treatment. Monitor! Monitor!

Choice of a maintenance agent should depend upon the experience (learning curve) with a particular agent or technique that the anesthesiologist has attained. Theoretical advantages and/or disadvantages may be advanced for any given agent or combination of agents.

All volatile anesthetic agents in current use cause myocardial depression and varying degrees of vasodilatation. Halothane produces the least decrease in systemic vascular resistance while isoflurane is the most potent vasodilator. The vasodilatation seen with isoflurane may prove harmful in the patient with combined IHSS and ischemic coronary artery disease. Outflow tract obstruction may be worsened by a decrease in preload, while at the same time a "steal phenomenon" (controversial) may divert blood away from coronary arteries with fixed obstruction.

Halothane may depress global myocardial contractility and thus decrease outflow tract obstruction, especially in the hyperdynamic heart. This will also decrease oxygen demand, a salutary effect in patients with ischemic coronary artery disease. For these reasons, it would be my choice for an inhalation agent. The electrophysiologic effects of halothane may lead to loss of normal sinus rhythm and thus hemodynamic impairment secondary to loss of atrial contraction.

Narcotic, nitrous oxide and/or narcotic oxygen technique may be quite satisfactory *if* the anesthesiologist prevents catecholamine-induced tachycardia. However, I believe that the combined technique of intravenous narcotics and an inhalation agent such as halothane and/or isoflurane provides the smoothest course. The clinician must be aware of the pharmacologic effects of these agents and potential hemodynamic consequences, and employ continuous monitoring of the effects they produce at any given time.

The geriatric patient, most likely to have the combined diseases of IHSS and CAD, when stressed increases his/her cardiac output by increasing stroke volume rather than increasing heart rate. These patients may be greatly compromised, however, in their ability to increase stroke volume. Left ventricular cavities in IHSS are small and resist diastolic filling due to decreased compliance and functional impairment. Ejection fractions may be supernormal and very little increase in systolic ejection volume may be possible. Homeostatic reflexes are diminished in the geriatric patient but should they result in release of catecholamines the coincidental increase in contractility would result in greater obstruction to the outflow tract as well as increased oxygen demand, which may be poorly tolerated in a patient with ischemic coronary artery disease.

If mitral regurgitation is an important component of the patient's disease, the clinician must be aware that conventional pharmacologic methods of reducing regurgitation may produce a paradoxical increase in regurgitation (Kaplan[16]). α-Adrenergic agonists, phenylephrine, titrated to produce a small increase in systemic vascular resistance may lessen the regurgitation that accompanies outflow tract obstruction. Hypertension should be avoided because of its effect on myocardial oxygen demand.

Mechanical positive pressure ventilation, especially when combined with positive end expiratory pressure (PEEP) may decrease venous return and result in hemodynamic deterioration due to the increase in outflow tract obstruction. A decrease in the systolic ejection murmur as heard via the esophageal stethoscope may occur during mechanical ventilation if it causes a decrease in venous return. The decrease in stroke volume due to decreased preload will reduce the amount of blood passing through the stenotic outflow tract and reduce the intensity of the murmur.

Ventilatory patterns should, therefore, be adjusted to minimize interference with venous return while providing adequate oxygenation and carbon dioxide elimination. End tidal carbon dioxide should be monitored to guide minute ventilation and prevent excess ventilation of dead space areas of the lung. Hypocarbia should be avoided, if possible, because of its effect on coronary arteries (vasoconstriction) and augmentation of hypokalemia. Serum potassium level should be measured frequently. Significant hypokalemia may precipitate supraventricular tachyarrhythmias and hemodynamic deterioration. The clinician needs to be aware that intravenous bolus doses of potassium in excess of 6 mEq may cause a marked secretion of epinephrine and increases in systemic vascular resistance.

During atrial cannulation the surgeon should make every attempt to avoid producing tachyarrhythmias or multiple extra systoles. Electrocardioversion should be used to terminate the tachyarrhythmias if they persist. The surgeon should be urged to use a single-stage atrial cannula to diminish manipulation of the atrium. A single-stage cannula may produce less trauma to the atrium and decrease the incidence of tachyarrhythmias following cardiopulmonary bypass.

Patients with IHSS may have marked hypertrophy of the ventricular free wall in addition to the septum. Protection of the hypertrophied myocardium with associated significant occlusive coronary artery disease during aortic cross clamping is of paramont importance.

Addition of nifedipine, a calcium channel blocker, to the cold potassium cardioplegia solution may provide better preservation of myocardial adenosine triphosphate (ATP), decrease muscle water content, and prevent reperfusion injury secondary to calcium flux. Reperfusion of the myocardium with perfusate containing high levels of catecholamines (epinephrine, norepinephrine, and vasopressin) secreted during cardiopulmonary bypass and deliberate hypothermia may cause an increased myocardial oxygen consumption and depletion of high-energy substrates (ATP) necessary for myocardial contraction and relaxation. Measurement of myocardial temperature throughout the procedure will help in determining the adequacy of cooling maneuvers in the hypertrophied heart. Both atrial and ventricular temperatures should be measured.

The clinician should maintain an adequate depth of anesthesia and analgesia during the cardiopulmonary bypass period to minimize catecholamine outpouring. Peak increases in catecholamines occur when the heart and lungs are excluded from the circulation (Reves et al.[17]). The increase in epinephrine exceeds that of norepinephrine. The increased catecholamine secretion during cardiopulmonary bypass causes a concomitant increase in vasopressin, which further augments peripheral and organ vasoconstriction.

Halothane or isoflurane may be added to the pump oxygenator since they have been shown to decrease or obtund catecholamine release and thromboxane production during cardiopulmonary bypass.

A properly performed and adequate myectomy is usually successful in relieving outflow tract obstruction. The efficacy of coronary artery bypass for the treatment of selected subsets of patients with ischemic coronary artery disease has been well documented.

Myectomy must be considered palliative treatment for patients with IHSS who are refractory to medical therapy. Although it may relieve outflow tract obstruction, myectomy does *not* alter the underlying process. Myectomy per se has not been shown to cause any significant impairment of global left ventricular function with the patient at rest or during exercise. Because patients with IHSS may have a broad spectrum of hypertrophic cardiomyopathy with dynamic and varying degrees of obstruction the need for reoperation may be as high as 10% (Edwards[18]).

Weaning From Cardiopulmonary Bypass

Many anesthesiologists use intravenous nitroglycerin during the rewarming phase of cardiopulmonary bypass to provide more uniform warming and decrease the degree of postbypass hypothermia. Surgeons also request intravenous nitroglycerin to minimize coronary vasospasm, dilate native coronary arteries, and increase graft runoff. Local injection of nitroglycerin into the saphenous vein graft has been shown to be more effective than intravenous nitroglycerin and produces minimal systemic symptoms.

If intravenous nitroglycerin is deemed absolutely necessary, the perfusionist should be directed to transfuse sufficient volume of perfusate to maintain adequate filling volumes (preload) to prevent outflow tract obstruction in patients who have undergone coronary artery bypass graft without myectomy.

Hemoglobin should be maintained at levels which do not require marked increases in heart rate to compensate for the anemia. The ideal hemoglobin/hematocrit level for an individual patient should be agreed upon preoperatively so that adequate quantities of packed red blood cells will have been typed and crossmatched. Decreases in hematocrit reading to the range of 21% to 25% will result in marked reduction in sinus venous rhythm due to vasodilatation and necessitate a compensatory increase in heart rate to maintain cardiac output and oxygen transport to the tissues. Thus, severe hemodilution may be deleterious to the patient with IHSS and those with a compromised myocardium secondary to ischemic coronary artery disease.

In the immediate period following cardiopulmonary bypass, even though adequate relief of the obstructive component of IHSS has been accomplished by myectomy, the hypertrophied ventricle remains noncompliant and the atria dilated. Supraventricular tachyarrhythmias slow junctional rhythm and varying degrees of heart block are not uncommon during this period. Surgeons may choose to place ventricular pacing wires to maintain adequate heart rate and cardiac output in patients with bradyarrhythmias and heart block. Since maintenance of atrial systole is necessary for adequate diastolic filling of the noncompliant ventricle(s), atrial or atrioventricular sequential pacing should be employed rather than ventricular pacing.

Paroxysmal supraventricular tachyarrhythmias are not uncommon during the immediate postoperative period in patients having coronary artery bypass graft in which cardiopulmonary bypass was employed. These arrhythmias are usually of the AV nodal reentrant type. Atrial pacing wires may be used for the following reasons:

1. To record an atrial electrogram for identification of the site of origin of the arrhythmia,

2. For temporary rapid atrial stimulation, which is usually effective in terminating an AV nodal reentrant tachycardia,

3. To decrease the degree of heart block and slow ventricular rate in patients with rapid atrial flutter.

If an atrial pacing wire was not placed during surgery, insertion of an esophageal ECG electrode in the intubated patient may be helpful in identifying the origin/etiology of the arrhythmia and choice of proper therapeutic intervention.

Verapamil has been shown to be useful in the treatment of patients with IHSS who have dysrhythmias that are refractory to multiple attempts at cardioversion/defibrillation and conventional pharmacologic agents during the immediate period following cardiopulmonary bypass. The side effects of hypotension need to be considered when using verapamil. The negative inotropic effect of verapamil combined with its ability to improve left ventricular compliance and therefore improve diastolic filling may offset the peripheral vasodilating effects in patients with IHSS.

Hypothermia should be avoided in the period following cardiopulmonary bypass. Hypothermia results in outpouring of catecholamines, shivering, increased production of carbon dioxide, and myocardial oxygen demands. Temperature should be measured at the nasopharyngeal or high esophageal area or by a temperature probe included in the urinary catheter (Foley catheter).

Choice of treatment of low cardiac output states and hypotension during the weaning from cardiopulmonary bypass and immediate postbypass period will depend upon the surgical procedure(s) performed.

If an adequate myectomy has relieved the outflow tract obstruction and filling volumes are adequate, small doses of inotropic agents may be tried to improve cardiac output. Since surgery does not correct the underlying disease process in IHSS, the clinician must be astute in monitoring the effect of any inotropic intervention. If inotropes are given via a central line and in dilute solution, they may be easily withdrawn from the tubing should hemodynamic deterioration occur subsequent to their use.

In patients who have not had a myectomy but only coronary artery bypass graft, positive inotropes, calcium chloride, and vasodilating agents such as nitroglycerine or nitroprusside should *not* be used to treat low cardiac output states. Titrated doses of phenylephrine and volume expansion should be the first-line treatment.

SUMMARY

There is no "one way" to manage patients with combined IHSS and ischemic coronary artery disease (CAD). Effects of anesthetic agents and pharmacologic and mechanical interventions need to be continuously monitored. A sound knowledge of the pathophysiologic process involved in IHSS and CAD is an absolute necessity for proper anesthetic management. Any given drug or technique may prove to be good at one time and bad at another. It is a series of bad choices that will get you and the patient into trouble, so know the odds before you place your bet, and you may never need to ask, "Why?"

Acknowledgment

I wish to thank Jill Belasco and Freda Cooper for their assistance in editing and preparation of this manuscript.

REFERENCES

1. Berger M, Rethy C, Goldberg E: Unsuspected hypertrophic subaortic stenosis in the elderly diagnosed by echocardiography. *Geriatr Soc* 1979; 27:178
2. Johnson RA, Haber E, Austen WG: *The Practice of Cardiology.* Boston, Little Brown & Co, 1980.
3. Starnes VA, Oyer PE, Miller C, et al: IHSS: Are there preoperative predictors of favorable outcome? *Circulation* 1985; 72 (suppl 3), Abstracts, No. 1782.
4. Duda AM, Gill CC, Kitazume H, et al: Surgical treatment of idiopathic subaortic stenosis with other cardiac pathology. *Cleve Clin Q* 1984; 51:27.
5. Silverman KJ, Hutchins GM, Weiss JL, et al: Catenoidal shape of the interventricular septum in idiopathic hypertrophic subaortic stenosis: Two dimensional echocardiographic confirmation. *Am J Cardiol* 1982; 49:27.
6. Spirito P, Maron BJ, Chiarella F, et al: Diastolic abnormalities in patients with hypertrophic cardiomyopathy: Relation to magnitude of left ventricular hypertrophy. *Circulation* 1985; 72:311.

7. Maron BJ, Epstein SE, Roberts WC: Hypertrophic cardiomyopathy and transmural infarction without significant atherosclerosis of the extramural coronary arteries. *Am J Cardiol* 1979; 43:1086.

8. Stewart S, Schreiner B: Coexisting idiopathic hypertrophic subaortic stenosis and coronary artery disease. *Thorac Cardiovasc Surg* 1981; 82:278.

9. Kerin NZ, Mori I, Edelstein J, et al: Evaluation of phentolamine as a provocative test for idiopathic subaortic stenosis. *Am Heart J* 1979; 97:204.

10. Gill CC, Duda AM, Kitazume H, et al: Idiopathic hypertrophic subaortic stenosis and coronary atherosclerosis. *J Thorac Cardiovasc Surg* 1982; 84:856.

11. Jeffery DL, Signorini W, Flemma RJ, et al: Left ventricular myotomy. *Chest* 1981; 80:550.

12. Frank MJ, Abdulla AM, Canedo MI, et al: Long term management of hypertrophic obstructive cardiomyopathy. *Am J Cardiol* 1978; 42:993.

13. Lown B, Temte JV, Reich P, et al: Basis for recurring ventricular fibrillation in the absence of coronary heart disease and its management. *N Eng J Med* 1976; 294:623.

14. Sobel BE, Dingell JV, Mock MB: *Electrophysiological Mechanisms Underlying Sudden Cardiac Death.* Mount Kisco, NY, Futura Publishing Co, 1982.

15. Bharati S, McAnulty JH, Lev M, et al: Idiopathic hypertrophic subaortic stenosis with split His bundle potentials, electrophysiologic and pathologic correlations. *Circulation* 1980; 62:1373.

16. Kaplan JA: *Cardiac Anesthesia.* New York, Grune & Stratton Co, 1979.

17. Reves JG, Karp RB, Buttner EE, et al: Neuronal and adrenomedullary catecholamine release in response to cardiopulmonary bypass in man. *Circulation* 1982; 66:49.

18. Edwards H, Mulder DG: Surgical management of subaortic stenosis. *Arch Surg* 1983; 118:79.

19. Braunwald E: *Heart Disease: A Textbook of Cardiovascular Medicine.* Philadelphia, WB Saunders Co, 1980.

23

Air Embolism and Subsequent Central Nervous System Dysfunction

A 44-year-old woman in otherwise good health had rheumatic mitral valve disease. Anesthesia was uncomplicated as was replacement of the mitral valve. After customary measures were used to eliminate air from the heart, cardiopulmonary bypass was discontinued without difficulty; however, air was seen in the aortic cannula after termination of cardiopulmonary bypass. In the intensive care unit the patient's emergence from anesthesia was slow during the next several hours. Upon full emergence the next day, the patient had left-sided paresis of the upper arm that ultimately resolved over the ensuing five weeks.

Recommendations by Nancy A. Nussmeier, M.D., and John P. McDermott, M.D.

ANALYSIS OF THE PROBLEM

Numerous studies suggest that intraoperative macroembolic events, including air and/or particulate emboli, are a major cause of postoperative focal neurologic deficits.[1-5] The risk of macroembolism of air is obviously greater in operations requiring opening of a cardiac chamber (valve replacement or repair, ventricular aneurysm resection, or closure of a septal defect) compared to coronary artery bypass grafting (CABG).[1, 5-8] Macroembolism of particulate debris from the surgical field, including calcium fragments, valve vegetations or intraventricular thrombus, also is more common during intracardiac surgery. However, some risk of embolism is also present in extracardiac operations (CABG), in which air or atherosclerotic debris may arise from the cannulated aorta and pass to the cerebral vessels.[1] Venting of the left atrium during CABG, still performed by some cardiac surgeons, may increase the likelihood of air embolization.[9] In any cardiac operation, macroembolization is most likely during aortic cannulation prior to initiation of cardiopulmonary bypass, and during the initial cardiac ejections on weaning from bypass, because the heart is not excluded from the circulation by the aortic cross clamp during these periods.[1, 2, 10]

The observation that the right cerebral hemisphere is more frequently involved in postoperative focal neurologic deficits supports the view that embolism from the surgical field causes such deficits.[1, 4] Thus, emboli pass up the first great vessel arising from the aorta, the right brachiocephalic (innominate) artery, causing unilateral focal ischemic injury. It is important to distinguish embolization from the surgical field from other sources of air or particulate matter, e.g., gaseous microemboli from the oxygenator, or platelet aggregates, fat and fibrin traveling via the cardiotomy suction. Microfilters in the arterial line and cardiotomy return would reduce air and particulate emboli from such sources, but they would have little impact on embolization directly from the surgical field. It is also important to distinguish focal neurologic deficits due to macroembolism from subtle and often transient changes in intellectual function that may be due to diffuse microembolism.[11] Finally, a rare cause of severe neurologic injury or death is massive air embolism resulting from technical accidents such as depletion of the oxygenator reservoir, line disconnection, runaway pump heads, or reversed connections to vent tubing. The causes, prevention, and management of massive air embolism due to perfusion accidents are reviewed elsewhere.[12, 13]

APPROACH TO THE PROBLEM

The approach to the problem should be considered in these ways:

Prevention

Prevention of air and particulate emboli from the aorta and cardiac chambers depends primarily upon fastidious surgical technique.[6, 12] Careful assessment of the aorta before cannulation and before clamping is imperative in order to avoid manipulation of areas of the aorta from which atheromatous debris may be dislodged. All air must be eliminated from the aortic cannula, which is primed with fluid from the cardiopulmonary bypass circuit. The attentive anesthesiologist will examine this cannula just before insertion, and inform the surgeon of any residual air bubbles. Following initiation of cardiopulmonary bypass, the ascending aorta is routinely clamped before opening any chamber of the heart, thereby excluding air from the circulation. Cardiac contractions are then eliminated by arresting the heart with cold cardioplegia solution, or by inducing ventricular fibrillation. During intracardiac repair, surgical vigilance is required to ensure removal of all tiny fragments of valve tissue, calcific debris, atherosclerotic plaque, etc. from the field. Following completion of the repair, air must be conscientiously eliminated, especially from the left side of the heart. This should be completed before termination of bypass, and before the first ventricular ejections.

The precise ritual or sequence used to evacuate air may vary substantially from hospital to hospital. However, several specific sites of entrapment must be addressed. Air is flushed from the pulmonary veins into the left atrium by vigorous lung inflations, often accompanied by tilting of the operating table from side to side. The left atrial vent is then removed and the site closed under a level of blood so that no air can be entrained. Before release of the aortic cross-clamp, the patient is placed in a steep Trendelenburg position. Many surgeons then further evacuate trapped air by elevating the left ventricle and inserting a large needle through its apex. Air is flushed through this apical needle by manual massage of the heart, accompanied by inflation of the lungs or impedance of venous return in order to fill the heart with blood. Simultaneously, a slotted needle attached to a suction vent is placed into the ascending aorta at its highest point, thus evacuating any residual aortic air. The patient should be in a head-down position and the pulmonary veins, left atrium, left ventricle, and aorta thoroughly evacuated of air when the cross-clamp is released. The aortic cannula and the epicardial coronary arteries should then be inspected carefully for the presence of air. If the aortic cannula does manifest bubbles, they should be evacuated with a fine needle, and the aorta and left ventricle should again be probed for air. Some clinicians prefer to keep the patient in Trendelenburg position for at least five to ten minutes after release of the cross-clamp because this keeps the carotid arteries in the most dependent position. Ejected residual air is thus likely to traverse the inside of the aortic arch rather than the carotid arteries, thereby avoiding embolism to the brain. [14]

Detection

Despite conscientious attempts to eliminate air and particulate matter from the heart, macroembolic events may still occur. [5-7] Intracardiac air can be trapped in atrial, ventricular, or aortic cul-de-sacs (such as the left atrial appendage or left ventricular trabeculae) and remain trapped, even though the heart is beating and cardiopulmonary bypass has terminated. Eventual embolization may occur at any time during the post-bypass period. The anesthesiologist can significantly influence the outcome by employing methods to detect and treat air emboli. The usual method of detection is direct observation of air in the aortic cannula or coronary grafts. Use of a Doppler ultrasonic flowmeter secured on the right brachiocephalic or carotid artery to detect air emboli has also been reported.[6, 10, 15] When bubbles are observed with Doppler monitoring, maneuvers to remove air should be reinstituted. In patients undergoing intracardiac operations, neurologic sequelae were reduced (compared to a historical control group) when repetitive surgical attempts to evacuate air were combined with Doppler technology to monitor embolization.[6]

Most recently, echocardiography has been used to detect air retained in cardiac chambers after cardiopulmonary bypass. The threshold dose of air detectable by transesophageal echocardiography (TEE) in the right side of the heart in dogs is 0.02 ml/kg, and in the left ventricle, 0.001 ml/kg.[16] Using M-Mode TEE in humans, Oka et al.[5] reported a remarkably high incidence of air emboli after completion of standard air evacuation maneuvers. Air emboli were detected in 79% of patients (n = 15) undergoing intracardiac procedures, and in 11% (n = 18) of patients undergoing CABG. Central nervous system dysfunction occurred in 23% of the patients with air emboli, and in none of those without air emboli. Although quantification of the amount of air embolized is not possible using TEE, qualitative estimates of embolization may be clinically useful.[5] In addition, recurrent showers of air emboli may be prevented by repeating maneuvers to evacuate air from the heart when indicated by TEE. Transesophageal monitoring is not the only approach to intraoperative echocardiographic detection of intracardiac air. Several investigators have used a sterile, hand-held phased-array transducer applied directly to the heart.[7, 17]

There are also indirect methods of detection of emboli. Clinical manifestations of coronary arterial embolism (such as ST-segment elevation, ventricular arrhythmias, or poor ventricular contraction) suggest that emboli may also travel to the heart. When intraoperative monitoring includes the mass spectrometer, air emboli originating from the right side of the heart are detectable by a sudden decrease in end tidal carbon dioxide and increase in end tidal nitrogen. If the right and left sides of the heart are communicating at any time during a procedure, e.g., during closure of a septal defect, air emboli may also originate from the left ventricle.

The presence of cerebral ischemia during and after macroembolism may be detected on an intraoperative electroencephalogram (EEG). Air embolism may manifest as flattening of the EEG waveform, with diminished high-frequency and increased low-frequency activity.[14, 18] Monitoring the EEG bilaterally may increase the chance of detecting hemispheric focal ischemia resulting from gaseous or particulate emboli. Asymmetric EEG depression, particularly of the right cerebral hemisphere, would suggest this diagnosis. Duration of ischemia on the EEG may be predictive of a postoperative cerebral deficit.[18, 19] Seizure activity, apparently indicating an acute ischemic episode, also may correlate with cerebral air embolism.[20] However, even dramatic changes on the EEG do not necessarily represent cerebral ischemia. For example, a flat or isoelectric EEG can occur in the presence of severe ischemia, hypothermia, high doses of barbiturates, or high concentrations of isoflurane. Thus, an abnormal intraoperative EEG may not be predictive of postoperative cerebral deficit. Unfortunately, the converse may also be true; a normal intraoperative EEG may not preclude postoperative neurologic deficit.

Treatment

The clinician should be attentive to the risk of macroembolic events during all intracardiac operations, even when there is no immediate direct or indirect evidence of emboli. As discussed, the surgeon should thoroughly evacuate air from the heart before permitting ejection. The use of nitrous oxide should be avoided during and after cardiopulmonary bypass because it would dramatically expand any retained air bubbles. Carotid compression during the initial cardiac ejections, when embolization is most likely to occur, may be of benefit; however, this technique incurs the risk of reducing cerebral blood flow.

An alternative approach to the problem of embolization is to provide cerebral protection against the resultant neuropsychiatric sequelae. Hypothermia is the classic form of protection used during cardiopulmonary bypass, in an attempt to prevent postoperative sequelae by reducing cerebral oxygen consumption. However, hypothermia is induced after initiation of bypass and reversed before the first attempt to terminate bypass. Embolization from the heart is unlikely during the hypothermic period, because the heart is excluded from the circulation by the aortic cross-clamp. During the periods of highest risk, aortic cannulation and weaning from bypass, the brain is invariably normothermic. Thus, hypothermia cannot provide cerebral protection during these vulnerable periods.

Pharmacologic protection of the brain during periods of risk may be a more viable option. Large doses of barbiturates in animals decrease the neurologic deficit and mortality from cerebral infarction induced by interruption of the middle cerebral artery.[21-23] The decrease in morbidity and mortality is associated with a measurable reduction in infarct size, which is attributable to a barbiturate-induced reduction of cerebral oxygen uptake in the area of ''relative vulnerability'' surrounding the infarct.[21-23] This form of protection can be demonstrated only when the barbiturate is administered before, during, or very shortly after the ischemic event.[24, 25] The maximum protective effect occurs at doses that abolish cortical electrical activity and result in a flat EEG.[26, 27]

In a recent study, a barbiturate provided cerebral protection in patients undergoing intracardiac surgery.[2] Eighty-nine patients were randomly assigned to receive sufficient thiopental to maintain EEG silence throughout the period of risk for embolic events. Approximately ten minutes prior to cannulation of the aorta, thiopental was administered to patients in the thiopental group in 50-to

100-mg increments until the EEG became isoelectric. Thiopental was then administered by continuous infusion, beginning at a rate of 500 μg/kg/minute. The rate of infusion was adjusted to maintain a burst suppression pattern having more than 60 seconds between bursts throughout the period of cannulation, cardiopulmonary bypass, and weaning from bypass. Thiopental administration terminated when cardiopulmonary bypass was discontinued. These patients received an average of 39.5 mg/kg of thiopental. Ninety-three control patients, also undergoing open-ventricle surgery, received only fentanyl, 20 to 40 μg/kg, during the same period.

On the first postoperative day, five (5.6%) patients who received thiopental and eight control (8.6%) patients exhibited clinical neuropsychiatric abnormalities. By the tenth postoperative day, all neuropsychiatric dysfunction had resolved in the group that had received thiopental, but persisted in seven (7.5%) of the eight patients in the control group. Thus, pretreatment with thiopental significantly lowered the incidence of persistent neuropsychiatric complications. Nussmeier et al. noted that the overall incidence of transient neuropsychiatric sequelae did not differ between the thiopental and control groups in this study. This result is consistent with the theory that barbiturate therapy does not decrease the frequency of embolization, but rather reduces its clinical expression, presumably by reducing the size of the resulting infarct. This is precisely the same phenomenon seen in animal models of barbiturate protection.

Cerebral protection with thiopental was not entirely benign. [2] Although all patients who received thiopental were successfully weaned from cardiopulmonary bypass, they required more frequent inotropic support than the control group. In addition, the large doses of thiopental led to longer sleeping times, delayed tracheal extubation, and obviously increased sedation during the first three postoperative days. These side effects were not considered prohibitive; however, the authors of the study suggested that other agents with less cardiac effects and duration of action should be examined under the same clinical circumstances. Other data reported in this study support the view that embolism is the most important cause of sensorimotor neurologic dysfunction following cardiopulmonary bypass. The authors found that the incidence of complications was significantly related to aortic valve replacement and to heavy calcification of replaced valves.

DISCUSSION

Neurologic complications are common following open-ventricle surgery. These complications are often caused by macroembolic events that produce focal ischemic injury. Prevention of embolization is critical, but even the most careful and repetitive evacuation of intracardiac air and particulate matter may not be adequate. Echocardiographic detection of intracardiac air and electroencephalographic detection of cerebral ischemia are possible; however, the clinical benefits of these technologies are not yet clearly demonstrated. Hypothermia as a form of cerebral protection is not present at the times when embolization is most likely to occur. Pharmacologic intervention is therefore the only means of cerebral protection available, and barbiturate adminstration the only therapy supported by both experimental and clinical studies. Patients undergoing intracardiac surgery may therefore benefit from thiopental adminstration before and during periods in which macroembolism is likely to occur. Experimental evidence suggests that treatment with thiopental might also be successful when initiated immediately after a suspected macroembolic event. [26, 27] Other drugs may provide cerebral protection by depressing the cerebral metabolic rate (isoflurane, etomidate, midazolam), by improving cerebral blood flow and reducing cerebral edema (mannitol, steroids), or by exercising calcium entry blocking properties (nimodipine). However, these drugs have not been studied in any human model of cerebral ischemia and therefore cannot be recommended at this time.

REFERENCES

1. Slogoff S, Girgis KZ, Keats AS: Etiologic factors in neuropsychiatric complications associated with cardiopulmonary bypass. *Anesth Analg* 1982; 61:903–911.
2. Nussmeier N, Arlund C, Slogoff S: Neuropsychiatric complications after cardiopulmonary bypass: Cerebral protection by a barbiturate. *Anesthesiology* 1986; 64:165–170.
3. Aberg T, Ronquist G, Tyden H, et al: Adverse effects on the brain in cardiac operations as assessed by biochemical, psychometric and radiologic methods. *J Thorac Cardiovasc Surg* 1984; 87:99–105.
4. Sotaniemi KA: Brain damage and neurological outcome after open-heart surgery. *J Neurol Neurosurg Psychiatry* 1980; 43:127–135.
5. Oka Y, Moriwaki KM, Hong Y, et al: Detection of air emboli in the left heart by M-mode transesophageal echocardiography following cardiopulmonary bypass. *Anesthesiology* 1985; 63:109–113.
6. Lawrence GH, McKay HA, Sherensky RT: Effective measures in the prevention of intraoperative aeroembolus. *J Thorac Cardiovasc Surg* 1971; 62:731–735.
7. Rodigas PC, Meyer FJ, Haasler GB, et al: Intraoperative 2- dimensional echocardiography: Ejection of microbubbles from the left ventricle after cardiac surgery. *Am J Cardiol* 1982; 50:1130–1132.
8. Nicks R: Arterial air embolism. *Thorax* 1967; 22:320–326.
9. Hughes D: Air embolism during cardiopulmonary bypass. *J Thorac Cardiovasc Surg* 1981; 82:639.
10. Krebber HJ, Hanrath P, Janzen R, et al: Gas emboli during open heart surgery. *Thorac Cardiovasc Surg* 1982; 30:401–404.

11. Taylor KM: Brain damage during open-heart surgery. *Thorax* 1982; 37:873–876.

12. Mills NL, Ochsner JL: Massive air embolism during cardiopulmonary bypass: Causes, prevention, and management. *J Thorac Cardiovasc Surg* 1980; 80:708–717.

13. Stoney WS, Alford WC, Burrus GR, et al: Air embolism and other accidents using pump oxygenators. *Ann Thorac Surg* 1980; 29:336–340.

14. Gomes OM, Pereira SN, Castagna RC, et al: The importance of the different sites of air injection in the tolerance of arterial air embolism. *J Thorac Cardiovasc Surg* 1973; 65:563–568.

15. Gallagher EG, Pearson DT: Ultrasonic identification of sources of gaseous microemboli during open heart surgery. *Thorax* 1973; 28:295–305.

16. Furuya H, Suzuki T, Okumura F, et al: Detection of air embolism by transesophageal echocardiography. *Anesthesiology* 1983; 58:124–129.

17. Duff HJ, Buda AJ, Kramer R, et al: Detection of entrapped intracardiac air with intraoperative echocardiography. *Am J Cardiol* 1980; 46:255–260.

18. Fritz H, Hossmann KA: Arterial air embolism in the cat brain. *Stroke* 1979; 10:581–589.

19. Rampil IJ, Holzer JA, Quest DO, et al: Prognostic value of computerized EEG analysis during carotid endarterectomy. *Anesth Analg* 1983; 62:186–192.

20. Stockard J, Calanchini P, Bickford R, et al: Electroencephalographic seizures during cardiopulmonary bypass. *J Neurol Neurosurg Psychiatry* 1974; 37:181–190.

21. Corkill G, Sivalingam S, Reitan JA et al: Dose dependency of the post-insult protective effect of pentobarbital in the canine experimental stroke model. *Stroke* 1978; 9:10–12.

22. Michenfelder JD, Milde JH, Sundt TM Jr: Cerebral protection by barbiturate anesthesia: Use after middle cerebral artery occlusion in Java monkeys. *Arch Neurol* 1976; 33:345–350.

23. Smith AL, Hoff JT, Nielsen SL, et al: Barbiturate protection in acute focal cerebral ischemia. *Stroke* 1974; 5:1–7.

24. Corkill G, Chikovani OK, McLeish I: Timing of pentobarbital administration for brain protection in experimental stroke. *Surg Neurol* 1976; 5:147–149.

25. Selman WR, Spetzler RF, Roski RA, et al: Barbiturate coma in focal cerebral ischemia: Relationship of protection to timing of therapy. *J Neurosurg* 1982; 56:685–690.

26. Michenfelder JD: The interdependency of cerebral functional and metabolic effects following massive doses of thiopental in the dog. *Anesthesiology* 1974; 41:231–236.

27. Kassell NF, Hitchon PW, Gerk MK, et al: Alterations in cerebral blood flow, oxygen metabolism and electrical activity produced by high dose sodium thiopental. *Neurosurgery* 1980; 7:598–603.

24

Bradycardia With Aortic Insufficiency: Indication for Pacing Swan-Ganz Catheter

A 70-year-old man with a long-standing history of hypertension and aortic valve insufficiency was scheduled for aortic valve replacement. He had periods of brady-cardia (40 to 50) documented on his hospital ECG. The anesthesiologist was con-sulted by the surgeon regarding the advisability of placing a pacing Swan-Ganz catheter as part of the perioperative management.

Recommendations by Kenneth D. Hall, M.D.

ANALYSIS OF THE PROBLEM

Bradycardia in a patient with aortic insufficiency may be disastrous.[1] During systole, blood may be injected from the left ventricle into the aorta in a normal fashion if no significant stenosis exists. In diastole, however, blood will rush back through the incompetent valve into the left ventricle, causing a profound and precipitous decrease in aortic root pressure. Therefore, coronary blood flow, which depends primarily upon mean diastolic aortic root pressure and coronary artery resistance, may be decreased, causing seriously compromised perfusion of the left ventricular myocardium. The Venturi effect of regurgitant blood may further decrease coronary blood flow.[2, 3] If the patient has concomi-tant coronary artery disease, the condition is even worse and severe myocardial ischemia may result. The slower the heart rate, the longer the diastolic time, and, due to the regurgitant flow, the greater the drop in mean diastolic pressure that then becomes rate dependent.

APPROACH TO THE PROBLEM

Pacing Pulmonary Artery Catheter

Although vagal blocking agents, such as atropine, in large doses (0.4 to 2 mg) may increase heart rate in β-blocked patients, they are uncertain, limited in degree, and transient. A much more dependable methodology is to place a pacing pulmonary artery (Swan-Ganz) catheter prior to anesthesia. A pulmonary artery catheter probably will be a part of the monitoring plan for the patient with valve surgery anyway and adding the pacing modality is very little extra trouble. These perform well and the rate can be adjusted moment-to-moment, providing precise control of heart rate independent of inotropic drug therapy. By 1985, about 20,000 pacing catheters were in use annually.[4] Atrial, ventricular, and atrioventricular (AV) sequential pacing was achieved in nearly 90% of patients in one series (65 patients).[5] Atrial pacing (and with second-or third-degree heart block, AV sequential pacing) resulted in better cardiac outputs than ventricular pacing.[6] As consultant in this case, the anesthesiologist should advise placement of a pacing catheter. The catheter should be placed in the awake patient before anesthesia, sedation, AM β-blockers, or other rate slowing agents are given. After successful pacing capability is achieved, intravenous anesthetics and β-blockers, if needed, can be administered safely. The case may then proceed as usual for valve surgery.

Anesthetic Management

Light premedication with supplemental oxygen and particular avoidance of bradycardiac drugs during preparation will prevent hypoxia in a possibly already compromised myocardium. Marked vasodilation should be avoided, as a reduction in systemic vascular resistance will worsen the already low mean diastolic perfusion pressure in the coronary arteries. In patients with aortic insufficiency accompanied by ventricular dysfunction, however, prudent use of venodilators (prazosin) for preload reduction or arteriole dilators (nifedipine) for afterload reduction has been shown to be beneficial.[7, 8] Avoidance of halothane, enflurane, isoflurane, and thiopental and the use of fentanyl rather than morphine might be preferable for the same reasons. With a nitrous oxide/narcotic technique, however, the systemic vascular resistance and pulmonary vascular resistance may increase sharply with surgical stimulation; judicious doses of sodium nitroprusside may be necessary to return these resistances to preincision levels (but no lower) in order to maintain an adequate forward cardiac output. The intra-aortic balloon pump cannot be used in patients with aortic insufficiency until after the valve is replaced, as it will only increase the regurgitant fraction and further stress an already compromised left ventricle. After valve replacement, vasodilators may be necessary to protect against hypertension and subsequent disruption of the new valve leaflets or suture line. The management from this point on becomes that of the patient with potential or actual left ventricular failure and pulmonary congestion but without the specific problems of regurgitant blood flow, and the intra-aortic balloon pump may now be used if needed.

DISCUSSION

Background

Aortic insufficiency is a fairly common disease with multiple etiologies and was responsible for about 1,500 deaths in the United States in 1970 (0.07% of all deaths).[9] Infectious diseases such as rheumatic fever and syphilis were among the leading causes of aortic insufficiency until about two decades ago when improvement in treatment of infectious processes reduced this incidence. Today metabolic, unrecognized congenital defects, and degenerative diseases have become the leading contenders.[10] Bicuspid aortic valves increase the likelihood of developing aortic insufficiency. Trauma is becoming another major factor.

Regardless of etiology, the most difficult problem in the treatment of aortic insufficiency is to decide when in the natural history of the disease aortic valve replacement should be considered. Too early a replacement may leave the patient exposed for many years to the hazards of an artificial valve, including thromboembolism, suture line disruption, and intrinsic valve mechanical failure. Heart failure and permanent myocardial damage occurs slowly in patients with aortic insufficiency (in contrast to those with aortic stenosis) and patients may be able to function adequately for many years without valve replacement.[2, 11] Unlike aortic stenosis, aortic insufficiency is rarely associated with syncope and sudden death.[3]

In asymptomatic patients less than 4% per year require valve surgery due to developing symptoms or ventricular dysfunction.[12] It is widely held, therefore, that the patient should be carefully observed for definitive signs of left ventricular failure or rapid progression of symptomatology before valve replacement is attempted.[13] Newer methods of more accurately defining early decreased ventricular function have included echocardiogram, preexercise and postexercise ejection fraction by radionuclide angiography, angiographic determinations of ventricular wall dimensions, and transesophageal echocardiography.[14–19]

Because of the remarkable 71% five-year survival probability with valve replacement patients aged 70 and over, the decision on when to operate may be easier in the elderly.[20]

Pathophysiology

Patients with aortic stenosis have pressure-overloaded left ventricles, whereas those with aortic insufficiency are volume overloaded. Blood flows backward into the left ventricle during diastole, increasing the left ventricular and diastolic volume, requiring a larger ejection on the next beat unless the heart fails. [21] The backward flow, or regurgitant fraction, depends upon the left ventricular compliance, peripheral vascular resistance, and heart rate. [22] If this regurgitant fraction is 60% or greater (considered a "severe" lesion), the backward flow may be 6L or more per minute and the left ventricle has to do that much extra nonproductive work. [23] Severe left ventricular hypertrophy results which increases the myocardial oxygen consumption, compromises coronary artery blood flow, and leads eventually to myocardial fibrosis and left ventricular failure.

Heart Rate

A relative tachycardia can, to a considerable degree, compensate and maintain a reasonable coronary blood flow, as well as probably decrease the regurgitant fraction. Some studies have shown a decrease in left ventricular end diastolic volume and stroke volume regurgitant fraction. However, due to the increased heart rate the minute volume regurgitant fraction is not significantly altered. [24] The normal awake patient does this reflexly and can tolerate exercise with its reflex tachycardia remarkably well in contrast to the patient with aortic stenosis. [25] In the patient who is heavily β-blocked (for coronary artery disease), and is anesthetized with rate-decreasing drugs such as fentanyl, efforts must be made to maintain a reasonable heart rate. Even patients who were atrially paced at rates up to 120 to 140 beats per minute showed no evidence of myocardial ischemia. In these patients, the decrease in diastolic coronary blood flow time was more than compensated for by the decrease in regurgitant fraction and increase in mean aortic root pressure due to the faster heart rate.

REFERENCES

1. Lowenstein E, Bland JHL: Anesthesia for cardiac surgery: Aortic valve disease. *Br J Haematol* 1970; 19:75–102.
2. Segal J, Harvey WP, Hufnagel C: A clinical study of one hundred cases of severe aortic insufficiency. *Am J Med* 1956; 21:200–210.
3. Goldschlager N, Pfeifer J, Cohn K, et al: The natural history of aortic regurgitation. *Am J Med* 1973; 54:577–588.

4. Gibberman R: Personal communication, American Edwards Laboratories, Santa Ana, Calif, 1985.
5. Zaidan JR, Freniere S: Use of a pacing pulmonary artery catheter during cardiac surgery. *Ann Thorac Surg* 1983; 35:633–636.
6. Zaidan JR, Waller JL, Lonergan JH: Hemodynamics of pacing after aortic valve replacement and coronary artery surgery. *Ann Thorac Surg* 1983; 36:69–72.
7. Jebavý P, Koudelková E, Henzlová M: Unloading effects of prazosin in patients with chronic aortic regurgitation. *Am Heart J* 1983; 105:567–574.
8. Shen WF, Roubin GS, Hirasawa K, et al: Noninvasive assessment of acute effects of nifedipine on rest and exercise hemodynamics and cardiac function in patients with aortic regurgitation. *J Am Coll Cardiol* 1984; 4:902–907.
9. Singer RB, Levinson L: Congenital and valvular heart disease, in *Medical Risks,* Lexington, Mass Lexington Books, 1976, pp 104–109.
10. Rahimtoola S: Valvular heart disease: The decision to treat. *Hosp Pract* 1984; 19:63–78.
11. Corrigan DJ: On permanent patency of the mouth of the aorta, or inadequacy of the aortic valves. *Edinburgh Med Surg J* 1832; 37:225–245.
12. Bonow RO, Rosing DR, McIntosh CL, et al: The natural history of asymptomatic patients with aortic regurgitation and normal left ventricular function. *Circulation* 1983; 68:509–517.
13. Bonow RO: Timing of operation for chronic aortic regurgitation: Influence of left ventricular function on clinical management. *Herz* 1984; 9:319–332.
14. Gaasch WH, Carroll JD, Levine HY, et al: Chronic aortic regurgitation: Prognostic value of left ventricular end-systolic dimension and end-diastolic radius/thickness ratio. *J Am Coll Cardiol* 1983; 1:775–782.
15. Huikuri HV, Ikäheimo MJ, Linnaluoto MK, et al: Value of isometric exercise testing in the optimal timing of aortic valve replacement in aortic regurgitation. *Eur Heart J* 1983; 4:632–638.
16. Bonow RO: *Aortic Regurgitation: Medical Assessment and Surgical Intervention.* Chicago, Year Book Medical Publishers Inc, 1983, pp 93–113.
17. Almeida P, Córdoba M, Javier G, et al: Relation of midwall circumferential systolic stress to equatorial midwall fibre shortening in chronic aortic regurgitation. *Br Heart J* 1984; 52:284–291.
18. Matsumoto M, Oka Y, Strom J, et al: Application of transesophageal echocardiography to continuous intraoperative monitoring of left ventricular performance. *Am J Cardiol* 1980; 46:95–105.
19. Schlüter M, Langenstein BA, Hanrath P, et al: Assessment of transesophageal pulsed Doppler echocardiography in the detection of mitral regurgitation. *Circulation* 1982; 66:784–789.
20. Glock Y, Pecoul R, Cerene A, et al: Aortic valve replacement in elderly patients. *J Cardiovasc Surg* 1984; 25:205–210.
21. Cowper W: Of ossifications or petrifactions in the coats of arteries, particularly in the valves of the great artery. *Philos Trans R Soc Lond* 1702; 23:1970–1977.
22. Schlant RC, Nutter DO: Heart failure in valvular heart disease. *Medicine (Baltimore)* 1971; 50:421–451.

23. Tyrrell MJ, Ellison RC, Hugenholtz PG, et al: Correlation of degree of left ventricular volume overload with clinical course in aortic and mitral regurgitation. *Br Heart J* 1970; 32:683–690.

24. Brawley RK, Morrow AG: Direct determinations of aortic blood flow in patients with aortic regurgitation. *Circulation* 1967; 35:32–45.

25. Judge TP, Kennedy JW, Bennett LJ, et al: Quantitative hemodynamic effects of heart rate in aortic regurgitation. Circulation 1971; 44:355–367.

25

Transverse Midventricular Rupture After Mitral Valve Replacement

A 65-year-old woman underwent mitral valve replacement for correction of long-standing mitral stenosis and heart failure. The induction, sternotomy, and bypass progressed well. The patient was weaned from cardiopulmonary bypass without major difficulty. About five minutes after bypass, the patient's hemodynamic status deteriorated with decreasing systemic and pulmonary arterial pressures, as well as decreasing cardiac output. Copious bright red blood filled the pericardium.

Recommendations by John H. Tinker, M.D., and Sandra L. Roberts, M.D.

ANALYSIS OF THE PROBLEM

Ventricular rupture is one of the most dreaded complications associated with mitral valve replacement (MVR). Fortunately it is also a rare occurrence. In the case above, it occurred five minutes following bypass. Unfortunately, at least in my experience (JHT), (n = 6), this was the case in only two. The other four patients suffered left ventricular ruptures either on their way to the intensive care unit (ICU) (n = 2) or during the first 12 (n = 1) to 24 (n = 1) hours after surgery. Of my six cases, only one patient survived the acute rupture, and that patient eventually succumbed in the intensive care unit to pulmonary complications.

APPROACH TO THE PROBLEM

First, think of the diagnosis when bright red blood appears—even if it is not (yet) copious—either at surgery or in the chest tubes postoperatively. The rupture, once it begins, will enlarge rapidly as the heart literally tears itself apart. Stopping all inotropes and emergency sternotomy must be done immediately. Repair requires bypass (see below).

If the rupture occurs while the heart is still cannulated for bypass, then a new dose of heparin must be remembered if protamine has been given and the patient placed back on bypass. This alone does *not* solve the problem. If the pump suction is providing most of the return to the pump oxygenator, a circuit may be established (especially if there is aortic valve incompetence due to surgical distortion) whereby there will be little or no systemic arterial pressure or blood flow except in the aorta itself. This must not be allowed to continue at normothermia or the patient will suffer irreversible brain damage. The surgeons must not spend a long time with the heart tilted anteriorly, using the pump suction, and, in essence, putting blood into the aorta (or the femoral artery) and taking it out of the pericardium. They must quickly clamp the aorta, cool the patient, and administer cold cardioplegia. Some surgeons are *not* aware of the fact that it is entirely possible, with the scenario described above, to have high pump flow with little or no arterial pressure and therefore little cerebral oxygen delivery. One of the patients in my "series" died as a result of a similar scenario despite efforts of a senior cardiac surgeon and even though the aortic cannula was fortuitously still in place.

Unfortunately, at least in my "series," a more likely scenario is that the chest will be already closed or, worse, that the patient will be somewhere else but in the operating room.

DISCUSSION

Pathophysiology of Ventricular Rupture After MVR

Surgical mitral valve disease was formerly nearly always rheumatic in origin. That is not to say that the pathophysiology of rheumatic mitral valve disease is understood, but the clinical features are well known. At present considerably more mitral operations (number unknown) are performed after posterior papillary muscle rupture/dysfunction or infarction renders the mitral valve relatively acutely insufficient. The origins of this process are nearly always ischemic rather than rheumatic. (Why the mitral valve should get tougher and tighter in the "rheumatic" process, vs. floppier in the other is food for thought!).

A very important point needs to be made about rheumatic-origin mitral (or other) valve disease. The disease is also *heart* disease. The ventricle is decidedly not normal. Mitral stenosis may have "protected" the gradually failing left ventricle from high filling pressures, but the "protection" does not stop the fundamental degenerative "rheumatic" process. Thus, patients with "long-standing" mitral stenosis nearly always have ventricular dysfunction. Also, again perhaps because of the aforementioned protection mitral stenosis affords against high ventricular filling pressures, these ventricles are *not* thick, are not usually hypertrophied.

As mitral stenosis progresses, the left atrium enlarges to potentially enormous size if the mitral valve is left untouched. The left atrium, of course, is really mostly posterior—and perhaps it is too simplistic a view to note—but it is of course attached to the left ventricle. Perhaps this affords a mechanical explanation why the posterior wall of the left ventricle in patients with large left atria *may* be exceedingly thin (as left ventricles go).

Experienced cardiac surgeons tell us that operating upon a ventricle that has been gradually failing for many years is fraught with real hazard. The tissue is friable; the cardiac "skeleton" is not firm; sutures do not hold well, and there is much calcification.

Summarizing the initial case, we have a patient with "long-standing" (years), presumably rheumatic (most occur in females) mitral stenosis, who was likely to have a greatly enlarged left atrium coupled to a poorly functioning, rheumatically "wheezing" left ventricle comprised of infirm tissue that was likely to be not very thick, especially posteriorly. By now, dear reader, you are saying, "Aha, for once we have a purely surgical complication—anesthesia is off the hook; this complication is due to improper placement of the mitral suture ring, or to excessive excision of the old mitral valve." No question, this *is* largely a surgical complication, but the anesthetist is not necessarily completely off the hook.

Preanesthetic Evaluation and Preparation

There is no sure way to predict even the likelihood of ventricular rupture after MVR—but we can, perhaps, identify those patients likely to be at highest risk. First, the size of the left atrium can be very roughly estimated by presence (how long?) of atrial fibrillation. Have there been embolic phenomena? If so, this usually means a larger left atrium. Next, we should work especially hard to ascertain degree of preoperative congestive failure. Left ventricular end diastolic pressure may be lower than would be present without a stenotic mitral valve interposed (of course this will yield a low output). Exercise tolerance is misleading also, because it seems that the high left atrial and pulmonary vascular pressures lead to "stiff" lungs and very early dyspnea, perhaps even before the relatively fixed, low cardiac output limits activity. What we are really saying here is that we have not been very successful preoperatively, in mitral stenosis patients, in predicting degree of post-bypass left ventricular dysfunction, using either clinical or catheterization data.

What about the patient who has *not* had "long-standing" mitral disease? Beware of these patients! While it is true that catheterization data does seem to give a better picture of ventricular function in these patients, a different problem enters the picture. Experienced cardiac anesthetists who have anesthetized many patients for valve replacements have *seen* many aortic valves, but seldom have they actually *seen* much of the mitral valve! The latter valve is difficult even for the surgeon to visualize. The larger the left atrium, in general, the easier it is for the surgeon to expose and operate upon the mitral valve. This is why a patient with recent acute ischemic mitral incompetence, who has a small left atrium, sends shivers up the experienced anesthetist's spine. The surgical assistant (who also seldom gets to see the mitral valve) must pull much harder on the mitral retractor to gain exposure when the left atrium is small, thus potentially exposing the heart to considerably greater trauma during the valve replacement itself.

In summary, *both* kinds of mitral replacements are potentially at risk. The rheumatic heart is thinner and more friable but exposure may be easier. The ischemic recently mitral-incompetent heart is thicker walled, but the posterior wall may be partly infarcted, and exposure can be exceedingly difficult. Preoperatively, these considerations should run through the anesthetist's mind during evaluation.

Preparation? Should digitalis be stopped or continued? Episodes of rapid atrial fibrillation may herald severe ventricular decompensation and thus provide a warning that this is a poor ventricle. Digitalis *must not be stopped* if it is clearly indicated for heart rate control in atrial fibrillation. When digitalis is given for acute relatively recent failure, again most anesthetists would continue it. When digitalis is present for no *recent* (weeks) reason, many advocate discontinuing it during the bed rest period (several days) that often accompanied the workup of these patients—at least in the days before DRGs. If this is done carefully, it is true that many "heart disease" patients taking digitalis can be weaned from it. Patients with severe mitral stenosis probably do *not* fall into this category. Our recommendation is to have a documented therapeutic digitalis blood level "aboard" for mitral valve replacement surgery.*

Anesthetic Management

We will only point out that which is relevant to mitral valve replacement in general and prevention of left ventricular (LV) rupture in particular. During the

---

*A major reason in the past for stopping digitalis was that toxicity was much more likely because there always seemed to be severe hypokalemia. Cardioplegia has ameliorated this problem, perhaps serendipitously.

prebypass period, trying hard to prevent increased LV failure virtually goes without saying. These patients have low cardiac outputs preoperatively and (at least with respect to brain, kidney, etc.) tolerate said low outputs relatively well. Measuring output carefully during this period is the only reliable way of getting an "under anesthesia" target to shoot for postbypass. Volatile agents are often poorly tolerated by these patients and it is here that the inherent fallacy of using a negative inotrope to control arterial pressure will be quickly impressed upon at least the thoughtful neophyte.

It is during the post-bypass and post-anesthesia period that we anesthetists can come in for our share of the blame for post MVR ventricular rupture. Slavish adherence to some "formula" for output, or arterial pressure, or LV preload, or peripheral vascular resistance can be contributory to disaster here. If the patient had been getting by with a cardiac index of 1.8 L/minute/m^2, then why push her higher? If her preoperative arterial pressures ran 80 to 90 mm Hg systolic, why push her beyond the cardiac anesthetist's magic 100 mm Hg mark?*

The patient in this case suffered ventricular rupture just a few minutes following separation from bypass. Was she being "whipped" by some "routine" formula usage of epinephrine or other inotrope? Was her preload pushed up to much higher levels than her "protected" ventricle had previously been "accustomed" to working against, in a misguided attempt to push her cardiac index above the magic 2.0 L/minute/m^2 mark? If so, did the increased preload exacerbate her failure, stretch further her already thin posterior ventricular wall, and perhaps result in increased exogenous catecholamine usage on top of it all? To be fair, there are plenty of *endogenous* catechols circulating at this juncture, and chronically failing hearts may be poorly responsive to catecholamines.

Let's summarize this part by saying that these patients do not need massive outputs to support other vital organ function and probably should not have their frail, thin-walled hearts excessively stretched or whipped.

What about those ruptures in JT's "series" that occurred after anesthesia, either in or on the way to the ICU? Were not those ruptures purely surgical complications? No again. If we simply turn off whatever anesthetics we are giving and transport the patients, we should not be surprised to find varying degrees of hyperdynamism and/or elevated preloads developing during transport. Hemodynamic control during transport and during the ICU stay is just as important in these patients as it was in the operating room. If these posterior wall sutures are going to tear through the ventricle, our surgical colleagues tell

*We are impressed by how many of us *say* absolute arterial pressure is not what is important —only O$_2$ delivery to tissues; yet in actual practice we feel uncomfortable till the actual pressure is over 100 mm Hg; never mind the cost in terms of oxygen demand.

us that the first 48 hours is critical, though 24 hours is the latest rupture in our "series."

Literature Review

Nili et al. in 1981 reported two cases and summarized the literature reports of 46 previously reported cases. The complication is rare: for example, two cases in the hospital of Nili et al.[1] over a 17-year period and 520 total cases of mitral replacement. The mortality is high, with the literature series (none large) averaging 65% ranging from 40% to 100%. These are all surgical reports. None specifically discusses the possible role that exogenous (or endogenous) catecholamines might have played, although Katske et al.[8] mention "transient hypertension" as a possible etiologic factor. Improper excision of the old valve, improper suture placement, or an improper alignment of the struts or the prosthesis are most commonly mentioned. Cobbs et al.[5] believe that too rapid emergence from bypass with ventricular distention may have played a role and consequently they recommend a 15- to 30-minute period of empty beating before trying to have the patient come off bypass. A reasonably complete review of the English language literature is provided.[1-14] Immediate sternotomy with manual posterior tamponade of the rupture is possible, but unlikely to be successful and should only be done by an experienced surgeon.

Should such a repair be effected, with multiple Teflon pledgets, etc., arterial pressure and cardiac filling pressure should be kept as low as compatible with vital organ function.

SUMMARY

Why spend so much time discussing an uncommon complication? First, it is a threat to any patient following MVR. Predicting which patients are at highest risk has not been possible, prospectively or retrospectively, for us. Second, it is an iatrogenic complication—any of which is high on our worry lists. Third, thinking about appropriately "gentle" postbypass management for mitral patients, plus the pathophysiology of mitral disease, plus the special features of preanesthetic evaluation was hopefully a useful excercise, particularly in this day when valve surgery constitutes such a diminishing portion of our practice.

Finally, where does the surgeon fit into all of this? Ventricular rupture after MVR is, assuredly, a surgical complication. Those posterior sutures must be placed with considerable expertise, at the proper location, depth, and tension. We have no intention of letting our surgical colleagues "off the hook" when one of these tragedies occurs, but we do believe that appropriately "gentle" postbypass and postoperative management of these patients is of value.

No "series" of these cases exists that could prove or disprove our contentions about either causation or management. Although that which seems logical today might prove ludicrous, dangerous, or both in the future, still in the absence of firmer guideposts, we find comfort in doing that which seems most logical.

REFERENCES

1. Nili M, Solomon J, Halevi A, et al: Left ventricular rupture after mitral valve replacement. *Scand J Thorac Cardiovasc Surg* 1981; 15:235–238.
2. Bortolotti U, Livi U, Mazzucco A, et al: Successful treatment of intraoperative rupture of the left ventricle after mitral valve replacement: Report of a case review of the literature. *Int Surg* 1981; 66:345–347.
3. Gosalbez F, de Linera FA, Cofino JL, et al: Isolated mitral valve replacement and ventricular rupture: Presentation of 6 patients. *Ann Thorac Surg* 1981; 31:105–110.
4. Bortolotti U, Thiene G, Casarotto D, et al: Left ventricular rupture following mitral valve replacement with a Hancock bioprosthesis. *Chest* 1980; 77:235–237.
5. Cobbs BW, Hatcher CR, Craver JM, et al: Transverse midventricular disruption after mitral valve replacement. *Am Heart J* 1980; 99:33–50.
6. Achatzy R, Dittrich H, Jelesijevic V, et al: Rupture of the ventricle following prosthetic replacement of the mitral valve. *Thorac Cardiovasc Surg* 1979; 27:48–50.
7. Nunez L, Gil-Aguado M, Cerron M, et al: Delayed rupture of the left ventricle after mitral valve replacement with bioprosthesis. *Ann Thorac Surg* 1979; 27:465–467.
8. Katske G, Golding L, Tubbs R, et al: Posterior midventricular rupture after mitral valve replacement. *Ann Thorac Surg* 1979; 27:130–132.
9. Bjork VO, Henze A, Rodriguez L: Left ventricular rupture as a complication of mitral valve replacement. Surgical experience with eight cases and a review of the literature. *J Thorac Cardiovasc Surg* 1977; 73:14–21.
10. Wolpowtiz A, Barnard MS, Sanchez HE, et al: Intraoperative posterior left ventricular wall rupture associated with mitral valve replacement. *Ann Thorac Surg* 1978; 25:551–554.
11. Sharratt GP, Ross JK, Monro JL, et al: Intraoperative left ventricular perforation with false aneurysm formation. *Br Heart J* 1976; 38:1154–1159.
12. Treasure RL, Ranier WG, Strevey TE, et al: Intraoperative left ventricular rupture associated with mitral valve replacement. *Chest* 1974; 66:511–514.
13. Zacharias A, Groves LK, Cheanvechai C, et al: Rupture of the posterior wall of the left ventricle after mitral valve replacement. *J Thorac Cardiovasc Surg* 1975; 69:259–263.
14. Roberts WC, Morrow AG: Causes of early postoperative death following cardiac valve replacement. *J Thorac Cardiovasc Surg* 1967; 54:422–437.

PART FOUR

Electrophysiologic Dysfunction

26

Paroxysmal Atrial Tachycardia in a Patient With Wolff-Parkinson-White Syndrome

A 24-year-old man with Wolff-Parkinson-White (WPW) syndrome was scheduled to have ablation surgery with intraoperative electrophysiologic mapping. Induction and sternotomy were uneventful, but immediately prior to mapping the patient developed paroxysmal atrial tachycardia with a rate of 250 beats per minute and blood pressure of 70/50 mm Hg.

Recommendations by Fiona M. Clements, M.D.

ANALYSIS OF THE PROBLEM

Wolff-Parkinson-White syndrome is a condition in which an accessory pathway or pathways connecting the atrium with the ventricle give rise to paroxysmal tachycardias. Such aberrant pathways are comprised of ordinary working myocardial tissue and are normally invisible to the naked eye. The arrhythmia associated with this condition is most frequently paroxysmal atrial tachycardia in which a reentry circuit is set up involving antegrade conduction from the atrium to the ventricle via the atrioventricular (AV) node and then retrograde conduction back to the atrium via the accessory pathway (Kent bundle). Such reciprocating tachycardias may sustain ventricular rates between 150 to 250 beats per minute and even higher. At rates of 250 beats per minute and above the risk of degeneration into atrial and ventricular fibrillation is markedly increased. Various authors report the incidence of atrial fibrillation in patients with WPW at 12% to 39%.[1]

Generally patients with WPW syndrome can be managed medically with antiarrhythmics, most frequently verapamil, disopyramide, quinidine, procainamide, propranolol, and, more recently, amiodarone. Selection of the most efficacious regimen usually requires thorough electrophysiologic evaluation to assess the effects of the various drugs on automaticity, refractoriness, and conduction in the reentry tachycardia circuit. Another approach to chronic management of these patients involves implantation of pacemakers, which may fire automatically during tachycardia, or may be patient-activated by means of a radio-frequency transmitter placed over the pacemaker. Pacing can terminate tachycardias by providing a stimulus to the reentry circuit when one limb of the circuit is refractory. In this way the circuit is interrupted and a normal sinus rhythm is reestablished.

A small fraction of patients with WPW are referred for surgical ablation of their accessory pathways. Since the initial report of successful surgical ablation in 1968, considerable experience has been gained and the indications for surgery now include: (1) patients with medically refractory reciprocating tachycardias; (2) patients with spontaneous atrial fibrillation who are at risk for sudden death; (3) patients with drug intolerance; and (4) young, otherwise healthy patients with symptoms that warrant more than minimal medical therapy.[2] In the Duke University series of 267 patients undergoing surgery for these indications, the mean age was 31 ± 27 years. A substantial number of these patients had associated abnormalities, including 19 patients with Ebstein's anomaly, and 12 with some mitral valve abnormality. The ablation of the accessory pathway(s), therefore, was often done in conjunction with some other corrective procedure, most frequently involving closure of an atrial-septal defect, tricuspid valve replacement, or mitral valve replacement. It is therefore emphasized that not all patients with WPW syndrome have otherwise normal hearts, and occasionally an unexpected anomaly, e.g., atrial-septal defect, may be discovered at the time of surgery. Furthermore, the morbidity and mortality of surgery were substantially affected by the presence of associated anomalies.[3]

By the time patients present for surgery, they are often extremely apprehensive, having endured a number of unpleasant experiences; multiple defibrillations are often recalled by many of them, and several lengthy electrophysiologic studies may have been performed. For many of them, anxiety has historically precipitated tachycardias. The heightened sympathetic activity associated with stress and anxiety has been observed to affect the susceptibility to develop and sustain tachycardia during electrophysiologic studies, and the administration of sedatives and general anesthesia, simply by diminishing sympathetic outflow, appears to make it more difficult to induce arrhythmias. The overall management of patients presenting for surgical ablation of their accessory pathways is significantly altered by the requirements of the surgeon. In order to locate the accessory pathway, after the chest is opened, intraoperative cardiac mapping will be performed with epicardial electrodes. At Duke University a hand-held probe electrode is moved over all areas of the heart to identify atrial and ventricular insertion sites of the pathway. Accurate mapping relies on specific electrophysiologic properties of the accessory pathway and the rest of the myocardium. For this reason, it is imperative that other conditions should not alter these properties. All antiarrhythmics are withdrawn at least five half-lives prior to surgery; the anesthesiologist is obviously prohibited from using similar drugs intraoperatively. It is worth noting specifically that blood levels of lidocaine following local infiltration for catheter placement can result in therapeutic levels 30 to 120 minutes after use. Nattel et al.[4] reported that patients achieved therapeutic plasma levels of lidocaine 40 minutes after tissue infiltration with approximately 4 mg/kg of lidocaine. This represents approximately 14 ml of 2% lidocaine. For patients undergoing surgery such blood levels would clearly persist during the mapping phase of surgery and even lower levels of lidocaine may interfere with conduction in the accessory pathway. Therefore, for the placement of arterial and central venous lines, it is wise to use procaine, 0.5% lidocaine, or preferably to insert them after induction of the anesthesia.

With the exception of antiarrhythmic therapy, other modalities of treatment for tachycardias are acceptable in patients undergoing ablative surgery. However, it is initially the goal to avoid dysrhythmia. To this end it is my practice to invest in a thorough and reassuring interview with the patient to allay anxieties as much as possible and to make use of a generous premedication incorporating a potent amnesic agent, e.g., lorazepam 0.06 to 0.08 mg/kg, so that in the event that defibrillation is necessary prior to induction, there will be no recall. Provided the patient is well sedated and comfortable, a radial arterial line is inserted with local anesthesia prior to surgery in addition to a peripheral intravenous line. Following induction of anesthesia, an internal jugular venous line is established with a 7.5 F introducer, for monitoring central venous pressure and for insertion of a pulmonary artery catheter for management after cardiopulmonary bypass. The use of a pulmonary artery catheter has been justified in the Duke series by the occurrence of low cardiac output following surgery in several patients. This accounted for almost every death in this series, which had an overall mortality of 4.1%, although when patients with additional cardiac abnormalities besides accessory pathways are excluded the mortality becomes 1.1%. It is important to be very careful to avoid touching the right atrium with the guide wire and dilator during placement of the central venous catheter. This avoids iatrogenic precipitation of tachycardia. Likewise, unless cardiovascular instability warrants placement of a pulmonary artery catheter prior to mapping, it is wise to avoid the chance of causing catheter-induced arrhythmias. If the accessory pathway is right-sided, i.e., connecting the right atrium to the right ventricle, it is specifically contraindicated to advance the pulmonary artery catheter prior to mapping since temporary ablation of a pathway has been observed to occur during electrophysiologic study when intra-atrial catheters may traumatize the pathway. Furthermore, the pulmonary artery catheter would be in the way of endocardial mapping of the right atrium, which is usually done in addition to epicardial mapping for right-sided pathways.

APPROACH TO THE PROBLEM

The tachycardia occurring immediately prior to mapping is most easily treated with immediate direct current (DC) cardioversion, since the heart has been exposed and sterile paddles are available; 20 to 30 joules are almost always effective in terminating the tachycardia. The occurrence of tachycardia at this stage is extremely common, since premature beats are frequently caused by the surgeon touching the heart with his hand or with a suction instrument. A ventricular heart rate of 250 beats per minute and above is almost always, as in this case, associated with hemodynamic compromise that mandates immediate therapy. In the event of failure to cardiovert, which would be extremely uncommon, the second step in this stiuation would be to institute cardiopulmonary bypass. Since mapping will include elicitation of tachycardia, and hemodynamic instability is anticipated, an aortic cannula will have already been placed; however, because of irritating the right atrium and interference with mapping of the right atrium, the venous cannula is not always placed prior to mapping but can easily be inserted without delay.

DISCUSSION

Not all tachycardias merit cardioversion. Indeed, during an operation of this kind, the need for several cardioversions may be anticipated, and, in order to avoid cumulative myocardial injury, it is appropriate to avoid cardioversion when possible. A working defibrillator should obviously be in the operating room at all times, equipped with both internal and external paddles. The ability to synchronize power discharge is obviously desirable. Vagal maneuvers may be tried when hemodynamic stability permits; carotid sinus massage will prolong AV nodal conduction and may sometimes terminate tachycardia. A reliable alternative to cardioversion is pacing. Introduction of a stimulus to the atrium at a time when one limb of the reentry circuit is refractory will interrupt the tachycardia. This can be achieved in several ways. Underdrive pacing, at a slow rate, will sooner or later result in a paced beat occurring at the appropriate time to interrupt the tachycardia. Overdrive pacing, at a rate 30 to 40 beats per minute faster than the tachycardia may do the same thing, or may entrain the atrium at the paced rate so that cessation of pacing is followed by resumption of normal rhythm. Finally, specialized pacing techniques, i.e., ramp pacing, burst pacing, can be employed by the electrophysiologist. When hemodynamic stability permits, pacing is the desirable alternative to cardioversion in the operating room setting. The electrophysiologist performing the mapping may be the appropriate person to terminate the tachycardia by using his equipment with epicardial electrodes. At Duke University an atrial and a ventricular electrode are sutured in place prior to mapping for the purposes of pacing and recording and are therefore available for tachycardia termination. Generally, pacing techniques are effective and can be tried once or twice before cardioversion when time allows. When epicardial electrodes are not available, endocardial or esophageal atrial electrodes may also be used. Sometimes the frequency of tachycardia occurrence, particularly in patients whose usual antiarrhythmics have been withdrawn, leads the electrophysiologist to leave a coronary sinus catheter in place following the preoperative electrophysiologic study. This quadripolar atrial catheter, brought out via the left subclavian vein, is then available during the preoperative phase and intraoperative time prior to sternotomy for use in case of tachycardia. Alternatively, the anesthesiologist may take the precaution of placing esophageal atrial electrodes in place following intubation. A variety of catheters designed for this purpose are commercially available and have been used in both awake and anesthetized patients. It is important to recognize, however, that effective pacing from the esophagus is feasible only with pulse durations of approximately 10 msec and above, and may require higher current amplitudes than are available with ordinary temporary pacemakers.[5] Therefore, either the electrophysiologist's equipment, which offers these capabilities, or a suitable specialized pacemaker must be available.

REFERENCES

1. Gallagher JJ, Pritchett El, Sealy WC, et al: The preexcitation syndromes. *Prog Cardiovasc Dis* 1978; 20:285–327.
2. Cox JL: The status of surgery for cardiac arrhythmias. *Circulation* 1985; 71:413–417.
3. Gallagher JJ, Sealy WC, Cox JL, et al: Results of surgery for pre-excitation caused by accessory atrioventricular pathways in 267 consecutive cases, in Josephson ME, Hein JJ, Wellens LC (eds): *Tachycardias: Mechanisms Diagnosis Treatment*. Philadelphia, Lea & Febiger, 1984, p. 259.
4. Nattel S, Rinkenberger RL, Lehrman LH, et al: Therapeutic blood lidocaine concentrations after local anesthesia for cardiac electrophysiologic studies. *N Engl J Med* 1979; 301:418–420.
5. Benson DW, Dunnigan A, Benditt DG, et al: Transesophageal cardiac pacing: History, application, technique. *Clin Prog Pacing Electrophysiol* 1984; 2:360–371.

27

Atrioventricular Block After Coronary Artery Bypass Grafting

A 50-year-old man underwent coronary artery bypass surgery. His induction, sternotomy, and bypass anesthetic courses were uneventful. The myocardial ischemic period (cross-clamp time) was two hours. During the cross-clamp period, rapid rises in myocardial temperatures required frequent infusions of hypothermic (4° C), hyperkalemic (30 mg/L) cardioplegia. With reperfusion of the heart, the rhythm indicated third-degree atrioventricular block.

Recommendations by Joannes H. Karis, M.D.

ANALYSIS OF THE PROBLEM

The decreased mortality following coronary artery bypass graft surgery (CABG) has been partially attributed to the advance of myocardial preservation. In spite of the improvement of the cardioplegic techniques, a high incidence of supraventricular arrhythmia and atrial-ventricular (AV) conduction blocks have been reported.[1-4] The incidence appears to have increased with the increasing numbers of grafts being placed and the concomitant increase in ischemic time required to make the anastomoses.

If the AV block is complete, cardiac output can be markedly decreased because of the lack of an "atrial kick." Skinner et al.[5] showed that just a prolongation of the timing between the atrial systole relative to the ventricular contraction can have serious hemodynamic consequences. This was clinically substantiated by Hartzler et al.[6] in patients following cardiac surgery with intact

1:1 conduction. These authors measured a mean increase of cardiac output of 18% in five patients by artificially shortening the AV interval through sequential pacing. Therefore, it must be concluded that damage to the atrial-ventricular conduction system resulting in AV block can markedly interfere with cardiac performance.

APPROACH TO THE PROBLEM

The prevention of the development of a third-degree AV conduction block should be considered. Preventive measures consist of (1) separate superior and inferior vena cava drainage; (2) use of a lower concentration of K^+ in the cardioplegic solution after initial cardioplegia is achieved with a high K^+ concentration; (3) maintaining the atrial temperature at a low level by the use of slush and/or a continuous flow of cold saline to the atrial wall, specifically the atrial septum. These measures are, however, time consuming and, to a certain degree, make the procedure technically more complex. Treatment of third-degree AV block is by pacing the atrium and ventricle via epicardial pacing electrodes with an AV sequential pacemaker. Fortunately, electrical pacing has become a reliable and easily used mode of treatment.[7] Ventricular pacing alone may be adequate but cardiac function will be supported (and in critical cases required) by sequential pacing. The optimal heart rate and optimal AV interval must be chosen on an individual basis as correlated with arterial pressure and cardiac output. A starting place is a heart rate of 80 beats per minute, with an AV interval of 150 msec. Frequently, conduction improves before the patient reaches the intensive care unit. If the natural heart rate is adequate to sustain acceptable hemodynamics, the pacer should be discontinued; alternatively, atrial pacing can be continued at the most appropriate rate for the particular patient.

DISCUSSION

In order to prevent changes in the atrial-ventricular conduction, we must have an understanding of the pathophysiology. Local trauma to the AV node or fibers of the conducting system are not uncommon following atrial-septal defect repairs. In patients operated on for CABG, there is no direct intracardiac manipulation and this etiology is unlikely. Ellis et al.[8] attributed the conduction system dysfunction to the repeated use of high K^+ (20 mEq/L) cardioplegic solutions. In a physical model Rosenfelt and Watson[9] showed that when venous return passed through the right side of the heart and then the left side, the mean septal temperature increased markedly (from 7° to 23° C). This illustrates that despite attempts to keep the heart cooled, the septal portion of the myocardium gradually rewarms. More recently Smith et al.[4] showed that while the aorta was still cross-clamped, the temperature of the atrial septum after an initial drop returned rapidly to the systemic perfusate temperature, which was significantly higher than the ventricular temperature. Atrial electrical and mechanical activity returned while the ventricle stayed quiescent. Since the atrial and AV nodal conducting system is most sensitive to ischemia (Bagdonas et al.[10]) and apparently least protected by the cold cardioplegia, Smith reasoned that ischemic injury was the major cause of the conduction disturbance. Perhaps damage to the conduction system in our case could have been prevented by excluding venous return to the right atrium by using a separate superior and inferior vena cava tube rather than a Sarns two-stage venous return cannula. Blood from the superior vena cava that is at or above perfusate temperature would then bypass the right atrium so that the atrial temperature would remain low. Hearse et al.[11] reported that augmented right atrial hypothermia also reduced the incidence of postbypass supraventricular arrhythmias. The fact that myocardial temperature in our patient kept rising rapidly indicated that the heart was not adequately isolated from its surrounding and/or that inadvertently more than an usual amount of the bypass perfusate was allowed to reach the heart.

REFERENCES

1. Michelson EL, Morganroth J, MacVaugh H: Postoperative arrhythmias after coronary artery and cardiac valvular surgery detected by long term electrocardiographic monitoring. *Am Heart J* 1979; 97:442–448.
2. Engelman RM, Rousou JH, Vertrees RA, et al: Safety of prolonged ischemic arrest using hypothermic cardioplegia. *J Thorac Cardiovasc Surg* 1980; 79:705–712.
3. O'Connell JB, Wallis D, Johnson SA, et al: Transient bundle branch block following use of hypothermic cardioplegia in coronary artery bypass surgery: High incidence without perioperative myocardial infarction. *Am Heart J* 1982; 103:85–91.
4. Smith PK, Buhrman WC, Levett JM, et al: Supraventricular conduction abnormalities following cardiac operations. *Thorac Cardiovasc Surg* 1983; 85:105–115.
5. Skinner NS, Mitchell JH, Wallace AG, et al: Hemodynamic effects of altering the timing of atrial systole. *Am J Physiol* 1963; 205:499–503.
6. Hartzler GO, Maloney JD, Curtis JJ, et al: Hemodynamic benefits of atrioventricular sequential pacing after cardiac surgery. *Am J Cardiol* 1977; 40:232–236.
7. Strickland RA, Reves JG: Uses of temporary pacemakers in the perioperative period. *Semin Anesthesia* 1983; 2:276–286.
8. Ellis RJ, Mavroudis C, Gardner C, et al: Relationship between atrioventricular arrhythmias and the concentration of K^+ ion in cardioplegic solution. *Thorac Cardiovasc Surg* 1980; 80:517–526.

9. Rosenfelt FL, Watson DA: Interference with local myocardial cooling by heat gain during aortic cross-clamping. *Ann Thorac Surg* 1979; 27:1:13–16.
10. Bagdonas AA, Stuckey JH, Piera J, et al: Effects of ischemia and hypoxia on the specialized conducting system of the canine heart. *Am Heart J* 1961; 61:206–281.
11. Hearse DJ, Braimbridge MV, Jynge P: *Protection of the Ischemic Myocardium: Cardioplegia*. New York, Raven Press, 1981.

PART FIVE

Ischemic Heart Disease

28

Mitral Insufficiency—Acute Rupture of the Papillary Muscle

A 50-year-old laborer without any significant medical history collapsed at work after complaining of chest pain. He had dyspnea, cyanosis, and was in shock. An ECG revealed acute infarction and emergency echocardiogram revealed a ruptured papillary muscle with mitral valve leaflet dysfunction. Because of worsening heart failure despite maximal medical management, including insertion of an intra-aortic balloon pump, vasodilator and inotropic drug therapy, emergency mitral valve replacement and coronary bypass operation were scheduled.

Recommendations by C. E. Henling, M.D.

ANALYSIS OF THE PROBLEM

This is a true cardiac emergency. Patients with acute myocardial infarction complicated by mitral valve incompetence from papillary muscle rupture are at risk of sudden deterioration and death.

APPROACH TO THE PROBLEM

This critically ill patient is best managed by institution of cardiopulmonary bypass and operative repair. The role of the anesthesiologist is to provide optimal conditions for safe and expeditious operation. In addition to the usual preoperative assessment, the anesthesiologist should note the medical support the patient is receiving and his hemodynamic response. The infusions and monitoring devices required should then be readied in the operating room to facilitate transfer. Monitoring should include electrocardiography to detect both arrhythmias and myocardial ischemia, an arterial line for continuous measurement of systemic pressure, and catheters for measuring filling pressures and cardiac output. Most likely a Swan-Ganz catheter has already been placed by the cardiologist for diagnostic and monitoring purposes. If not, and if provision can be made for expeditious placement in the operating room, this should be done, because measurement of cardiac output and systemic resistance is required for optimal management. However, operation should not be unnecessarily delayed in the hemodynamically compromised patient. A pulmonary artery thermistor or left atrial line can be placed intraoperatively or a Swan-Ganz catheter can be placed postoperatively.

When the patient arrives in the operating room, if he is not already intubated, he should be given oxygen by mask. Induction and intubation then should proceed with the usual precautions taken in patients with a full stomach. Suction should be readily available to clear edema fluid and secretions. Unless the patient is moribund, induction can usually be carried out with etomidate (0.2 to 0.3 mg/kg) and succinylcholine (1.5 to 2.0 mg/kg). Etomidate has less effect on myocardial function and systemic resistance than either thiopental or ketamine. After intubation, ventilation with 100% oxygen should be continued. Nitrous oxide is best avoided not only because of its potential to depress the circulation and increase pulmonary vascular resistance, but also because it limits the inspired oxygen concentration that can be used in this patient with impaired pulmonary function. Anesthesia can be maintained with carefully titrated doses of diazepam or midazolam for amnesia, fentanyl or sufentanil for analgesia, and pancuronium or vecuronium for muscle relaxation. These anesthetics do not depress the myocardium. Their combination may slightly decrease peripheral resistance[1] but will not blunt the vasoconstrictive response to surgical stimuli. Vasoconstriction will cause a fall in cardiac output and a worsening of pulmonary congestion, changes that will be missed if only the systemic arterial pressure is monitored. Treatment is increasing the infusion of vasodilator.[2] Potent inhalation agents should not be used because their depressant effect on the myocardium is greater than any benefit they may offer through sympathetic blockade or afterload reduction. Further anesthesia can be administered once the patient has been placed on cardiopulmonary bypass.

Operation consists of mitral valve replacement and, if possible, coronary artery bypass grafting. After the aortic cross-clamp is removed, intra-aortic balloon pumping should be resumed. Vasopressor or vasodilator support can then be added as indicated by the measurement of pressures, resistances, and output. Need for support will be determined primarily by the extent to which the myocardium has been injured by the infarction and further injured or salvaged by the operation.

DISCUSSION

Background

There are two mitral papillary muscles: the posteromedial, which receives its blood supply from the posterior descending coronary artery, and the anterolateral, which is supplied by the left anterior descending diagonal and by circumflex marginal coronary arteries. The papillary muscles are particularly vulnerable to ischemia. The vessels perfusing them are end arteries that must first traverse the entire thickness of the left ventricular wall and are exposed to the full magnitude of systolic pressures.

Mitral insufficiency will occur in 60% to 70% of patients with acute myocardial infarction.[3] However, it is usually transient and hemodynamically insignificant. Acute severe mitral insufficiency due to ischemic papillary muscle rupture is a rare complication. Incidence of patients dying with acute myocardial infarction is less than 1%.[4] Papillary muscle rupture most often occurs two to seven days after the infarction and may be complete or involve only one or several heads of the muscle.[5]

Pathophysiology

With the onset of mitral valvular insufficiency from papillary muscle rupture, left ventricular output suddenly becomes divided between forward flow into the high pressure aorta and retrograde flow into the lower pressure left atrium. An acute volume load is placed on the left ventricle, consisting of the usual pulmonary venous return plus the volume of blood that had been ejected into the left atrium during the previous systole. An acute pressure load is placed on the right ventricle. The limited ability of the left atrium to distend to accommodate the increased volume forces blood back into the pulmonary veins and causes acute pulmonary hypertension. The results are biventricular failure, a sharp decrease in effective (forward) cardiac output, and acute pulmonary edema.

The degree of hemodynamic deterioration depends upon the site of rupture and the extent to which myocardial function has been impaired by the infarction (Fig 28–1). In many cases the infarction is not large and circulatory collapse is almost wholly the result of disruption of the mitral valve rather than myocardial injury.[6, 7] However, untreated mitral insufficiency can extend myocardial damage and result in irreversible myocardial failure. Mitral insufficiency decreases left ventricular afterload, but increases preload, and reflexly increases heart rate and contractility. Myocardial oxygen demand increases at the same time that oxygen supply is further compromised by hypotension and hypoxemia.

PAPILLARY-MUSCLE RUPTURE

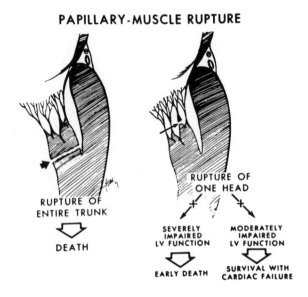

FIG 28–1.
The mitral valve leaflets are tethered by chordae tendineae to two papillary muscles. Rupture of a papillary muscle trunk disrupts the support of both leaflets, resulting in massive regurgitation and, without urgent repair, death. Rupture of one or several heads is more common, and outcome depends on both the extent of disruption and the extent of infarction. (From Roberts WC, Perloff JK: Mitral valvular disease: A clinicopathologic survey of the conditions causing the mitral valve to function abnormally. *Ann Intern Med* 1972; 77:939–975. Used by permission.)

Preoperative Assessment

As in this case, patients with papillary muscle rupture complicating acute myocardial infarction will often complain of chest pain at the time of rupture, rapidly followed by shock and pulmonary edema. A systolic murmur may be unimpressive or even absent if regurgitation is massive and left ventricular function poor. The differential diagnosis includes papillary muscle dysfunction and rupture of the ventricular septum. Diagnosis can be made by echocardiography and catheterization of the right side of the heart. Echocardiography will show a flail leaflet and allows assessment of left ventricular wall motion. Catheterization of the right side of the heart will demonstrate a large V wave in the pulmonary wedge tracing. Catheterization with a Swan-Ganz catheter carries little risk and is also extremely valuable in assessing the response to therapy. Although coronary angiography is useful in defining coronary anatomy, coronary bypass grafting can be performed empirically when the patient's hemodynamic condition precludes catheterization.

Perioperative Management

The goals of therapy in this patient are to restore normal hemodynamics and limit further myocardial injury. Medical treatment alone cannot restore valvular integrity but may improve his condition by increasing the ratio of forward to retrograde cardiac output and improving myocardial perfusion. Vasodilators, the intra-aortic balloon pump (IABP), and inotropic drugs were rational agents to use.

The ratio of forward to retrograde flow is determined by (1) the relationship between the aortic impedance and the compliance of the left atrium, and (2) the size of the regurgitant orifice. Arterial dilation will decrease aortic impedance by decreasing systemic vascular resistance, which is usually abnormally high due to reflex sympathetic activation. Forward flow will increase, improving systemic perfusion, and retrograde flow will decrease, reducing pulmonary congestion and ventricular size. Venodilation will further reduce pulmonary congestion and ventricular size. As the ventricle becomes smaller, so does the regurgitant orifice, limiting the area available for regurgitation.[8] Thus, dilators with equivalent effects on arteries and veins (sodium nitroprusside) may be more effective than drugs that are predominantly venodilators (furosemide, nitroglycerin) or arterial dilators (hydralazine). But, while vasodilators can be lifesaving, their effectiveness is limited by the development of systemic hypotension and worsening of myocardial ischemia. The IABP, by deflating in systole, will act like vasodilators to reduce aortic impedance and increase forward cardiac output. But the balloon, by inflating in diastole, will also improve myocardial perfusion and may improve myocardial function and survival.[9]

The use of vasodilators and the IABP may obviate the need for inotropic support. When inotropic agents are required, those that increase contractility without increasing systemic vascular resistance are the most logical choices. Examples are low-dose dopamine, dobutamine,and amrinone. But even agents with potent α-activity, such as epinephrine and norepinephrine, may so improve contractility that forward cardiac output increases. Undesirable vasoconstriction accompanying their inotropic effects can be mitigated by the use of vasodilators. Drugs that are pure vasoconstrictors should be avoided as they will only increase regurgitant flow. Inotropic agents will have a variable effect on myocardial oxygen balance because of their opposing effects to increase contractility, decrease ventricular size, and improve cardiac output.

When medical therapy is successful, operation might be postponed until after the acute phase of the infarction. However, further deterioration often occurs abruptly and without warning.[6, 7] When medical therapy is unsuccessful, as in this case, an urgent operation clearly offers the only hope of survival.

Outcome

The major cause of postoperative morbidity in patients with papillary muscle rupture is low cardiac output. The major causes of mortality are left ventricular failure and recurrent infarction.[6] Perioperative mortality is 30% to 50%,[6, 10] but compares favorably to an early mortality of 80% to 90% in patients who do not have operations.[11] Often the extent of infarction is not great, so that prognosis is good once the hemodynamic abnormality has been corrected.[4, 6, 7] Still, because of underlying coronary disease, long-term survival is not as great as in patients with mitral regurgitation of other etiologies.

REFERENCES

1. Tomicheck RC, Rosow CE, Philbin DM, et al: Diazepam-fentanyl interaction: Hemodynamic and hormonal effects in coronary artery surgery. *Anesth Analg* 1983; 62:881–884.
2. Stone JG, Faltas AN, Hoar PF: Sodium nitroprusside therapy for cardiac failure in anesthetized patients with valvular insufficiency. *Anesthesiology* 1978; 49:414–418.
3. Heikkila J: Mitral incompetence complicating acute myocardial infarction. *Acta Med Scand* 1969; 475(suppl):7–149.
4. Cederqvist L, Soderstrom J: Papillary muscle rupture in myocardial infarction. *Acta Med Scand* 1964; 176:287–292.
5. Wei JY, Hutchins GM, Bulkley BH: Papillary muscle rupture in fatal acute myocardial infarction. *Ann Intern Med* 1979; 90:149–153.
6. Nishimura RA, Schaff HV, Shub C, et al: Papillary muscle rupture complicating acute myocardial infarction: Analysis of 17 patients. *Am J Cardiol* 1983; 51:373–377.
7. Nunley DL, Starr A: Papillary muscle rupture complicating acute myocardial infarction: Treatment with mitral valve replacement and coronary bypass surgery. *Am J Surg* 1983; 145:574–577.
8. Yoran C, Yellin EL, Becker RM: Dynamic aspects of acute mitral regurgitation: Effects of ventricular volume, pressure and contractility on the effective regurgitant orifice area. *Circulation* 1979; 60:170–176.
9. Weiss AT, Engel S, Gotsman CJ, et al: Regional and global left ventricular function during intra-aortic balloon counterpulsation in patients with acute myocardial infarction shock. *Am Heart J* 1984; 108:249–254.
10. Clements SD, Story WE, Hurst JW, et al: Ruptured papillary muscle, a complication of myocardial infarction: Clinical presentation, diagnosis, and treatment. *Clin Cardiol* 1985; 8:93–103.
11. Sanders RJ, Neubuerger KT, Ravin A: Rupture of papillary muscles: Occurrence of rupture of the posterior muscle in posterior myocardial infarction. *Dis Chest* 1957; 31:316–323.

29

Pulmonary Shunting After Coronary Artery Bypass Surgery

A 50-year-old man operated on for correction of three vessel coronary artery disease had an uneventful induction and bypass. Immediately after coming off cardiopulmonary bypass, the PaO_2 dropped to 60, with inspired O_2 of 100%. The anesthesia machine, inspired oxygen, inflation of the lungs were all checked and found to be normal. The low PaO_2 persisted. Blood pressure at this time was 90/60mm Hg. The heart rate, central venous pressure (CVP), and pulmonary artery diastolic pressure (PAD) were normal.

Recommendations by Gerald Bushman, M.D.

ANALYSIS OF THE PROBLEM

Pulmonary dysfunction following cardiopulmonary bypass (CPB) has been recognized since the advent of extracorporeal circulation. Episodes of "pump-lung" syndrome have become far less frequent as the understanding of the physiologic and mechanical aspects of cardiopulmonary bypass has grown. However, when it occurs, pulmonary dysfunction following cardiopulmonary bypass remains a major contributor to postoperative morbidity. Etiologies of pulmonary complications are multifactorial and may relate to indigenous patient factors such as preexisting pulmonary disease; mechanical aspects of cardiopulmonary bypass such as inadequate left atrial venting resulting in pulmonary venous distention; or physiologic responses to cardiopulmonary bypass, as seen in the leukocyte sequestration injury typically observed in histologic sections of lung following cardiopulmonary bypass.

Hypoxemia in the cardiac patient following cardiopulmonary bypass must

229

be evaluated with respect to the usual and more common causes of hypoxia in the anesthetized patient as well as by analyzing the impact of cardiopulmonary bypass and cardiac surgery on the cardiorespiratory system of the patient with cardiac disease. A physiologic classification of the causes of hypoxia would include decreased inspired oxygen content, presence of an anatomical "shunt", the exacerbation of "physiologic" intrapulmonary shunt, or the creation of a diffusion barrier at the capillary level.

Decreased Fraction of Inspired Oxygen

Hypoxemia due to inadequate oxygen delivery to the patient's lungs is usually the result of mechanical malfunction of the anesthesia machine or circuit or due to failure in the oxygen supply system or its various connections. These mishaps can be minimized by meticulous preanesthetic checks of the anesthesia apparatus and oxygen supply system, and the appropriate use of such devices as oxygen and end-tidal CO_2 monitors, pulse oximetry, precordial and esophogeal stethoscopes, and, most importantly, continuous observation of the anesthetized patient.

Anatomical Shunt

In healthy adults, up to 3% of the cardiac output enters the left ventricle without having passed through the pulmonary capillary bed. The anatomical shunts normally consist of the bronchial and pleural circulations that arise from systemic circulation and drain into the left atrium via the pulmonary veins, and the thebesian vessels that originate from and empty into the left heart. In some diseases, this amount of shunted blood may increase. For example, bronchitis or pleuritis may increase shunt flow to 10% of the cardiac output. Portal hypertension may promote esophageal to mediastinal to bronchial to pulmonary vein pathways that contribute desaturated blood to the left atrium. Intrapulmonary arteriovenous connections, which are present and normally closed, may open in the face of acute pulmonary hypertension and increase the amount of anatomical shunt.

An unusual cause of anatomical shunt in adult patients following CPB is the presence of an intracardiac shunt that was previously unsuspected. Pathologic studies demonstrate that up to 25% of adults who have autopsies have a patent foramen ovale and thus a potential site for intracardiac shunting. Any physiologic situation that causes right atrial pressure to exceed left atrial pressure in the patient with an intracardiac communication may lead to right-to-left shunting with resulting arterial hypoxemia.

Right and left atrial pressures are determined by the compliances, contractility, and preloading of the atria and their respective ventricles. These factors are known to be altered following cardiopulmonary bypass (CPB) and cardiac surgery.

Many normal patients demonstrate an increase in pulmonary vascular resistance, right ventricular end diastolic pressure, and right ventricular end diastolic volume following cardiopulmonary bypass. The use of positive pressure ventilation and positive end expiratory pressure (PEEP) may significantly worsen these changes, further increasing the right atrial pressure. In patients with chronic obstructive pulmonary disease with right ventricular hypertrophy or strain, inadequate myocardial protection of the right ventricle during cardioplegic arrest may contribute to high right atrial pressures following CPB.

Patients undergoing aortic valve replacement for aortic insufficiency may have dilated, hypertrophied left ventricles that will generate adequate cardiac output with low left atrial pressure following valve replacement. After CPB, volume replacement may be easily accommodated by the left side of the heart with minimal increases in left atrial pressure, but may significantly increase right atrial pressure.

These examples of physiologic patterns have in common an increase in right atrial pressure relative to left atrial pressure after CPB and thus put the patient with a potential intracardiac shunt at risk for arterial desaturation.

Ultimately, verification of right-to-left shunting as the cause of hypoxemia requires either indicator dilution curves, echocardiography, or heart catheterization with measurements of oxygen saturations. The indicator dilution method allows discovery of shunts as small as 5% of systemic flow and may be done in the operating room or at the bedside. Commonly, an indicator dye is injected into central venous circulation while blood is withdrawn from a peripheral arterial catheter and monitored by a densitometer (Fig 29–1). Premature appearance of the indicator is seen in the left circulation when a right-to-left shunt is present. Shunts may be visualized at the atrial or ventricular level using echocardiography and rapid injection of an agitated fluid. Oximetry may be useful in the patient who has a left atrial catheter in place via the pulmonary vein. If pulmonary venous blood is highly oxygenated in the presence of systemic arterial desaturation, a source of right-to-left intracardiac shunting should be sought.

In evaluating the patient with an intracardiac shunt, it is important to remember that the commonly used method of determining cardiac output by thermodilution may be misleading. In this technique a cold solution is injected into the right atrium via the proximal port of a pulmonary artery catheter, and a thermistor at the tip of the catheter evaluates the change in temperature, deriving flow or "cardiac output." If part of the cold injectate is shunted through a right-to-left intracardiac shunt, the thermistor may give a falsely elevated estimation of cardiac output, since it "interprets" the smaller change in temperature as increased forward flow.

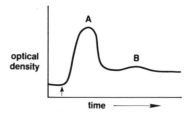

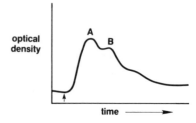

FIG 29–1.
Top, normal. Arrow represents injection of indicator dye into central circulation. *A* is the initial passage of dye throughout systemic circulation. *B* is recirculation of dye. **Center,** left-to-right shunt. Injection followed by initial passage *(A)* of dye and early recirculation *(B)* due to short-circuit back to pulmonary circulation. **Bottom,** right-to-left shunt. Injection followed by a premature appearance of dye *(A)* in systemic circulation without passing through pulmonary circulation.

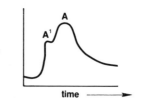

Physiologic Shunt

Physiologic or intrapulmonary shunting accounts for only 1% to 2% of the cardiac output of the healthy, awake, upright person. This shunting is different from anatomical shunting in that it occurs within the lung and is due to ventilation/perfusion (V/Q) mismatching that occurs even in the absence of pulmonary dysfunction, causing a small amount of pulmonary blood flow not to be exposed to gas exchange at the alveolus.

The distribution of pulmonary blood flow is primarily determined by gravity. In the upright lung, the absolute pressure in the pulmonary artery decreases 1 cm H_2O per centimeter vertical distance up the lung. This allows division of the lung into four separate compartments, based on the relationships between pulmonary artery pressure, pulmonary venous pressure, and alveolar pressure (Fig 29–2).

Zone I.—Alveolar pressure exceeds pressure in the pulmonary artery and pulmonary venous pressure; therefore, pulmonary blood vessels are collapsed and no blood flow occurs. Zone I lung is believed by some to be present only in pathologic states (such as hypovolemia or increased alveolar pressure associated with positive pressure ventilation) and to not exist in the normal patient.

Zone II.—At some vertical level, pulmonary artery pressure becomes positive and as it exceeds alveolar pressure, blood flow will occur. However, the blood flow is intermittent and depends on the relationship of pulmonary artery

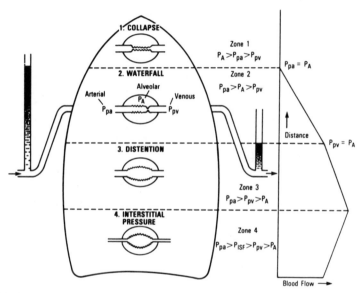

FIG 29–2.
Distribution of pulmonary blood flow in the upright lung. Zone I lung has no blood flow because alveolar pressure exceeds pulmonary artery pressure and intra-alveolar vessels are collapsed. In Zone II, pulmonary arterial pressure is greater than alveolar pressure and alveolar pressure exceeds pulmonary venous pressure. Blood flow at any time is determined by the difference in arterial and alveolar pressures. Pulmonary pressures increase down Zone II and in Zone III arterial and venous pressures exceed alveolar pressure. Blood flow in Zone III is therefore determined by the arterial-venous pressure difference. In Zone IV interstitial pressure increases, exceeding alveolar and venous pressures. Thus flow is related to the arterial-interstitial difference in pressures. (From Benumof JL: The pulmonary circulation, in Kaplan JA (ed): *Thoracic Anesthesia.* New York, Churchill Livingstone Inc, 1983. Used by permission.)

pressure to alveolar pressure during the cardiac and respiratory cycles ("waterfall" or "sluice" effect).

Zone III.—As pulmonary venous pressure becomes positive down the lung, both pulmonary artery and pulmonary venous pressures will always exceed alveolar pressure; therefore, blood flow is continuous. Its magnitude depends on the difference in the pulmonary artery and pulmonary venous pressures.

Zone IV.—If pulmonary venous pressure becomes high (such as in mitral stenosis or left atrial distention during cardiopulmonary bypass), fluid may translocate out of the pulmonary capillary into the interstitial compartment. If the interstitial fluid hydrostatic pressure exceeds pulmonary venous pressure, blood flow in the lower lung actually decreases. Thus, pulmonary blood flow increases down the lung unless Zone IV lung occurs.

Ventilation is also affected by gravity. Pleural pressure becomes more positive down the lung; the total gradient from the apex to the base is about 7 to 8 cm H_2O. Since alveolar pressure is the same down the lung, changes in the transpulmonary distending pressures (alveolar pressure minus pleural pressure) cause basilar alveoli to be compressed and apical alveoli to be well expanded. Therefore, a tidal volume is preferentially distributed to the more compliant basilar alveoli, which in the upright lung occupy the steep portion of the pressure-volume curve (Fig 29–3).

Although ventilation and perfusion increase with lung dependency, there is not perfect matching of their distributions. Blood flow increases more rapidly down the lung than does ventilation, causing apical alveoli to be relatively un-

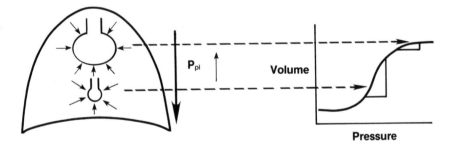

FIG 29–3.
Pleural pressure is greatest in the dependent portions of the upright lung. Transpulmonary distending pressures (Pa-Ppl) therefore also demonstrate a gradient down the lung. Ventilation is preferentially distributed to the compressed, compliant basilar alveoli that occupy the favorably steep portion of the pressure-volume curve.

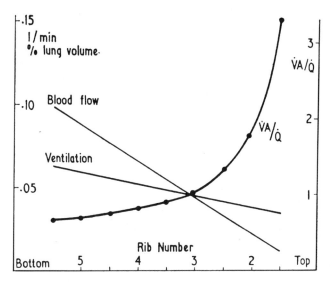

FIG 29–4.

Ventilation and blood flow (left vertical axis) and the ventilation-perfusion ratio (right vertical axis) are shown as a function of lung dependency in the upright lung. Blood flow and ventilation increase down the lung, but blood flow increases more than ventilation. Thus the ventilation-perfusion (V/Q) ratio decreases with lung dependency. (From West JB: *Ventilation/Blood Flow and Gas Exchange,* ed 3. Oxford, England, Blackwell Scientific Publications, 1977. Used by permission.)

derperfused (V/Q > 1) relative to their ventilation, and basilar alveoli to be overperfused (V/Q <1) (Fig 29–4).

The contribution of intrapulmonary shunting to systemic blood flow is quite small in the healthy awake person. However, in the anesthetized patient and particularly in the patient with cardiac and possibly pulmonary disease following cardiopulmonary bypass, other factors may become operative in increasing the amount of ventilation/perfusion mismatching that occurs.

Functional residual capacity (FRC) is the lung volume that exists at end-expiration when there is no air flow. Any deviation from functional residual capacity results in increased pulmonary vascular resistance and may decrease pulmonary blood flow (Fig 29–5). Functional residual capacity is decreased by assuming a supine position, and the induction of anesthesia causes further decreases in FRC in patients who spontaneously breathe as well as those having controlled ventilation. These decreases in functional residual capacity correlate well with V/Q mismatching after anesthesia and surgery and are easily demonstrated by widened alveolar-arterial gradients in patients postoperatively.

Regional alveolar hypoxia, regardless of the cause, results in hypoxic pulmonary vasoconstriction (HPV). This response of the pulmonary circulation acts to limit the deleterious effect of regional hypoxia by decreasing circulation to the affected area of the lung, improving overall ventilation and perfusion matching. This protective reflex may be inhibited or negated by various factors occurring during the course of an anesthetic, especially conditions that cause vasodilation (intravenous vasodilators, volatile anesthetics, respiratory or metabolic alkalosis) or increases in pulmonary artery pressure (volume overload, vasopressors, pulmonary embolism, mitral stenosis, large areas of hypoxic lung segments). Inhibition of HPV can therefore contribute to arterial desaturation by increasing venous admixture.

The interaction of physiologic shunt with cardiac output is relatively complex. Early studies predicted an indirect relationship between cardiac output (CO) and physiologic shunt, i.e., decreasing cardiac output would cause greater venous desaturation and greater amounts of venous admixture (physiologic shunt), reducing the patient's PO_2. However, cardiac output itself has been shown to have a direct relation with physiologic shunt in normal and diseased lungs. If the patient has a significant physiologic shunt and cardiac reserve is adequate, cardiac output will be high, ensuring good oxygen delivery to the tissues. If the patient is hypovolemic with decreasing cardiac output, the shunt will remain small as long as there are not regionally atelectatic or diseased areas of lung. There is little wasted pulmonary perfusion, V/Q is greater than 1, and areas of Zone I lung (essentially "dead space" lung) probably exist. Therefore, the rationale for improving cardiac output in the compromised patient is not to improve his PaO_2, but to improve oxygen

FIG 29–5.
Relationship of pulmonary vascular resistance to lung volume demonstrates that resistance is lowest at FRC. Above FRC intra-alveolar vessels are compressed by the alveoli, and below FRC hypoxic pulmonary vasoconstriction occurs. In both instances pulmonary vascular resistance is increased. (From Benumof JL: The pulmonary circulation, in Kaplan JA (ed): *Thoracic Anesthesia.* New York, Churchill Livingstone Inc, 1983. Used by permission.)

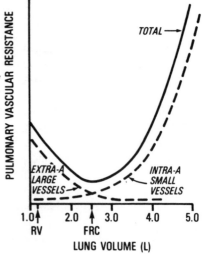

delivery to the tissues. The PaO_2 has not been found to consistently reflect the change in venous admixture associated with change in cardiac output in patients with normal or diffusely diseased lungs. In contrast, changes in cardiac output in the patient with a diseased region of lung vary indirectly with changes in venous admixture. For example, hypovolemia with decreased cardiac output in the patient with a diseased lobe of lung due to cancer will greatly increase the already present shunt. Improving cardiac output alone will increase the PaO_2 significantly.

Intrapulmonary shunting, therefore, represents a spectrum of ventilation and perfusion abnormalities. In the worst case, absolute shunt units with perfusion but no ventilation, (V/Q = O) oxygen is deleterious in that it does not improve the PaO_2 but increases the venous admixture by promoting absorption atelectasis in other alveolar units with low V/Q ratios. This atelectasis may be refractory to even high levels of PEEP, but becomes responsive if nitrogen (i.e., room air) is added to the inspired gases. Thus, decreasing the fraction of inspired oxygen (FIO_2) may improve ventilation and perfusion matching by allowing nitrogen to splint open marginally functional alveoli.

In summary, the patient undergoing cardiopulmonary bypass is at risk for numerous events affecting V/Q matching, acutely in the operating room and later in the postoperative course. Pulmonary vascular resistance is known to increase following cardiopulmonary bypass. The relation of this acute change to the release of vasoactive mediators, such as catecholamines and various prostaglandins is unclear. Changes in lung volumes such as functional residual capacity occur during anesthesia and surgery with the patient in the supine position despite positive-pressure ventilation. Administration of volatile anesthetics or vasodilators commonly causes increases in the alveolar-arterial gradient by inhibiting hypoxic pulmonary vasoconstriction. Increases in pulmonary artery pressure (e.g., overzealous volume loading) also can increase admixture by negating hypoxic pulmonary vasoconstriction to atelectatic areas of lung. Atelectasis in the operating room is commonly seen when the pleurae are opened and fluid and blood accumulate in the pleural sacs. Hemodynamic instability can cause decreases in PaO_2, especially if there is an atelectatic lobe of lung. Adminstration of 100% oxygen with the patient on cardiopulmonary bypass has been reported to cause increased venous admixture following cardiopulmonary bypass, presumably by promoting absorption atelectasis.

Despite the apparently endless opportunities to disrupt V/Q relationships, patients with uncomplicated conditions usually show only a transient modest increase in shunting following cardiopulmonary bypass. The etiology of this change seen in the operating room is not clear, but it is likely multifactorial. In the postoperative period, however, modest increases in admixture are seen for one to ten days postoperatively. Measurements indicating decreased functional residual capacity and lung compliance correlate well with roentgenographic findings of atelectasis and increased alveolar-arterial gradients as determined by blood gas analysis. In the absence of hemodynamic instability, these abnormalities of gas exchange rarely delay ventilatory weaning and extubation of patients with uncomplicated conditions.

Diffusion Block

A category of V/Q mismatching that deserves separate comment is the concept of alveolar diffusion block, most commonly manifested as interstitial and alveolar pulmonary edema. The net transcapillary flow of fluid is governed by the balance of pulmonary capillary hydrostatic pressure and interstitial hydrostatic pressure, and capillary colloid osmotic and interstitial colloid osmotic pressures. In addition, the pulmonary lymphatics remove the slow transudation of fluid and can clear significantly more fluid from the interstitial space than is usually required. However, if increases in pulmonary capillary hydrostatic pressure or decreases in pulmonary capillary colloid osmotic pressure cause more fluid to be transudated than can be removed, the interstitial fluid compartment and eventually the alveolar space will become edematous. This can also occur if the integrity of the capillary membrane becomes impaired or if pulmonary lymphatic flow is decreased. Therefore, pulmonary edema increases venous admixture by causing areas of microatelectasis and diffusion block both of which behave as shunt units, that is, V/Q approaches 0.

The most impressive cases of diffusion block following cardiopulmonary bypass occur in the setting of "pump-lung" syndrome, in which diffuse lung water leakage occurs into the interstitial and alveolar spaces. The alveolar-capillary membrane in the post-CPB lung has been shown to become more permeable to large proteins and smaller low molecular weight dextrans for up to seven days postoperatively. The decrease in colloid oncotic pressure, often seen during the operative period, and high pulmonary vascular pressures may play contributing roles in the presentation similar to that of adult respiratory distress syndrome (ARDS). The type of oxygenator used during cardiopulmonary bypass has also been implicated in creating fibrin, bubble emboli, and blood trauma, all of which may lead to pulmonary vasculitis and capillary leakage. Some patients do therefore demonstrate an ARDS-type pulmonary dysfunction immediately after exposure to CPB. Typically, oxygenation is poor and pulmonary edema is present. Pulmonary compliance and functional residual capacity are diminished.

The significance of CPB-related pulmonary dysfunction as a common event in the acute setting of the operating room is unclear, since a recent study demonstrated only transient, self-limiting increases in shunt following CPB and could find no relation in the magnitude of this shunt to the duration of CPB or the type of oxygenator.

APPROACH TO THE PROBLEM

In evaluating the patient with arterial hypoxemia immediately following cardiopulmonary bypass an orderly process should be initiated (Fig 29–6). It must first be ascertained that the anesthesia circuit is functioning properly, that oxygen delivery is sufficient, and that both lungs are adequately ventilated. Errors in blood gas sampling techinque should be ruled out and a repeat sample sent for analysis while further evaluation of the patient is in progress. The surgeon should evacuate the pleural cavities of any blood or fluid and consider opening the pleura if there is a doubt about "inadvertent" pleurotomy.

If these and other mechanical causes of hypoxemia are ruled out, the evaluation consists of ruling out the previously described causes of increased intrapulmonary shunting following cardiopulmonary bypass.

When hypoxemia is severe and otherwise unexplained, the cardiac team should verify that no intracardiac shunt exists. Digital examination by the surgeon of the right atrium may indicate an atrial-septal defect or patent foramen ovale. Dye dilution curves and oxygen saturation analysis of pulmonary venous blood may be useful in diagnosing right-to-left shunts.

More commonly, modest hypoxemia acutely following cardiopulmonary bypass is the end result of derangements in V/Q matching, with increases in venous admixture, increased pulmonary vascular resistance that may be associated with right ventricle failure, diffusion block due to interstitial or alveolar pulmonary edema, leaky capillary syndromes following cardiopulmonary bypass, or exacerbation of premorbid pulmonary conditions such as bronchospasm. Treatment of the hypoxemia in these cases is directed at reversing, if possible, the underlying causes.

The use of PEEP in patients following cardiopulmonary bypass deserves mention, because it has potentially therapeutic as well as detrimental effects. Positive end expiratory pressure recruits atelectatic areas, increasing the functional residual capacity and compliance. However, alveoli may be overdistended or disrupted, and cardiac output may be impaired due to decreased venous return. The use of PEEP in patients with uncomplicated conditions following cardiopulmonary bypass may not be warranted since low levels (3 to 6 cm) do not significantly improve gas exchange in the lungs, while higher levels (6 to 9 cm) may impair cardiac performance. In patients with compliant lungs on controlled ventilation, PEEP may also induce a discrepancy between measurements of pulmonary capillary wedge pressure (PCWP) and left atrial pressure. In most patients with pulmonary failure, however, PEEP usually improves the total static compliance of the lung, corresponding with maximum oxygen transport ($CO \times PaO_2$) and the lowest dead space to tidal volume ratio.

Optimal PEEP has recently been redefined to be the quantity of PEEP re-

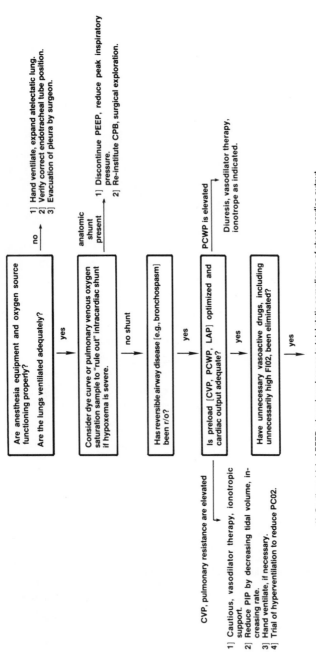

FIG 29–6.

Patient care decision plan used in the diagnosis and treatment of hypoxemia following cardiopulmonary bypass. *PEEP* = positive end expiratory pressure. *CVP* = central venous pressure. *PCWP* = pulmonary capillary wedge pressure. *LAP* = left atrial pressure. *PIP* = peak inspiratory pressure. *FIO₂* = fraction of inspired oxygen.

quired to restore intrapulmonary shunt to 15%. Restoration of pulmonary function by the therapeutic use of PEEP occasionally requires hemodynamic intervention to maintain cardiac output, allowing higher levels of PEEP and lower FIO_2 than would otherwise be indicated on the basis of cardiac function.

DISCUSSION

Hypoxemia in the period following cardiopulmonary bypass may endanger the patient's convalescence. There are multiple causes of hypoxemia. A systematic approach to the diagnosis leads to a logical treatment plan.

REFERENCES

1. Andersen NB, Ghia J: Pulmonary function, cardiac status, and postoperative course in relation to cardiopulmonary bypass. *J Thorac Cardiovasc Surg* 1970; 59:474–483.
2. Anyanwu E, Dittrich H, Gieseking J, et al: Ultrastructural changes in the human lung following cardiopulmonary bypass. *Basic Res Cardiol* 1982; 77:309–322.
3. Benumof JL, Pirlo AF, Johanson I, et al: Interaction of Pvo_2 with Pao_2 on hypoxic pulmonary vasoconstriction. *J Appl Physiol* 1981; 51:871–874.
4. Berryhill RE, Benumof JL: PEEP-induced discrepancy between pulmonary arterial wedge pressure and left atrial pressure: The effects of controlled vs. spontaneous ventilation and compliant vs. noncompliant lungs in the dog. *Anesthesiology* 1979; 51:303–308.
5. Bushman GA, Hall KD, Reves JG, et al: Development of acute intrapulmonary shunt following cardiopulmonary bypass abstract. *Anesthesiology* 1985; 63(suppl 2A):A569.
6. Byrick RJ, Kolion M, Hart JT, et al: Hypoxemia following cardiopulmonary bypass. *Anesthesiology* 1980; 53:171–174.
7. Byrick RJ, Noble WH: Postperfusion lung syndrome: Comparison of Travenol bubble and membrane oxygenator. *J Thorac Cardiovasc Surg* 1978; 76:685–693.
8. Cheney FW, Colley PS: The effect of cardiac output on arterial blood oxygenation. *Anesthesiology* 1980; 52:496–503.
9. DeLeon RS, Paterson JL, Sykes MK: Changes in colloid osmotic pressure and plasma albumin concentration associated with extracorporeal circulation. *J Anaesth* 1982; 54:465–473.
10. Dobbinson TL, Miller JR: Respiratory and cardiovascular responses to PEEP in artificially ventilated patients after cardiopulmonary bypass surgery. *Anaesth Intensive Care* 1981; 9:307–313.
11. Douglas MD, Downs JB, Shook D: Response of pulmonary venous admixture: A means of comparing therapies? *Chest* 1980; 77:764–770.
12. Downs JB, Mitchell LA: Pulmonary effects of ventilatory pattern following cardiopulmonary bypass. *Crit Care Med* 1976; 4:295–300.

13. Gallagher TJ, Civetta JM, Kirby RR: Terminology update: Optimal PEEP. *Crit Care Med* 1978; 6:323–326.

14. Kaplan JE, *Thoracic Anesthesia.* New York, Churchill Livingstone Inc, 1983.

15. Lynch JP, Mhyre JG, Dantzker DR: Influence of cardiac output on intrapulmonary shunt. *J Appl Physiol* 1979; 46:315–321.

16. Morthy SS, Losasso AM, Gibbs PS: Acquired right to left intracardiac shunts and severe hypoxemia. *Crit Care Med* 1978; 6:28–31.

17. Pennock JL, Pierce WS, Waldhausen JA: The management of the lungs during cardiopulmonary bypass. *Surg Gynecol Obstet* 1977; 145:917–927.

18. Rackow EC, Fein LA: Fulminant noncardiogenic pulmonary edema in the critically ill. *Crit Care Med* 1978; 6:360–363.

19. Rea HH, Harris EA, Seelye BA, et al: The effects of cardiopulmonary bypass upon pulmonary gas exchange. *J Thorac Cardiovasc Surg* 1978; 75:104–120.

20. Royston D, Minty BD, Higenbottam TW, et al: The effect of surgery with cardiopulmonary bypass on alveolar-capillary barrier function in human beings. *Ann Thorac Surg* 1985; 40:139–143.

21. Shapire BA, Cane RD, Harrison RA, et al: Changes in intrapulmonary shunting with administration of 100% oxygen. *Chest* 1980; 77:138–141.

22. Stanley TH, Liu WS, Gentry S: Effects of ventilatory techniques during cardiopulmonary bypass on post-bypass and postoperative pulmonary compliance and shunt. *Anesthesiology* 1977; 46:391–395.

23. Suter PM, Fairley HB, Isenberg MD: Optimum end-expiratory airway pressure in patients with acute pulmonary failure. *N Engl J Med* 1975; 292:284–289.

24. Svennevig JL, Lindberg H, Geiran O, et al: Should the lungs be ventilated during cardiopulmonary bypass? Clinical, hemodynamic, and metabolic changes in patients undergoing elective coronary artery surgery. *Ann Thorac Surg* 1984; 37:295–300.

25. Tonnesen AS, Gabel JC, McLeavey CA: Relation between lowered colloid osmotic pressure, respiratory failure and death. *Crit Care Med* 1977; 5:239–240.

26. Turnbull KW, Miyagishima RT, Gerein AN: Pulmonary complications and cardiopulmonary bypass: A clinical study in adults. *Can Anaesth Soc J* 1974; 21:181–194.

30

Coronary Artery Bypass Grafting in a Patient With Kidney Transplant

A 45-year-old man was scheduled to have coronary bypass surgery for three-vessel coronary artery disease. He had a right kidney transplant and was receiving prednisone; he had normal renal function. Preoperative consultation centered on discussions covering the optimal perfusion pressure and urine output during cardiopulmonary bypass (CPB).

Recommendations by Mark Hilberman, M.D.

ANALYSIS OF THE PROBLEM

The issues include:

1. What is the risk of a perioperative cardiac death in such a patient? Is this the dominant cause of death, or are the patient's other obvious complicating medical conditions more important?

2. What are the most important antecedents to acute renal failure (ARF) in the cardiac surgical patient? How should we apply information derived from normal patients undergoing heart surgery to the immune suppressed patient with a functioning denervated kidney in place?

3. Will the problems of infection control and wound healing in the immune suppressed host—so important in overall morbidity and mortality in this patient population—prove more important as a cause of postoperative problems

than either the potential cardiac or renal complications evident in the case presentation?

APPROACH TO THE PROBLEM

The intraoperative management of this patient should be like any other with regard to use of vasoactive drugs during cardiopulmonary bypass. The denervated kidney could have jeopardized renal blood flow if excessive α-adrenergic drugs were used. Adequate pump flow and relative hypothermia should be established. Prophylactic administration of diuretics should be used (see discussion below).

DISCUSSION

Perioperative Cardiac Complications

Renal transplant recipients coming to cardiac operation can be expected to have a relatively high risk for perioperative cardiac complications. Routine coronary arteriographic studies performed at the Cleveland Clinic have demonstrated a high frequency of significant coronary artery disease (CAD) and ventricular dysfunction in renal transplant candidates and recipients.[1] English investigators have demonstrated severely impaired exercise tolerance associated with impaired ventricular performance in comparable patients.[2] The degree and severity of CAD is substantially higher in diabetics than in nondiabetics with end-stage renal disease.[3] Despite the high incidence of CAD that accounted for 8% of the deaths in renal transplant recipients, the majority of deaths appeared to be consequent to immune suppression or renal failure.[1]

Despite the prevalence of CAD in these patients, only a limited subset of renal transplant recipients come to cardiac operation. Case reports identify approximately 24 patients who have undergone cardiac operations subsequent to renal transplantation.[4–8] The largest series derives from 2,000 renal transplant procedures performed at the University of Minnesota, 14 patients (0.7%) came to cardiac surgery.[8] The two postoperative deaths (14%!) were due to cardiac dysfunction and arrhythmias. Thus, in the limited experience reported to date, postoperative cardiac complications resulted in adverse outcomes more frequently than ARF, infection, or wound-healing problems.

Finally, it has recently been documented that, in the absence of left main disease, patients with multiple-vessel disease AND poor ventricular function received the greatest relative benefit from surgical therapy.[9, 10] In most centers this has resulted in a dramatic worsening in the ventricular performance of patients presenting for CABG.

These factors are important for postoperative renal graft survival, as data summarized in the subsequent section clearly indicate that impaired cardiac performance in the postoperative period represents a substantially greater threat to renal function than cardiopulmonary bypass per se.

Acute Renal Failure and Cardiac Operations

General Issues

The incidence of ARF following cardiac surgery is substantially lower than that reported during the mid 1960s when this complication was a frequent and more important contributor to postoperative morbidity and mortality. We have recently completed a series of investigations related to renal function and the development of ARF following cardiac surgery.[11–14] These studies, and substantial work by other investigators, have recently been summarized.[15] Denervation will eliminate the sympathetically mediated renal vasoconstriction that accompanies atrial hypotension. During hemorrhagic shock (low atrial pressures) but not cardiogenic shock (high atrial pressures), these reflexes severely restrict renal blood flow. In addition, the autoregulatory ability of the kidney, largely under extrarenal control, will be substantially reduced. At perfusion pressures below approximately 60 mm Hg, renal vasoconstriction is eliminated, and renal vasodilation is maximal (passively). Transplantation thus eliminates one source of potential renal ischemia, but still leaves the kidney vulnerable to renal ischemia consequent to poor systemic perfusion with the usual elevation of circulating vasoconstrictor hormones from endogenous or exogenous sources. Postoperative ARF generally developed following a complex series of events. The most important single factor was severely depressed postoperative cardiac performance. The results of these studies would appear generally applicable to the renal transplant patient. In the small group of patients in which bypass events resulted in ARF, good postoperative cardiac performance resulted in high survival rates. The majority, who developed ARF as a consequence of a protracted treated variant of cardiogenic shock, had a very high mortality. The ARF was very uncommon following CABG only.[11, 12, 15]

Cardiopulmonary Bypass

These studies were conducted at Stanford University with nonpulsatile CPB flows of 1.6 to 1.8 L/kg/minute, at temperatures of 30°C, and moderate hemodilution (hematocrit readings in the mid 20s). Both normal controls and patients who exhibited renal dysfunction (RD) or ARF had mean bypass pressures of approximately 50 mm Hg; early bypass pressures between 30 and 40 mm Hg were standard and usually untreated. No relation could be established between perfusion pressure or CPB urine flow and renal outcome. The RD/ARF patient group actually had higher CPB blood flow than those with normal postoperative renal function. The CPB duration was substantially longer (160 vs. 110 minutes). Perioperative quantification of renal and cardiac function indicated that prolonged CPB times usually did not result in ARF but were implicated statistically because they were associated with longer and more complex procedures resulting in poorer postoperative cardiac function. In one patient a five-hour (300 minute) CPB run did appear to cause ARF.[11,12,15]

The decline in perfusion pressure early in CPB diminishes glomerular ultrafiltration pressure directly and probably reduces renal blood flow. However, renal blood flow appears adequate to maintain renal cellular integrity. In the transplanted kidney, α-adrenergic agents administered to elevate perfusion pressures during CPB will result in renal vasoconstriction. It is not clear whether the net effect upon the kidney will be detrimental or beneficial. Given the extensive and detailed documentation of our experience with renal function in the context of low flow CPB, there would appear no justification for altering usual regimens for this patient, except that vasoconstrictive drugs should be avoided altogether or used exceedingly sparingly. An efficient and experienced surgeon should perform the procedure, both to avoid excessively prolonged CPB and to minimize aortic cross-clamp time with the inevitable (at present) ischemic depression of cardiac function that follows, even with good cardioplegic protective regimens.

Postoperative Cardiac Performance

Patients who exhibited postoperative RD or ARF exhibited marked depression of cardiac performance early in the postoperative period when compared to those who did not exhibit such signs.[11, 12] The RD group differed from the ARF group by showing substantial hemodynamic recovery during the first postoperative week.[12] Some patients developed ARF following withdrawal of hemodynamic support several days postoperatively. This observation led to a change in philosophy regarding maintenance of postoperative inotropic or vasodilator support. Specifically, withdrawal of drug support is not regarded as an indication of patient improvement unless hemodynamic function is clearly adequate (not marginal) following such withdrawal. Some patients merit prolonged (weeks) intravenous inotropic support; this subgroup, though small, will be benefited by the introduction of potent oral inotropic drugs that may be taken with existing oral vasodilators. In the renal transplant recipient who undergoes cardiac operation, it may be important to remove monitoring catheters early to avoid potential infection and to administer dopamine or epinephrine using noninvasive indicators of cardiac function. Maintenance of good cardiac performance AND the avoidance of infection are dominant concerns in the postoperative management of this patient.

Vasoactive Drugs

Dopamine is a potent inotropic drug and tubular inhibitor of solute transport (diuretic) that remains the agent of choice for inotropic support in these patients. It does not appear to cause selective renal vasodilation in postoperative patients with depressed cardiac performance. In addition, its range of inotropic effectiveness without excessive renal vasoconstriction may extend to 20 μg/kg/minute.[13]

In some patients epinephrine infusion may be indicated in the early postoperative period. We documented improved renal function with epinephrine in one patient whose glomerular filtration rate and renal blood flow doubled with administration of epinephrine at 0.04 μg/kg/minute (unpublished data, 1978). Subsequent clinical experience indicates that epinephrine may be safely used at infusion rates between 0.02 and 0.07 (perhaps as high as 0.1 μg/kg/minute). Therefore, as soon as possible, the treatment of these patients is changed to maintenance dopamine infusions.

Sodium nitroprusside is a direct renal vasodilator that can substantially improve renal blood flow in proportion to its effect upon cardiac output. The usual clinical measures of renal function (urine flow and glomeruler filtration rate) are not improved by this drug. However, in the hemodynamically marginal patient, the improvement in renal blood flow obtainable with this agent may be critical. Reports of diminished renal blood flow in humans made hypotensive with this agent are explainable by a sympathetically mediated renal vasoconstriction triggered by atrial hypotension. Such a response would not be present in the denervated kidney. Monitoring of cardiac output is the best technique for estimating the effects upon renal blood flow of nitroprusside's opposing effects of direct renal vasodilation and declining arterial perfusion pressure.[14]

Diuretic Prophylaxis

It has been conclusively demonstrated that diuretic administration prior to or following a complete renal ischemic insult dramatically decreases the degree and duration of the consequent ARF. By contrast, we were unable to demonstrate a relationship between urine flow during cardiopulmonary bypass and subsequent renal outcome. Despite this discrepancy, the relative benefits of prophylactic diuretic administration in this patient population outweigh any risks. Mannitol (0.5 to 1.0 gm/kg) is an appropriate component of the priming solution, with furosemide administration indicated for oliguria once CPB perfuson pressures exceed 50 mm Hg. Furosemide is also indicated for postoperative oliguria and should be administered concurrently with correction of any underlying hemodynamic problems.[15]

Infection Control

Infection remains the leading cause of death following renal transplantation.[16] Thus, despite the absence of complications due to infection or wound healing problems in the CABG/renal transplant patients reported to date,[4–8] meticulous attention to sterile technique is clearly warranted. This is true during and following placement of intravascular monitoring catheters. Airway management must be oriented toward minimizing aspiration or infection. The susceptibility of individual patients to catastrophic infections justifies the use of sterile endotracheal tubes, breathing circuits, and bacterial filters. It should be recognized that the latter practice has not been provable by recent patient studies. [17,18] Nonetheless, I believe the cost/benefit ratio favors meticulous attention to any and all acts that limit nosocomial infections in this patient population.

The use of prophylactic antibiotics during cardiac surgery is well established. The infection pattern in an individual hospital may warrant the prophylactic use of potentially nephrotoxic antibiotics. The nephrotoxicity of these agents is enhanced by poor renal perfusion, and their administration during or immediately after CPB or during periods of depressed cardiac performance should be avoided. The same caution may well apply to the administration of the nephrotoxic immune suppressive drug, cyclosporin A.

Immunosuppressive Drug Therapy

Immunosuppressive drug therapy will obviously need to be maintained during the perioperative period and should pose no particular problems. Steroid doses are normally increased somewhat to cover the operative stress. [16] It would seem prudent to time cyclosporin A administration so that peak levels are not encountered during CPB and the immediate postoperative period.

Summary

The patient with a normally functioning kidney transplant may be safely managed during cardiac surgery with preservation of renal function. Attention to details of cardiac management is of highest priority, but renal protection is a major concern.

REFERENCES

1. Braun WE, Phillips D, Vidt DG, et al: Coronary arteriography and coronary artery disease in 99 diabetic and nondiabetic patients on chronic hemodialysis or renal transplantation programs. *Transplant Proc* 1981; 13:128–135.
2. Bullock RE, Amer HA, Simpson I, et al: Cardiac abnormalities and exercise tolerance in patients receiving renal replacement therapy. *Br Med J* 1984; 289:1479–1484.
3. Braun WE, Phillips HB, Vidt DB, et al: Coronary artery disease in 100 diabetics with end-stage renal failure. *Transplant Proc* 1984; 16:603–607.
4. Lamperti JJ, Conn LH, Collins JJ Jr: Cardiac surgery in patients undergoing renal dialysis or transplantation. *Ann Thorac Surg* 1975; 19:135–41.

5. Beauchamp GD, Sharma JN, Crouch T, et al: Coronary bypass surgery after renal transplantation. *Am J Cardiol* 1976; 37:1107–1110.

6. Chawla R, Gailiunas P Jr, Lazarus JM, et al: Cardiopulmonary bypass surgery in chronic hemodialysis and transplant patients. *Trans Am Soc Artif Intern Organs* 1977; 23:694–697.

7. Monson BK, Wickstrom PH, Haglin JJ, et al: Cardiac operation and end-stage renal disease. *Ann Thorac Surg* 1980; 30:267–272.

8. Bolman RM III, Anderson RW, Molina JE, et al: Cardiac operations in patients with functioning renal allografts. *J Thorac Cardiovasc Surg* 1984; 88:537–543.

9. The Veterans Administration Coronary Artery Bypass Surgery Cooperative Study Group: Eleven-year survival in the Veterans Administration randomized trial of coronary bypass surgery for stable angina. *N Engl J Med* 1984; 311:1333–1339.

10. Bonow RO, Kent KM, Rosing DR, et al: Exercise-induced ischemia in mildly symptomatic patients with coronary-artery disease and preserved left ventricular function. *N Engl J Med* 1984; 311:1339–1345.

11. Hilberman M, Myers BD, Carrie BJ, et al: Acute renal failure following cardiac surgery. *J Thorac Cardiovasc Surg* 1979; 77:880–888.

12. Hilberman M, Derby GC, Spencer RJ, et al: Sequential pathophysiological changes characterizing the progression from renal dysfunction to acute renal failure following cardiac operation. *J Thorac Cardiovasc Surg* 1980; 79:838–844.

13. Hilberman M, Maseda J, Stinson EB, et al: The diuretic properties of dopamine in patients after open-heart operation. *Anesthesiology* 1984; 61:489–494.

14. Maseda M, Hilberman M, Derby GC, et al: The renal effects of sodium nitroprusside in postoperative cardiac surgical patients. *Anesthesiology* 1981; 54:284–288.

15. Hilberman M: The kidneys: Function, failure, and protection in the perioperative period, in Ream AK, Fogdall RP (eds): *Acute Cardiovascular Management.* Philadelphia, JB Lippincott Co, 1982; pp 806–829.

16. Strom TB, Tilney NL, Merrill JP: Renal transplantation: Clinical management of the transplant recipient, in Brenner BM, Rector FC Jr, (eds): *The Kidney.* Philadelphia, WB Saunders, 1981, pp 2618–2658.

17. Garibaldi RA, Britt MR, Webster C, et al: Failure of bacterial filters to reduce the incidence of pneumonia after inhalation anesthesia. *Anesthesiology* 1981; 54:364–368.

18. Feeley TW, Hamilton WK, Xavier B, et al: Sterile anesthesia breathing circuits do not prevent postoperative pulmonary infection. *Anesthesiology* 1981; 54:369–372.

31

Anesthetic Management of the Patient With Dynamic Coronary Stenosis

A 56 year-old woman with coronary artery disease underwent coronary bypass surgery. She had a history of chest pain with emotional stress and with exertion that was relieved by nitroglycerin. Angiography revealed a single lesion that caused a 90% reduction in the diameter of the proximal circumflex coronary artery. She had no symptoms of congestive heart failure. Anesthesia was induced with fentanyl (10 μg/kg), diazepam (0.2 mg/kg) and pancuronium (0.1 mg/kg). Laryngoscopy and intubation increased systolic blood pressure by 20% to 160 mm Hg and increased heart rate by 20% to 95 beats per minute. New 2-mm depression of the ST segment of electrocardiogram lead V_5 was noted. This sign of myocardial ischemia resolved as heart rate and blood pressure returned to control values following intubation. A nitroglycerin infusion (1.0 μg/kg/minute) was begun. Following skin incision 15 minutes later, systolic blood pressure increased to 160 mm Hg and heart rate to 95 beats per minute, but no ST segment depression was noted. The pulmonary artery wedge pressure was 6 to 8 mm Hg throughout.

Recommendations by Charles W. Buffington, M.D., and Alan Levine, M.D.

ANALYSIS OF THE PROBLEM

Myocardial ischemia occurred during laryngoscopy but failed to occur during skin incision, even though blood pressure and heart rate increased to the same extent during these two stresses. Nitroglycerin clearly accounts for the difference, but via what mechanism?

APPROACH TO THE PROBLEM

We carefully question any patient with coronary artery disease about the circumstances that produce angina. A history of pain at rest with preserved exercise capacity, pain with emotional stress, or a variable exercise threshold for pain suggests dynamic stenosis.[1]

We attempt to avoid myocardial ischemia during anesthesia in patients with dynamic stenosis by a combination of two strategies. Nitroglycerin is administered to block stenosis vasoconstriction. Then blood pressure and heart rate are adjusted to avoid hypotension and/or tachycardia. Specifically, mean arterial pressure is kept above heart rate.[2] We do not worry about moderate levels of hypertension unless the increase in blood pressure is accompanied by left ventricular failure. The choice of anesthetic agent and depth of anesthesia is probably less important than hemodynamic control and nitroglycerin administration.

We continue all cardiac medications until surgery but usually reduce by half the final dose of β-blocking drugs if surgery is to follow within two hours. On arrival in the operating room, electrocardiographic monitoring including a V_5 lead is begun and arterial pressure determined, usually with an intra-arterial catheter. An intravenous nitroglycerin infusion is begun at a rate of 1 μg/kg per minute. Should mean arterial pressure fall, preload is augmented by mild head-down tilt or fluid administration. Occasionally, phenylephrine infusion is required as well. The importance of maintaining arterial pressure during nitroglycerin infusion has been stressed previously.[3] Heart rate is kept below mean arterial pressure by administration of propranolol (up to 0.1 mg/kg intravenously, in divided doses) in patients with normal left ventricular filling pressures and no current symptoms of congestive heart failure. The constrictor effect of propanolol on large coronary arteries is effectively antagonized by nitroglycerin.

Intraoperative Coronary Spasm

Coronary spasm represents a dynamic event that may suddenly compromise myocardial blood supply. Spasm that occurs during anesthesia is best recognized by the sudden onset of ST-segment change. Elevation occurs if ischemia is transmural. Depression occurs if occlusion is incomplete or collateral flow provides enough blood so that only subendocardial ischemia results. This evidence of ischemia is not preceded by alterations in blood pressure or heart rate.[4] The periods of spasm are usually one to five minutes long and tend to reoccur unless treatment is begun. Intravenous nitroglycerin is effective therapy for coronary spasm,[4] and intravenous verapamil has been recently advocated.[5] Large doses of nitroglycerin (2 to 3 μg/kg per minute) may be required.

DISCUSSION

Clinical Presentation

Patients with rigid coronary stenoses develop angina during exercise because coronary flow cannot rise enough to satisfy the enhanced myocardial oxygen demand. These patients give a history of reproducible angina with exertion. In contrast, angina at rest in a patient who does *not* develop angina during exercise suggests true coronary spasm.[6]

The patient in this case had a history of angina both with exertion and during emotional stress while at rest. Pain during exercise is consistent with severe narrowing of at least one coronary artery. Pain during emotional stress probably resulted from sympathetic constriction at a compliant coronary stenosis. Although constriction occurred at the site of the single, severe stenosis in this patient, other patients with multivessel disease may have both types of lesions.

Pathophysiology of Dynamic Coronary Stenosis

An emerging concept is that a large fraction of coronary stenoses are not "fixed" but, rather, are subject to dynamic changes in stenosis caliber. Coronary spasm is an extreme example of such dynamic behavior. However, between coronary spasm and fixed coronary stenosis is a continuum of dynamic behavior[7] that needs better understanding if the anesthetic management of patients with coronary artery disease is to be improved.

Coronary spasm has been recognized as a cause of myocardial ischemia.[8–11] True coronary spasm is not common. Heupler, for example, found an incidence of symptomatic coronary spasm of 0.1% in 28,000 patients undergoing cardiac catheterization for suspected atherosclerotic heart disease.[9] In addition to such vasospastic events, vasotonic mechanisms may involve a large fraction of stenoses and thus contribute importantly to ischemia during anesthesia.[12–15]

Central to a discussion of vasotonic angina is the concept of compliant coronary stenosis. Such stenoses usually have an eccentric atheroma that bulges into the lumen of the vessel. In contrast, fixed lesions are usually concentric.[1] Since an eccentric atheroma involves only one side of the vessel, an arc of relatively normal wall is left. A recent postmortem study found that 45% of moderate and severe stenoses had an arc of at least 90 degrees of normal arterial wall.[16] The presence of normal wall makes the stenosis compliant and thus subject to active and passive changes in caliber.

The remaining normal wall at the site of an eccentric coronary stenosis is influenced by factors that alter the tone of epicardial coronary vessels. Importantly, the degree of contraction and relaxation of smooth muscle appears to be normal, but the geometric arrangement of the atheroma amplifies the resulting change in coronary resistance.[12] For example, sympathetic stimulation produces a 10% to 15% reduction in normal vessel circumference. Such a reduction affects the resistance of an unstenosed epicardial vessel only slighty,[17] but a similar change at the site of an eccentric stenosis can cause a dramatic increase in resistance. Brown and associates have shown that isometric handgrip, a potent sympathetic stimulus, increased stenosis resistance by an average of 240% in patients with coronary artery disease.[18] This twofold to threefold increase in stenosis resistance was completely abolished by sublingual nitroglycerin during a repeated handgrip.

It is likely that sympathetic activation during anesthesia produces vasoconstriction at the site of compliant, eccentric coronary stenoses. Such vasoconstriction decreases coronary blood flow. Thus, a decrease in oxygen supply occurs during a period of enhanced oxygen demand. In the present case, administration of nitroglycerin abolished stenosis vasoconstriction and permitted adequate coronary flow to meet the increase in oxygen demand associated with skin incision.

Pharmacology of Large Coronary Vessels

Recent studies have focused on the response of large coronary arteries to physiologic stimuli and pharmacologic agents. Although much of the information is derived from nondiseased human and animal epicardial vessels, these findings probably apply directly to the normal wall segment of an eccentric stenosis. An important exception is the case of true coronary spasm in which an abnormal vascular response to vasoconstrictor substances is implicated.

The coronary arterial system decreases in lumen area from the left main coronary artery (4 to 5 mm in diameter) to small arterioles. For the purposes of study, however, an arbitrary division into large vessels and arterioles is usually made. Large vessels are epicardial vessels greater than 0.6 mm in diameter that can be identified on a coronary angiogram. Vessels 2 to 3 mm in diameter can be dissected free of the epicardium in animals for direct study.

Although these large vessels respond to vasoconstrictor and vasodilator substances in a fashion similar to the arteriolar bed, certain differences exist. Arteriolar vessels are surrounded by metabolically active myocardial cells, whereas epicardial vessels are isolated from such metabolic stimuli. A therapeutic dose of nitroglycerin selectively dilates large coronary vessels without significant effect on arterioles.[19] In contrast, adenosine, dipyridamole, and chromonar selectively dilate arterioles without an effect on large arteries. Sodium nitroprusside and the calcium channel blockers dilate vessels of both sizes.

Large Vessel Constriction

Coronary vasoconstriction mediated by α-receptors has been demonstrated both in dogs[20] and in humans.[18] This constriction appears to be balanced by β-receptor mediated vasodilation.[21] Administration of propranolol decreases the diameter of normal vessels[1] and potentiates vasoconstriction caused by the cold pressor test in patients with coronary artery disease.[22] Propranolol has also been reported to worsen coronary spasm in humans.[23] Although direct blockade of β-receptors may unmask α-mediated constriction, recent evidence in dogs suggests that an indirect effect via myocardial β-receptors is responsible for the effects on large vessels seen with propranolol.[24] Blockade of myocardial β-receptors reduces heart rate and contractility. Reduced myocardial metabolism and coronary flow cause a reduction in large vessel diameter.

Ergonovine is the most potent known constrictor of large coronary arteries[1] and is used as a provocative test for coronary spasm during cardiac catheterization.[25] Ergonovine contracts coronary arteries by a serotonergic mechanism,[26] that is potentiated, in vitro, by removal of endothelium.[27] This observation suggests that endothelial cells may play an important role in mediating the effects of humoral factors. In addition, endothelial cells produce a polypeptide vasoconstrictor that is unaffected by all currently known pharmacologic inhibitors and antagonists and may be important in the regulation of vascular smooth muscle contractility.[28]

Thromboxane A_2 is a potent coronary vasoconstrictor that is liberated by platelets during aggregation. Thromboxane A_2 apparently stimulates a specific thromboxane receptor that is dependent on an inward calcium flux.[29] Calcium antagonists noncompetitively inhibit thromboxane-induced vasoconstriction.

Large Vessel Dilators

The prostaglandins E_1 and I_2 are potent dilators of large coronary vessels. The "nitro" drugs including nitroglycerin,[19, 30, 31] sodium nitroprusside, and isosorbide dinitrate effectively antagonize vasoconstrictor substances[32] and cause a net vasodilation of 20% to 30% as well.[1] The arteriolar dilators, verapamil, diltiazem, hydralazine, and dipyridamole have no effect on the diameter of normal epicardial vessels. However, diltiazem does block sympathetically mediated constriction,[33] and nifedipine prevents constriction in response to the cold pressor test in patients with coronary artery disease.[34] One drawback of agents that cause arteriolar vasodilation is the potential for transmural coronary steal in the setting of severe stenosis.[35] A second problem is that dilation of the distal bed can cause collapse of a compliant stenosis and passively increase resistance at the site of the stenosis.[36] The effects of anesthetics on large vessel diameters have not been investigated with the exception of isoflurane.

Isoflurane does not dilate epicardial vessels, although it decreases coronary resistance at the arteriolar level.[37]

Coronary Artery Spasm

True coronary spasm probably involves an abnormal response to vasoconstrictor stimuli,[10, 38, 39] although a host of mechanisms appear to be possible.[21] During spasm, coronary flow is transiently decreased to very low levels and myocardial ischemia ensues.[40] Coronary spasm has been successfully treated with nifedipine[41] and verapamil[42] as well as nitroglycerin.[8]

Summary

There is a growing awareness that dynamic events at the site of coronary artery stenosis can influence the likelihood of myocardial ischemia in patients with coronary artery disease. Although true coronary spasm is not common, dynamic sympathetic constriction probably occurs during the stress of anesthesia and surgery. Such constriction dramatically increases the resistance to flow at the site of severe, eccentric stenoses. The most rational approach to management of these patients is a combination of hemodynamic control and stenosis vasodilation with nitroglycerin.

REFERENCES

1. Brown BG, Bolson EL, Dodge HT: Dynamic mechanisms in human coronary stenosis. *Circulation* 1984; 70:917–922.
2. Buffington CW: Hemodynamic determinants of ischemic myocardial dysfunction in the presence of coronary stenosis in dogs. *Anesthesiology* 1985; 63:651–662.
3. Miller RR, Awan NA, DeMaria AN, et al: Importance of maintaining systemic blood pressure during nitroglycerin administration for reducing ischemic injury in patients with coronary disease. *Am J Cardiol* 1977; 40:504–508.
4. Buffington CW, Ivey TD: Coronary artery spasm during general anesthesia. *Anesthesiology* 1981; 55:466–469.
5. Nussmeier NA, Slogoff S: Verapamil treatment of intraoperative coronary artery spasm. *Anesthesiology* 1985; 62:539–541.
6. MacAlpin RN, Kattus AA, Alvaro AB: Angina pectoris at rest with preservation of exercise capacity. *Circulation* 1973; 47:946–958.
7. Maseri A, Severi S, De Nes M, et al: "Variant" angina: One aspect of a continuous spectrum of vasospastic myocardial ischemia. *Am J Cardiol* 1978; 42:1019–1033.
8. Prinzmetal M, Kennamer R, Reuben M, et al: Angina pectoris: I. A variant form of angina pectoris. *Am J Med* 1959; 27:375–388.
9. Heupler FA Jr: Syndrome of symptomatic coronary arterial spasm with nearly normal coronary arteriograms. *Am J Cardiol* 1980; 45:873–881.

10. Maseri A, Chierchia S: Coronary artery spasm: Demonstration, definition, diagnosis, and consequences. *Prog Cardiovasc Dis* 1982; 25:169–192.
11. Hillis LD, Braunwald E: Coronary-artery spasm. *N Engl J Med* 1978; 299:695–702.
12. MacAlpin RN: Contribution of dynamic vascular wall thickening to luminal narrowing during coronary arterial constriction. *Circulation* 1980; 60:296–301.
13. Gorlin R: Dynamic vascular factors in the genesis of myocardial ischemia. *J Am Coll Cardiol* 1983; 1:897–906.
14. Pepine CJ, Feldman RL: Dynamic coronary blood flow reduction: Supply side considerations. *Int J Cardiol* 1983; 3:3–13.
15. Epstein SE, Talbot TL: Dynamic coronary tone in precipitation, exacerbation and relief of angina pectoris. *Am J Cardiol* 1981; 48:797–803.
16. Freudenberg H, Lichtlen PR: Das normale wandsegment bei koronarstenosen—eine postmortale studie. *Z Kardiol* 1981; 70:863–869.
17. Kelley KO, Feigl EO: Segmental α-receptor-mediated vasoconstriction in the canine coronary circulation. *Circ Res* 1978; 43:908–917.
18. Brown BG, Lee AB, Bolson EL, et al: Reflex constriction of significant coronary stenosis as a mechanism contributing to ischemic left ventricular dysfunction during isometric exercise. *Circulation* 1984; 70:18–24.
19. Hintze TH, Vatner SF: Comparison of effects of nifedipine and nitroglycerin on large and small coronary arteries and cardiac function in conscious dogs. *Circ Res* 1983; 52(suppl 1):139–146.
20. Vatner SF, Pagani M, Manders WT, et al: α-Adrenergic vasoconstriction and nitroglycerin vasodilation of large coronary arteries in the conscious dog. *J Clin Invest* 1980; 65:5–14.
21. Shepherd JT, Vanhoutte PM: Spasm of the coronary arteries: Causes and consequences (the scientist's viewpoint). *Mayo Clin Proc* 1985; 60:33–46.
22. Kern MJ, Ganz P, Horowitz JD, et al: Potentiation of coronary vasoconstriction by β-adrenergic blockade in patients with coronary artery disease. *Circulation* 1983; 67:1178–1185.
23. Robertson RM, Wood AJJ, Vaughn WK, et al: Exacerbation of vasotonic angina pectoris by propranolol. *Circulation* 1982; 65:281–285.
24. Vatner SF, Hintze TH: Mechanism of constriction of large coronary arteries by β-adrenergic receptor blockade. *Circ Res* 1983; 53:389–400.
25. Heupler FA, Proudfit WL, Razavi M, et al: Ergonovine maleate provocative test for coronary arterial spasm. *Am J Cardiol* 1978; 41:631–640.
26. Brazenor RM, Angus JA: Ergometrine contracts isolated canine coronary arteries by a serotonergic mechanism: No role for α-adrenoceptors. *J Pharmacol Exp Ther* 1981; 218:530–536.
27. Lamping KG, Marcus ML, Dole WP: Removal of the endothelium potentiates canine large coronary artery constrictor responses to 5-hydroxytryptamine in vivo. *Circ Res* 1985; 57:46–54.
28. Hickey KA, Rubanyi G, Paul RJ, et al: Characterization of a coronary vasoconstrictor produced by cultured endothelial cells. *Am J Physiol* 1985; 248:C550–C556.

29. Smith EF III, Lefer AM, Nicolaou KC: Mechanism of coronary vasoconstriction induced by carbocyclic thromboxane A_2. *Am J Physiol* 1981; 240:H493–H497.

30. Feldman RL, Pepine CJ, Conti CR: Magnitude of dilatation of large and small coronary arteries by nitroglycerin. *Circulation* 1981; 64:324–333.

31. McGregor M: The nitrates and myocardial ischemia. *Circulation* 1982; 66:689–692.

32. Angus JA, Brazenor RM, Le Duc MA: Responses of dog large coronary arteries to constrictor and dilator substances: Implications for the cause and treatment of variant angina pectoris. *Am J Cardiol* 1983; 52:52A–60A.

33. Hossack KF, Brown BG, Stewart DK, et al: Diltiazem-induced blockade of sympathetically mediated constriction of normal and diseased coronary arteries: Lack of epicardial coronary dilatory effect in humans. *Circulation* 1984; 70:465–471.

34. Gunther S, Green L, Muller JE, et al: Prevention by nifedipine of abnormal coronary vasoconstriction in patients with coronary artery disease. *Circulation* 1981; 63:849–855.

35. Gross GJ, Warltier DC: Coronary steal in four models of single or multiple vessel obstruction in dogs. *Am J Cardiol* 1981; 48:84–92.

36. Santamore WP, Kent RL, Carey RA, et al: Synergistic effects of pressure, distal resistance, and vasoconstriction on stenosis. *Am J Physiol* 1982; 243:H236–H242.

37. Sill JC, Bove AA, Nugent M, et al: Effects of isoflurane on proximal and distal coronary vasculature in intact dogs. *Anesthesiology* 1985; 63:A11.

38. Freedman B, Richmond DR, Kelly DT: Pathophysiology of coronary artery spasm. *Circulation* 1982; 66:705–709.

39. Kalsner S, Richards R: Coronary arteries of cardiac patients are hyperreactive and contain stores of amines: A mechanism for coronary spasm. *Science* 1984; 223:1435–1437.

40. Ricci DR, Orlick AE, Doherty PW, et al: Reduction of coronary blood flow during coronary artery spasm occurring spontaneously and after provocation by ergonovine maleate. *Circulation* 1978; 57:392–395.

41. Antman E, Muller J, Goldberg S, et al: Nifedipine therapy for coronary-artery spasm. *N Engl J Med* 1980; 302:1269–1273.

42. Johnson SM, Mauritson DR, Willerson JT, et al: A controlled trial of verapamil for Prinzmetal's variant angina. *N Engl J Med* 1981; 304:862–866.

32

Development of Ischemic Electrocardiographic Changes During Monitoring Procedures

A 62-year-old, 65-kg man had a history of severe three-vessel coronary disease and unstable angina. Sixty minutes prior to coming to the induction room, he was premedicated with diazepam 10 mg orally, morphine 7 mg intramuscularly (IM), and scopolamine 0.3 mg IM. On arrival, he complained of chest pain and the ECG showed 2-mm ST elevation in lead II.

Recommendations by Carolyn J. Wilkinson, M.D.

ANALYSIS OF THE PROBLEM

The development of ischemia prior to anesthesia induction necessitates prompt action since it is possible that prolonged ischemia may lead to infarction.

APPROACH TO THE PROBLEM

Time is important: decreasing the duration of ischemia is the goal. Specific steps are: (1) reassurance and patient comfort; (2) electrocardiograph (ECG) monitoring; (3) pharmacologic treatment to decrease myocardial O_2 consumption and optimize supply; (4) establishment of venous access; and (5) a decision regarding the necessity to institute further invasive monitoring while the patient is awake.

DISCUSSION

Background

Although the death rate from coronary artery disease is declining, presumably because of changes in lifestyle, new drugs, and the use of high technology in the diagnosis and treatment of cardiac disease, it is unclear whether the incidence of myocardial infarctions is also declining. In recent years, however, anesthesiologists have accepted increasing responsibility for limiting ischemia and infarction in patients requiring coronary artery bypass operations.

Data from the Texas Heart Institute have shown a threefold increase in perioperative myocardial infarction when ischemia was documented before cardiopulmonary bypass.[1] These data also showed for the first time a significant difference among anesthesiologists in frequency of postinduction ischemia and perioperative myocardial infarction.

In 1912, James Herrick pointed out in his classic article on "Clinical Features of Sudden Obstruction of the Coronary Arteries"[2] that although permanent occlusion of a coronary artery might cause myocardial infarction, it did not always cause death. He also emphasized the need for a classification of patients into subgroups of coronary artery disease with the hope of employing more rational therapy. It was not until 1980, however, that DeWood showed objective angiographic evidence of total coronary occlusion in almost 90% of patients during the first few hours after onset of symptoms of acute transmural myocardial infarction.[3] He also showed a lesser frequency of total obstruction when angiographic studies were performed 12 to 24 hours after onset of symptoms. This finding suggests that temporary stasis with either coronary spasm or thrombus formation with subsequent recannulation or both may occur in a substantial number of patients with transmural infarction.

We have now learned to analyze coronary artery disease according to clinical subsets (chronic stable angina, unstable angina, Printzmetal's angina, etc.) and realize that treatment cannot be stated in general terms. The prognosis is worse for some subsets than for others.

We can further analyze ischemic syndromes by considering the electrocardiogram. It must be remembered that ischemia, as an electrocardiographic term, refers to myocardial cellular changes that may not necessarily result from decreased blood supply. Although ST-segment depression and T-wave inversion are nonspecific electrocardiographic changes indicating possible ischemia, these same changes may occur with electrolyte imbalance, pericardial disease, and digitalis therapy. The ST-segment elevation is more ominous and represents transmural myocardial injury, with obstruction or spasm of large epicardial coronary arteries. Evidence of a new Q wave or elevation of myocardial specific isoenzyme, CK-MB, implies an infarction has occurred. Significant subendocardial ischemia is defined as greater than 1 mm of horizontal or downsloping ST-segment depression measured at a point 0.06 seconds from the J-point. Elevation of ST-segments greater than 1 mm indicates significant transmural ischemia.

Anatomical severity of coronary artery disease is the most important factor predisposing to myocardial infarction and death. The term, "severe triple-vessel disease," implies greater than 75% cross-sectional narrowing of the three major coronary arteries. "Unstable angina" is a clinical syndrome of new onset or increased frequency or duration of ischemia chest pain. Its sequelae are intermediate between chronic stable angina and acute myocardial infarction. During pain, the ECG may show transient ST-T wave changes indicating ischemia or ST elevation indicating spasm or injury. These changes return to baseline when the pain disappears or necrosis occurs. Although tissue necrosis may occur in patients with unstable angina, it is of insufficient amount to be detected by present clinical tests.

To be effective, therapeutic interventions must reduce the determinants of myocardial oxygen consumption (heart rate, contractility, and wall tension) and increase oxygen supply (coronary blood flow). For the sake of discussion, we will assume the above patient has good ventricular function but continuous, unremitting pain. An organized and immediate plan of appropriate management is imperative.

Evaluation and Management

Reassurance by an attentive, sympathetic physician or nurse may be just as important as drugs in relieving the patient's anxiety. If the ambient temperature is cold, warm blankets will help make the patient comfortable, but they are of little value in reducing the increased oxygen consumption induced by shivering. Excitement should be avoided but surgeons and perfusionists should be alerted to the change in the patient's status. While reassuring and talking with the patient, the anesthesiologist should look for clinical signs of pallor, sweating, or shortness of breath and at the same time apply a blood pressure cuff and electrocardiographic leads. An assistant must be available. One individual, while carefully observing electrocardiographic and hemodynamic changes, should administer oxygen, narcotics, and the necessary vasoactive or antiarrhythmic drugs, while the other inserts intravenous and arterial catheters for infusions and monitoring. The blood pressure, heart rate, and rhythm should be noted and a complete ECG tracing (seven-lead) should be quickly reviewed. Anterior-lateral wall ischemia implies involvement of a large area of myocardium vital for pumping. Bundle-branch block and premature ventricular contractions may be associated findings. Prognosis is better if signs of inferior ischemia are present because the apical or undersurface of the heart involves a smaller area of myocardium for pumping. If ischemia develops in the area supplied by the right coronary artery, sinus node dysfunction and atrioventricular block may occur.

Severe bradyarrhythmia, with atrioventricular block and hypotension, may necessitate insertion of a pacing pulmonary cathether. Depending upon the hemodynamic state, narcotics should be given for pain relief as soon as possible. Local anesthesia must be used when catheters are inserted. Although celerity is important, the anesthesiologist with an overzealous interest in or anxiety about the technical aspects of radial and pulmonary arterial catheterization must not forge ahead with these procedures and cause undue pain and anxiety for the patient.

Placing the patient in the Trendelenburg position during the insertion of central venous catheters may precipitate or aggravate preexisiting pulmonary edema. This position may be deleterious to a patient with angina because it increases preload, which may cause an increase in myocardial oxygen demand. Rao et al. reported a substantial reduction in perioperative myocardial reinfarction in patients undergoing noncardiac surgery: they implied that the use of aggressive monitoring with pulmonary artery catheterization leading to early detection and treatment of hemodynamic alterations was responsible for this benefit.[4] There are no data indicating that the insertion of a pulmonary artery catheter prior to anesthesia decreases (or increases) the hazards of ischemia in patients with unstable angina. Although we recommend its insertion prior to anesthesia, in some circumstances, it may be better judgment to proceed with anesthesia and insert the catheter after the patient is asleep.

Hemodynamic stabilization and amelioration of acute myocardial ischemia is now a possible goal. Any intervention that attains these goals is likely to be clinically beneficial. The following are some of the adjuvants to be considered in the care of a patient with symptoms and electrocardiographic findings of an impending myocardial infarction:

Time

"Tincture of time" in the conventional sense is to be avoided. Effectiveness of drugs in limiting ischemia and necrosis seems to correlate inversely with the time of application after the onset of ischemia.[5,6] Although not a drug, time is of the essence and may have an important influence on outcome.

Oxygen

Arterial hypoxemia is present in many patients with ischemic heart disease, presumably because of imbalance in ventilation perfusion ratios resulting from left ventricular failure. Although there is little clinical evidence that patients with normal arterial oxygen saturation benefit from an increase in whole blood oxygen content by 0.3% for each 100 mm Hg increase in arterial

PO_2, there is some evidence that administering oxygen to attain arterial oxygen tensions above the normal physiologic range may decrease myocardial ischemia in dogs with an evolving myocardial infarction.[7] Administration of oxygen is the standard of care and every effort should thus be made to restore arterial oxygen saturation to normal. Certainly, hypoxia, shock, and respiratory depression are indications for its use.

Narcotics

Narcotics should be administered as soon as possible after hemodynamic stability is established. Although morphine does not have a pronounced effect on the myocardium, it may produce hypotension in patients with acute myocardial infarction by decreasing arteriolar resistance and increasing venous capacitance. Meperidine has a myocardial depressant effect in addition to vagolytic effects that may cause a deleterious increase in ventricular rate in patients with atrial flutter or fibrillation. Fentanyl or its analogues, sufentanil and alfentanil, may be appropriate choices for relief of pain, although bradycardia and hypotension are not uncommon after their administration. The combination of diazepam and fentanyl may precipitate significant hypotension in patients with a compromised ventricle.

Nitroglycerin

Intravenous nitroglycerin requires careful hemodynamic and electrocardiographic monitoring. It is almost always used in the management of unstable angina. The mechanism of its beneficial effect is believed to be an increase in collateral blood flow to the ischemic myocardial area and a reduction in myocardial oxygen demand, secondary to a decrease in left ventricular wall tension. Since spasm of a major coronary artery may be present in some patients, a coronary vasodilator like nitroglycerin may produce favorable effect on flow, myocardial ischemia, and infarct size. The response of ischemia is variable depending on the hemodynamic state of the patient and the dose of nitroglycerin. Although it may be ineffective in decreasing ST-segment elevation in some patients with severe coronary artery spasm, it may decrease the accompanying hypertension.

Nitroprusside

The effects of intravenous nitroprusside are also closely related to the hemodynamic status of the patient. Chiariello et al. found that nitroprusside actually augmented ST-segment elevations in the nonfailing ischemic heart.[8] His work suggests that a "coronary steal" may divert flow from a maximally dilated ischemic area of myocardium to vessels that supply normal myocardium and can be vasodilated. Parenterally administered vasodilators (other than nitrates) may intensify acute ischemic injury when given after the onset of an infarction. There is little evidence that they limit infarct size and should be avoided unless specifically indicated. Nitroprusside is most often used in the management of left ventricular failure when systemic hypertension complicates infarction. In this circumstance, cardiac output and peripheral vascular resistance must be calculated before nitroprusside can be rationally used.

Calcium-Channel Blocking Agents

Agents that reduce the flux of calcium across the cell membrane may protect the ischemic myocardium by enhancing collateral blood flow to the ischemic zone, alleviating coronary spasm, reducing myocardial oxygen demand, and protecting ischemic cells from the harmful effects of entry of calcium.

Nifedipine is the calcium-channel blocker of choice and appears to have hemodynamic effects in acute infarction similar to other vasodilators, causing increases in cardiac output and decrease in systemic vascular resistance. An intravenous form is still unavailable. If the capsule is broken, it can be administered nasally or sublingually. Care must be taken to avoid hypotension if the patient is receiving other vasodilators.

β-Adrenergic Blocking Agents

In the absence of left ventricular failure, heart block, asthma, or other contraindications, propranolol has been used to reduce heart rate, arterial pressure, and (myocardial) contractility. Although the negative chronotropic and inotropic effects of β-blockers may reduce myocardial oxygen consumption and improve oxygen supply in an ischemic zone of myocardium, their use is not advocated as standard therapy in the treatment of acute myocardial ischemia or injury. Propranolol has been reported to increase symptoms of myocardial ischemia in patients with coronary artery spasm by allowing more intense α-adrenergic vasoconstriction when β-receptors are blocked.[8] Esmolol, a new, experimental β-blocker, with a shorter duration of action, may prove to be of value in managing hypertension or tachycardia in these patients.

Intra-aortic Balloon Counterpulsation

The need for insertion of the intra-aortic balloon immediately prior to surgery is questionable. Although deflation of the balloon during systole will reduce the afterload on the left ventricle and diastolic inflation will increase arterial and coronary perfusion pressure (thereby improving the oxygen supply-demand ratio and affecting acutely ischemic myocardium favorably), immediate surgery, institution of cardiopulmonary bypass, and reperfusion of the heart is preferable.

Inotropic Agents

Stimulation of myocardial contractility and acceleration of heart rate are not desirable during myocardial ischemia. The overall effect of inotropes on ischemic injury, however, will depend on the net changes in the balance of myocardial oxygen supply and demand. They should be reserved for patients with evidence of pump failure and used to ensure coronary and cerebral blood flow.

Summary

A clearer picture of the pathophysiology, clinical course, and modes of therapy for unstable angina has evolved in the last ten years. With recent evidence that spasm may be an important physiologic mechanism and that necrosis may occur in some of these patients, new challenges confront the anesthesiologist. Perioperative myocardial ischemia does lead to postoperative transmural myocardial infarction. The anesthesiologist has the responsibility to prevent it by appropriate monitoring and therapeutic intervention.

REFERENCES

1. Slogoff S, Keats AS: Does perioperative myocardial ischemia lead to postoperative transmural myocardial infarction? *Anesthesiology* 1985; 62:107–114.
2. Herrick JB: Clinical features of sudden obstruction of the coronary arteries. *JAMA* 1912; 59:2015–2020.
3. DeWood MA, Spores J, Notske R, et al: Prevalence of total coronary occlusion during the early hours of transmural myocardial infarction. *N Engl J Med* 1980; 303:897–902.
4. Rao TK, Jacobs KH, El-Etra AA: Reinfarction following anesthesia in patients with myocardial infarction. *Anesthesiology* 1983; 59:499–505.
5. Kaplan JA: Nitroglycerin infusion during coronary artery surgery. *Anesthesiology* 1976; 45:14–21.
6. Yusef S, Ramsdale D, Peto R: Early intravenous atenolol in suspected acute myocardial infarction. *Br Med J* 1975; 1:117–119.
7. Maroko PR, Radvany P, Braunwald E, et al: Reduction of infarct size by oxygen inhalation following acute coronary occlusion. *Circulation* 1975; 52:360–368.
8. Chiariello M, Gold HK, Robert CL, et al: Comparison between the effects of nitroprusside and nitroglycerin on ischemic injury during acute myocardial infarction. *Circulation* 1976; 54:766–773.
9. Yasue H, Omote S, Takizawa A, et al: Pathogenesis and treatment of angina pectoris at rest as seen from its response to various drugs. *Jpn Circ J* 1978; 42:1.

33

Bronchospasm in Patient With Coronary Artery Bypass Graft

A 45-year-old man with an apparent history of asthma underwent three-vessel coronary artery bypass grafting. He had an uneventful induction; anesthesia consisted of fentanyl, pancuronium, and enflurane. As the surgeon was preparing the aorta for cannulation, he found that the lungs were in his way. Compliance was significantly decreased. The value for Pa_{O_2} was 190 with fraction of inspired oxygen (FIO_2) of 1.0 and the Pa_{CO_2} was 60. Hemodynamics were normal.

Recommendations by Richard E. Buckingham, Jr., M.D.

ANALYSIS OF THE PROBLEM

Bronchospasm occurring during general anesthesia, while not commonly seen, does occur and may present the anesthesiologist with both diagnostic and therapeutic problems. In the majority of the cases, the diagnosis is easily made and the problem relatively easily treated. Patients undergoing cardiac surgery may be somewhat more likely to develop bronchospasm because of drugs that they have been taking to treat their cardiac problems, i.e., β-adrenergic blockers. Also, cardiac patients developing bronchospasm while under anesthesia will present more difficult management problems because of the interaction between the drugs used to treat this condition and the cardiovascular system.

Before any therapy can be initiated, the problem must be defined. A decrease in pulmonary compliance and the retention of CO_2 can have many

265

causes. Mechanical causes of the patient's difficulties should be ruled out. These include kinked endotracheal tube, mainstem bronchus intubation, bevel of the endotracheal tube against the tracheal wall, cuff over-inflated, cuff herniated over the end of the tube, mucus plug, secretions, foreign bodies in the airway, etc. Stiffness of the chest wall secondary to light anesthesia or inadequate muscle relaxation should be ruled out. Tension pneumothorax should also be in the differential diagnosis as it can mimic bronchospasm. In the absence of a mechanical problem (or problems), air trapping and wheezing are enough to make the diagnosis of bronchospasm. However, it should be kept in mind that wheezing is a noise made by turbulent air flow and that if the bronchospasm is quite severe, there may be so little air flow that the wheezes generated are not loud enough to be heard through the chest or esophageal stethoscope.

In order to understand bronchospasm, we must look at the factors and drugs that affect bronchiolar tone. As with most other systems of the body, there exists a homeostatic mechanism responsible for the muscle tone in the walls of the bronchi, the tone of which ultimately determines the caliber of the lumen. Under normal conditions this tone is controlled by the autonomic nervous system, with parasympathetic and α-adrenergic stimulation causing bronchoconstriction, while β-adrenergic stimulation (specifically β_2) causes bronchodilatation. These effects are mediated through cyclic adenosine monophosphate (cAMP) and cyclic guanosine monophosphate (cGMP) as shown in Figure 33–1. β_2-Stimulation increases the amount of cAMP by enhancing the action of the enzyme, adenyl cyclase. α-Adrenergic stimulation has an inhibitory effect on adenyl cyclase. Cholinergic stimulation increases cGMP, which causes bronchoconstriction. Substances such as histamine and slow-reacting substance of anaphylaxis (SRS-A) can act directly on bronchi to cause bronchoconstriction without going through cAMP or cGMP. Finally, the diameter of the lumen can also be affected by other factors besides bronchiolar muscular tone such as edema of the mucosal cells lining the bronchi. Table 33–1 lists the factors and drugs responsible for bronchodilatation as well as likely mechanisms, while Table 33–2 lists the factors and drugs likely to cause bronchoconstriction with probable mechanisms.

Knowing what causes bronchoconstriction enables the clinician to take steps to avoid this management problem, and knowledge of bronchodilatation enables him to deal with the constriction of the airway, should it occur.

Anesthesiologists are usually alerted to the possibility of bronchospasm by hearing wheezes through the esophageal stethoscope, by observing that the lungs tend to remain inflated (or having the surgeon point this out), and/or by noticing that the inspiratory pressure necessary to ventilate the patient has increased. Occasionally deteriorating blood gases may be the first clue. Once there is suspicion that ventilation is compromised, a diagnostic routine should be initiated.

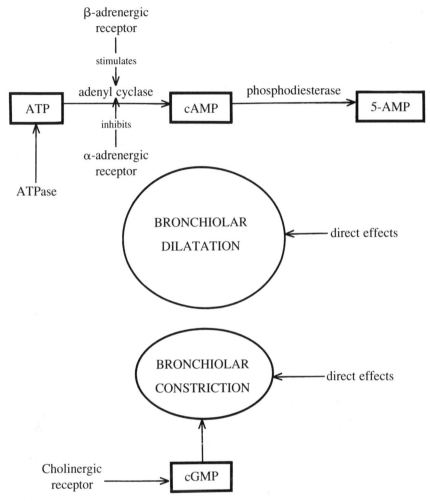

FIG 33–1.
Factors and drugs that affect bronchiolar tone. Under normal conditions, tone is controlled by the autonomic nervous system, with parasympathetic and α-adrenergic stimulation causing bronchoconstriction, while β-adrenergic stimulation causes bronchodilatation. These effects are mediated through cyclic adenosine monophosphate (cAMP) and cyclic guanosine monophosphate (cGMP). ATP = adenosine triphosphate.

APPROACH TO THE PROBLEM

The first things to be done include making a rapid observation of the surgical field (especially if the chest is open) and disconnecting the patient from the ventilator, switching to the "bag and educated hand" method of ventilation.

TABLE 33–1.

Bronchodilatation

FACTOR OR DRUG	MECHANISM
Sympathetic nervous system	Increases adenyl cyclase activity
Metabolic products CO_2 Lactic acid	Relax bronchiolar musculature (direct effect)
β_2-agonists Epinephrine Isoproterenol Ephedrine Terbutaline Metaproterenol Isoetharine Albuterol	Increase adenyl cyclase activity
Muscarinic cholinergic blockers Atropine Scopolamine	Block formation of cGMP
α-adrenergic blockers Phentolamine Phenoxybenzamine	Block inhibitory effect of α-stimulation on adenyl cyclase (same effect as stimulating adenyl cyclase)
Methylxanthines Caffeine Theobromine Theophylline Aminophylline	Increase cAMP by inhibiting its breakdown by phosphodiesterese
Steroids Prednisolone Hydrocortisone Methylprednisolone Prednisone Beclomethasone	Enhance sympathetic effects; block ATPase, thereby allowing more ATP to be available to form cAMP; block mediator release from mast cells, and decrease edema formation
Cromolyn sodium	Blocks mediator release (most effective if given before insult occurs)
Prostaglandins E_1 and E_2	Increase adenyl cyclase activity
Lidocaine (nebulized)	Blocks local reflexes
Inhaled general anesthetics Diethyl ether Halothane	Relax bronchiolar musculature (direct effect) and block local reflexes
Ketamine	Sympathetic stimulation

TABLE 33–2.

Bronchoconstriction

FACTOR OR DRUG	MECHANISM
Parasympathetic nervous system	Increases cGMP activity
α-adrenergic nervous system	Inhibits adenyl cyclase
Brain stem reflexes	Increase cGMP activity
Local reflexes	Increase cGMP activity

α-agonists
  Acetylcholine
  Pilocarpine
  Carbachol
	Inhibit adenyl cyclase

β-blockers
  Propranolol
  Metoprolol
	Decrease adenyl cyclase activity

Muscarinic cholinomimetics
  Neostigmine
  Pyridostigmine
  Physostigmine
  Edrophonium
	Increase cGMP activity

Mast-cell mediators
  Serotonin
  SRS-A
  Histamine
  Kinins
	Act directly on the bronchiolar musculature

Histamine-releasing drugs
  Morphine
  Meperidine
  D-tubocurarine
  Trimethaphan
  Metocurine
	Release histamine that acts directly on the bronchiolar musculature

Vagomimetic drugs
  Thiopentone
  Phenylephrine
  Methoxamine
	Increase cGMP activity

Prostaglandins F_{2a} and D_2	Inhibit adenyl cyclase

From this we will be able to ascertain:

1. Are the surgeons doing something that might be causing the problem?

2. Has the inspiratory pressure necessary to ventilate the patient increased?

3. Does the bag fill slowly on exhalation?

4. If exhalation is retarded by maintaining a positive pressure on the bag, is more complete and rapid emptying of the lungs obtained?

5. Do the lungs look as if they are trapping air?

While ventilating by hand, both sides of the patient's chest should be auscultated and the sounds compared with those heard after intubation. The presence or absence of wheezes and/or rhonchi should be noted. Air should be removed from the endotracheal tube cuff and the breath sounds checked. The tube should be suctioned to assure patency and to make sure that the problem is not simply one of secretions in the trachea either causing the problem directly or being the initiating irritant in reflex bronchospasm.

Another problem to be considered is "light" anesthesia or inadequate muscle relaxation, i.e., the patient is "fighting." In its simplest form, light anesthesia or inadequate muscle relaxation can be thought of as a "mechanical problem." The gases are not going in and out of the patient's tracheal-bronchial tree because he is resisting. An additional dose of a muscle relaxant will eliminate this cause while at the same time aid in making the diagnosis. A more difficult problem is bronchospasm brought on by "light" anesthesia. This will be discussed later.

This rapid diagnostic routine will rule out mechanical causes of respiratory difficulties. In the absence of mechanical problems, air trapping and wheezing are enough to make the diagnosis of bronchospasm, and the clinician can then proceed with definitive therapy.

There are many ways of treating bronchospasm under anesthesia. There is no "right" way or preferred way. As there can be many different precipitating causes of bronchospasm, so too can there be many different responses to therapy. Successful relief of the bronchospasm is the measure of a good method of treatment.

First, we must rule out bronchospasm brought on by light anesthesia. This is reflex bronchospasm caused by local stimulation of the upper or lower airway, traction on the hilum of the lung, or more complicated reflexes such as those from coronary or pulmonary vessels or from the carotid sinus. The easiest way of eliminating this cause is to deepen the anesthesia with a dose of fentanyl. Of course, once initiated, bronchospasm may not disappear with removal of the precipitating factor. In other words, light anesthesia may have caused the bronchospasm but more definitive therapy will be required to eliminate it. But, if the wheezing does disappear, then we have not only treated the patient but made the diagnosis.

If we still have evidence of bronchospasm, our treatment should include placing the patient on 100% O_2 and humidifying the inspired gas. Possible irritants or precipitating causes should be eliminated. Suctioning the endotracheal tube, as mentioned in our diagnostic routine, may have already initiated therapy by getting rid of reflex-inducing irritant material from within the trachea. This should be repeated as necessary. Any inhalational anesthetic should be discontinued, as all of them have been reported to cause bronchospasm on occasion. If the patient is not receiving halothane (the general anesthetic of choice for asthmatics), it can be started provided that the cardiovascular status is stable enough to tolerate it. Atropine and lidocaine can either be given intravenously or nebulized into the anesthesia circuit in order to block cholinergic-mediated bronchoconstriction and local reflexes. A β_2-agonist can be instilled directly into the anesthesia circuit from a pressurized cartridge, [1] i.e., isoproterenol or isoetharine. If no response is seen, aminophylline 3 to 5 mg/kg should be started in a rapid infusion (over a 20-minute period) in order to reach a rapid blood level. Steroids can then be administered intravenously, even if the bronchospasm is starting to show signs of abating.

The technique for treating bronchospasm under anesthesia is much the same as treating asthma in the unanesthetized patient; the clinician keeps trying different therapies until the bronchospasm is broken. The treatment cascade described here can be stopped at the time that the wheezing and air trapping disappear.

DISCUSSION

Cardiac anesthesiologists treat patients who may be more apt to develop bronchospasm. Left-sided heart failure with its associated interstitial edema may already have the patient compromised and suffering from "cardiac asthma." Cardiac patients are frequently taking β-blockers that make them more susceptible to bronchospasm. Heart surgery requires the use of an endotracheal tube, which is probably the most potent stimulus to bronchospasm unleashed by the anesthesiologist. Coronary bypass patients in particular tend to be older and frequently have a smoking history, thus, they tend to have chronic lung disease and/or an irritable bronchial tree from chronic bronchitis.

Cardiac anesthesiologists face limitations that usually do not concern other physicians treating asthma or other anesthesiologists treating intraoperative bronchospasm. These limitations focus on the heart, which may be failing, have a compromised blood supply, and/or be electrophysiologically irritable. One of the hallmarks of therapy in the asthmatic is the administration of a catecholamine such as epinephrine or a more selective β_2-agonist. Giving a drug that may increase blood pressure and/or heart rate in cardiac patients may be contraindicated. Added to this is the increased likelihood of arrhythmias in cardiac patients, especially if the patients are receiving halothane anesthesia.

Other drugs useful in the treatment of asthma such as atropine have cardiac effects that may be undesirable.

Prevention of bronchospasm is probably the easiest form of treatment. During the preanesthetic visit, information can be obtained about asthma, seasonal allergies, smoking, chronic bronchitis, and heart failure that will put the anesthesiologist on his guard. If it is possible without affecting the patient's cardiac problems, discontinuation of β-blockers should be considered in susceptible patients in order to make them less prone to developing intraoperative bronchospasm. In patients who are having elective procedures, it may be possible to delay their surgery until an acute infection has subsided or until the patient has had time to benefit from a "stop-smoking" program. Patients with chronic lung disease may benefit from pulmonary medicine consultation, chest physiotherapy, therapy with intermittent positive pressure breathing etc. provided that their surgery is not of an urgent nature. The patient may be treated with a bronchodilator and should certainly be started on incentive spirometry prior to surgery.

If an asthmatic history is obtained, the anesthesiologist should be well aware of the psychological factors involved in this disease and should provide reassurance and psychological support in order to decrease the likelihood of a susceptible patient coming into the operating room. Naturally, premedication can be just as important in this respect. Because of its histamine- releasing effects, morphine should be avoided. Atropine decreases airway resistance and blocks cholinergic bronchoconstriction. An antihistamine can be added to the preoperative medications to protect against histamine-induced bronchospasm as well as to provide additional sedation.

Cromolyn sodium, a drug that inhibits the release of mediators from mast cells can be given prior to surgery. This drug, which comes in powder form, is now much easier to prescribe as inhalers are now available with the powder suspended in the propellant.

As previously mentioned, we should think of bronchospasm occurring during anesthesia in many of the same ways that we would think of asthma in the unanesthetized individual. While anesthesiologists do have the disadvantage of doing many things to a patient that may precipitate bronchospasm, they do have one advantage—no psychological factors to treat once the patient is anesthetized, i.e., the anesthesiologist need only worry about pathology, physiology, and pharmacology.

There are many treatment modalities in asthma, all having a logical basis for their use. The individual physician develops a progression of treatment modalities based on his experience and keeps on adding additional modes of therapy until the bronchospasm is broken. With some patients, the first treatment tried may solve the problem; with others, several therapies or combinations of therapies may be used before the bronchospasm ends. A physician's experience will dictate what therapies he uses, in what order, and for what length of time before trying something different. To further complicate matters, what works in one patient may not work in another, so it is a good idea to have many methods of treatment in one's armamentarium.

One form of therapy that was popular in years past but has now "fallen by the wayside" is the use of helium in the inspired mixture. The use of helium as a therapeutic gas[2] was first proposed by Barach in 1938. In the same year Eversole discussed the experience of the Lahey Clinic using helium in anesthesia.[3] In 1946, Doll[4] discussed the use of helium in treating asthmatics. Even as late as 1954, helium was being advocated by Green and Day for use in patients with respiratory obstruction.[5] Why do we now find no references to helium in modern anesthesia texts? The two most likely reasons are: (1) Helium is entirely inert; the basis for its clinical use depends on its physical properties of low specific gravity and rapid rate of diffusion. Early advocates of the use of helium failed to take into consideration that in streamlined or laminar flow, it is *viscosity* that is important, and the viscosity of a mixture containing 80% helium and 20% oxygen is 1.11 compared with 1.00 for air. Therefore, helium mixtures offer no advantage whatsoever until the flow becomes turbulent. Once turbulent flow is initiated, it is the *density* of the gas that is important. The mixture of helium and oxygen is one third as dense as air. If there was not enough turbulence, then helium would offer no advantage, and physicians using it would become disenchanted with its use. (2) Physicians like to "cure" disease states with some active form of treatment. Helium does not treat the underlying condition causing the patient's respiratory difficulties. It may get more oxygen into the alveoli and more CO_2 out, but over the years, physicians have preferred to diagnose a medical problem and then administer something that acts directly on that condition. Helium, while perhaps helping the patient's ventilation and gas exchange did not treat the disease and, therefore, lost its appeal to physicians trained more and more to intervene in the disease process. In other words, helium does have something to offer the patient who develops bronchospasm under anesthesia, but it should be considered as an adjunct—something to buy some time while more definitive measures are undertaken.

Diethyl ether is considered the best general anesthetic for relaxing bronchial smooth muscle, but, unfortunately, it is not available for safe use in open heart surgery. Enflurane has been recommended for use in bronchospasm, but there are reports of its causing the condition.[6] Halothane is probably the agent of choice in the asthmatic patient.[7] The important thing to remember is that any anesthetic may precipitate bronchospasm, so unless the clinician can be sure that the bronchospasm is in response to "light" anesthesia (in which case, he would want to deepen it), it is best to discontinue the agent being used and try something else.

If the clinician is going to discontinue inhalational general anesthesia, a switch to ketamine presents some interesting possibilities for the cardiac anesthesiologist. It has been touted for bronchospasm[8] and has no myocardial depressant effects. However, the increase in heart rate and blood pressure seen with this drug might contraindicate its use in borderline compensated cardiac patients.

A most interesting way of treating bronchospasm occurring while the patient is under anesthesia was first proposed by Gold in 1975.[9] He used an isoproterenol (Isuprel) inhaler inserted into a ''T'' piece connected between the endotracheal tube and the anesthesia circuit. This arrangement would lend itself to the administration of almost all of the β_2 drugs that are available in aerosol form for asthmatics. Also available in this form are steroids, i.e., beclomethasone.

From this discussion, it is obvious that there are many different drugs available to us for the treatment of bronchoconstriction. Anesthesiologists, especially those doing cardiac cases, should not only be aware of the type of patient who is likely to develop bronchospasm under anesthesia but also of what drugs and interventions may precipitate this condition. They should understand the pathology, physiology, and pharmacology involved in order to make intelligent interventions into the process. Finally, anesthesiologists should be familiar with many different treatment modalities so that if one does not work, another can be tried, because, in the final analysis, whatever works is the ''drug of choice.''

REFERENCES

1. Gold MI: A convenient and accurate nebulizer. *Anesthesiology* 1967; 28:1102–1103.
2. Barach AL: Use of helium as a new therapeutic gas. *Proc Soc Exp Biol Med* 1938; 32:462–464.
3. Eversole UH: The use of helium in anesthesia. *JAMA* 1938; 110:878–880.
4. Doll R: Helium in the treatment of asthma. *Thorax* 1946; 1:30–38.
5. Green R, Day BL: Preoperative administration of helium in respiratory obstruction. *Lancet* 1954; 266:602–603.
6. Lowry CJ, Fielden BP: Bronchospasm associated with enflurane exposure: Three case reports. *Anaesth Intensive Care* 1976; 4:254–258.
7. Gold MI: Anesthesia for the asthmatic patient. *Anesth Analg* 1970; 49:881–888.
8. Rajanna P, Reddy JN, Gupta PK: Ketamine for the relief of bronchospasm during anesthesia. *Anaesthesia* 1982; 37:1215.
9. Gold MI: Treatment of bronchospasm during anesthesia. *Anesth Analg* 1975; 54:783–786.

34

Patient With Full Stomach, Failed Angioplasty for Acute Myocardial Infarction

Immediately following dinner one evening, a 60-year-old executive suffered an acute myocardial infarction. At cardiac catheterization an occluded left anterior descending coronary artery could not be opened by balloon angioplasty. Chest pain persisted, and the electrocardiogram continued to show changes compatible with acute myocardial infarction. The patient was scheduled to have emergency coronary artery bypass surgery.

Recommendations by Daniel M. Thys, M.D., and Fred Kahan, M.D.

ANALYSIS OF THE PROBLEM

This case represents a "new" type of emergency, the anesthetic management of a patient requiring revascularization who has an acute myocardial infarction with a full stomach.

APPROACH TO THE PROBLEM

Appropriate monitoring consists of ECG, radial artery and pulmonary artery catheterization, and, after induction, transesophageal echocardiography. A rapid-sequence induction with airway precautions should be employed. The specific agents for this are discussed below.

DISCUSSION

General Considerations

In recent years, a better understanding of the pathophysiology of acute myocardial infarctions (AMI) has led to the introduction of a variety of new therapeutic approaches. It is now well established that, in most patients, acute transmural infarctions are caused by coronary thrombi, usually located in close proximity to atherosclerotic plaques. The mechanisms by which thrombosis occurs have not yet been completely elucidated, but degeneration of atherosclerotic intima with exposure of collagen and platelet activation is a likely explanation. It remains unclear whether or not coronary spasm is important in the evolution from coronary atherosclerosis to acute myocardial infarction.[1]

The prognosis in patients with AMI is primarily determined by two major factors:

1. The infarct size, which determines the severity of left ventricular functional impairment.

2. The extent of obstructive lesions in the coronary arteries perfusing the nonischemic viable myocardium.

Conventional therapy of AMI has been aimed at the prevention and treatment of dysrhythmias, the optimization of myocardial O_2 balance by analgesics and β-blockers, and the correction of hemodynamic disturbances. However, even with the application of these therapeutic regimens, the mortality of AMI has remained high, and therefore other management options have been explored.[2]

The search for alternative therapies of AMI was stimulated by numerous animal experiments in which it was shown that ischemic damage was partially reversible. For instance, Reimer et al. demonstrated in dogs that as the duration of coronary artery occlusion increased, a "wave-front" of cell death progressed from subendocardium to subepicardium.[3] If reperfusion was accomplished within 40 minutes after occlusion, 60% to 70% of the area at risk could be salvaged. If, on the other hand, reperfusion was delayed until three hours after occlusion or if microvascular damage was extensive, leading to a "no-reflow phenomenon," salvage of ischemic myocardium was limited.

While in these laboratory experiments the period during which myocardial salvage could be achieved appeared very short, the same was not necessarily true in man. Indeed, since coronary artery disease is a chronic disease, extensive collateral circulation to the ischemic area has usually developed by the time of the myocardial infarction. In addition, not all infarcts result in total coronary occlusion. For these reasons it has been suggested that, in man, myocardial salvage is possible for a period as long as six hours after occlusion.

Four methods are currently in use to achieve myocardial reperfusion in humans; these are discussed below.

Intravenous Thrombolytic Therapy

A number of investigators have attempted to improve coronary perfusion of infarcted myocardium by intravenous administration of large doses of streptokinase (0.5 to 1.5 million units). Success rates with this therapy have greatly varied from study to study (10% to 96%) and have been markedly influenced by a number of methodological factors.[4] Indeed, while in some studies preinfusion angiograms were available, in others they were not. The timing of the postintervention angiography also varied from study to study.

Interpretation of recanalization rates is further complicated by the observation that incomplete obstruction of infarct-related vessels occurs in 5% to 33% of patients and by the fact that a number of spontaneous recanalizations are known to occur.

Complications associated with intravenous infusion of streptokinase are primarily related to bleeding. More recently, the introduction of newer agents with a greater degree of clot selectivity (such as acylated plasmin streptokinase and recombinant tissue plasminogen) has increased the potential of intravenous thrombolytic therapy. In one prospective and randomized clinical trial, results obtained with plasminogen were far superior to those obtained with placebo, while clinically significant fibrinolysis was not elicited in any patient.[5]

Intracoronary Thrombolytic Therapy

Intracoronary infusion of streptokinase or urokinase has been found effective in the recanalization of completely obstructed infarct-related vessels in 60% to 94% of cases.[6] One group of investigators was even able to demonstrate a significant improvement in left ventricular function after recanalization with intracoronary streptokinase.[7] While only a few complications have been attributed to the intervention itself, most are related to the failure of the therapy. Recanalization fails in 20% to 40% of cases, and reocclusion or reinfarction is observed in 20% of patients in whom therapy was initially successful. In addition, myocardial revascularization is often required due to severe residual stenosis or a persistently unstable clinical course.

Angioplasty, Alone or in Combination With Thrombolytic Therapy

The high incidence of recanalization failure and of coronary reocclusion after thrombolytic therapy has led some investigators to combine this therapy with percutaneous transluminal coronary angioplasty (PTCA).[8] More recently, PTCA alone has also been evaluated in the therapy of acute myocardial infarction. In a group of 11 patients, Holmes et al. achieved reperfusion with PTCA alone in 91% of patients.[9] In their small nonrandomized trial, the PTCA success rate compared favorably with the 80%, 82%, and 72% success rates obtained in patients treated with angioplasty followed by streptokinase, streptokinase alone, and streptokinase followed by PTCA, respectively. The authors' conclusion, however, was that angioplasty was particularly helpful in patients with severe residual stenosis after intracoronary administration of streptokinase and in patients in whom streptokinase failed to reopen the occluded artery. Complications related to the use of PTCA during the acute phase of a myocardial infarction include the rupture of plaques secondary to vessel wall trauma or to subintimal hemorrhage. Plaque rupture can possibly result in propagation of thrombi and further myocardial damage.

Surgical Reperfusion

Surgical revascularization to improve myocardial perfusion is the most aggressive therapy in acute myocardial infarction. In a series of 701 patients, DeWood et al. reported a surgical mortality of 5.2% in transmural infarctions and 3% in the nontransmural group.[10] The transmural group was further divided according to the time between onset of symptoms and reperfusion. The early reperfusion group (reperfusion accomplished in less than six hours after onset of symptoms) had a 3.8% mortality versus the late reperfusion group (more than six hours) with an 8% mortality. Similar trends were noted in long-term mortality. These authors advocated surgery as a primary treatment of myocardial infarction since their patients had a lower mortality than those treated by conventional therapy. In their community, the latter group had a mortality rate of 11.5%.

Whether surgery reduces infarct size and improves ventricular function was investigated by Van Haecke et al.[11] They used thallium myocardial scintigraphy and radionuclide ventriculography to assess infarct size and ventricular function in patients who had undergone surgical versus conventional medical treatment of infarctions. At late follow-up (> two months), patients who had early revascularization (< four hours after onset of symptoms) had significantly smaller infarcts and higher ejection fractions than those who underwent late revascularization or medical therapy.

The role of surgical revascularization in the management of the patient with AMI has, however, been challenged by a number of authors. Spencer, in a recent editorial, questioned the scientific value of the data of DeWood and associates and wondered whether the patients survived the AMI because of the surgical intervention or in spite of it.[12]

Less controversial is the use of surgical revascularization in patients with postinfarction angina, a clinical syndrome that suggests extension of the infarct. Nunley et al. reported on 15 patients with postinfarction angina who were operated upon within 24 hours after the AMI.[13] One operative death occurred in this group.

In the present case, angioplasty was selected as the primary method of reperfusion. Whether it was combined with thrombolytic therapy is not obvious from the case report. Unfortunately, angioplasty failed; ischemic changes persisted, and surgery was now urgently required.

The literature contains few reports describing the morbidity and mortality of surgical therapy under similar circumstances. Pelletier et al. have recently related their experience with emergency myocardial revascularization after failure of PTCA.[14] Although a few of their patients had preoperative signs of myocardial infarction, most had undergone elective angioplasty. In their study, coronary occlusion was the most common indication (23 of 35 patients) for emergency surgery, and in most patients the operation was begun within 60 minutes after termination of PTCA. Other indications were arterial wall dissection without occlusion (4 of 35 patients), coronary perforation (1 of 35 patients), and intractable angina without angiographic changes (7 of 35 patients). Of the 13 patients with preoperative signs of myocardial infarction, 6 had a normal electrocardiogram without signs of infarction at the end of the surgery. No intraoperative or postoperative deaths were observed, but in three patients new postoperative myocardial infarctions were diagnosed. Based on these results, Pelletier et al. recommend surgical treatment on an emergency basis following failure of PTCA.

In a different report, Brahos et al. relate their experience with 68 patients requiring urgent (within 24 hours) myocardial revascularization after PTCA.[15] Five patients in this series were operated upon after initial treatment of an AMI with emergency PTCA and streptokinase infusion. All five of these patients survived, but three other patients had cardiac-related deaths manifested by progressive and refractory low-output syndrome.

Brahos and associates further observed that patients undergoing emergency revascularization after failed PTCA had greater requirements for intra-aortic balloon pump support, lidocaine, and inotropic infusions than did a group of patients undergoing surgery on a nonemergent basis. The patients operated upon under emergency circumstances also suffered more postoperative complications.

In conclusion, it appears that surgery can be indicated in the immediate postinfarction period. Whether it has a role to play in the primary treatment of AMI remains to be proved. Current evidence would suggest, however, that if treatment of an AMI with angioplasty alone or in combination with thrombolytic therapy fails, emergency surgical revascularization is of benefit. Under these circumstances, a higher incidence of intraoperative and postoperative complications can be expected.

Patient Evaluation

Initial patient evaluation should begin with a brief review of the history of the present illness and a physical examination. The duration of the anginal symptoms will provide information about reversibility of the myocardial damage and will, to a certain degree, determine the amount of salvage that can be expected after reperfusion. The presence of symptoms or physical findings consistent with failure (bibasilar rales, S_3, jugular venous distention, etc.) and the spread of ST-segment elevation on ECG relate to the extent of myocardial damage already present. Since anterior infarcts frequently give rise to varying degrees of AV block and intraventricular block, the ECG should also carefully be evaluated for evidence of conduction disturbances.

While the patient is still in the catheterization laboratory, his hemodynamic status should be assessed. Heart rate, rhythm, and intra-arterial blood pressure should be measured and a pulmonary artery catheter (a pacing catheter in the presence of conduction disturbances) should be inserted to obtain filling pressures and cardiac output measurements. Prior to transfer of the patient to the operating room, the conventional therapies of AMI should be instituted. These include oxygen administration, analgesics, nitrates, antiarrhythmics, and possibly β-blockers or calcium-channel blocking agents. If hemodynamic instability is present, more aggressive therapy with inotropes and vasodilators should be pursued prior to transfer. In view of our patient's intractable pain, with or without hemodynamic instability, the insertion of an intra-aortic balloon is recommended.[16] During stabilization, a brief review of underlying medical disorders, previous surgical exposure, and laboratory parameters should be performed. Hypertension, diabetes, chronic obstructive lung disease, and peripheral vascular disease frequently coexist with ischemic heart disease and can influence the anesthetic management. Electrolyte disturbances can promote ventricular irritability and should be treated.

If the patient received thrombolytic therapy in combination with the angioplasty, coagulation disturbances may be present and may influence the choice of central venous access routes. While the patient is still in the catheterization suite, 30 ml of 0.3M sodium citrate can be administered orally. There is evidence that even with partially digested foodstuffs, this nonparticulate antacid reduces gastric pH effectively and lessens the extent of pulmonary injury should aspiration occur.[17] Additionally, the patient should receive metoclopramide 10 to 20 mg intravenously (injected slowly to avoid anxiety in the patient), as this has been shown to be effective in reducing gastric volume by increasing gastric motility and emptying.[18,19] The clinician must remember, however, that metoclopramide is a dopamine antagonist and that its use in combination with dopamine is not recommended.

Although cimetidine and anticholinergics have been demonstrated to be effective in decreasing both pH and gastric volume, a slow onset of action is expected with these drugs. They are unlikely to produce much benefit under the existing postprandial conditions. Furthermore, in this patient the clinician should be particularly careful with cimetidine since significant bradyarrhythmias have been reported after its intravenous administration. [20]

Anesthetic Management

Monitoring

As outlined in the previous section, a number of monitoring modalities will already have been applied before arrival in the operating room. Monitoring of the ECG in this patient should consist of lead II and V_5. Elevation of the ST segment in V_5 would be suggestive of lateral extension of the infarct, while ST-segment depression might reflect reciprocal changes or lateral ischemia. Detection of rhythm disturbances will be facilitated by the monitoring of lead II.

Although pulmonary artery catheterization in the present case entails a number of risks, particularly if coagulation is disturbed, the benefits seem to far outweigh the risks. Indeed, hemodynamic instability is to be expected and appropriate treatment with inotropes and vasodilators can only be achieved if essential flow and resistance parameters are known. [21] An additional benefit of the pulmonary artery (PA) catheter might reside in its ability to provide information on ventricular compliance. Indeed, Kaplan et al. have demonstrated that ischemia can be recognized by the appearance of large V waves on the pulmonary capillary wedge tracing before ECG changes have occurred. [22] If a pacing catheter were inserted, it can also be used to record intracardiac ECGs and to trigger the IABP. [23]

In our experience, the most useful monitoring technique to use in this patient with an extending myocardial infarction is undoubtedly two-dimensional transesophageal echocardiography (2D-TEE). Numerous investigators have indeed demonstrated that segmental wall motion abnormalities are sensitive and specific markers of ischemia or infarction. [24] In acute myocardial infarction, it has been demonstrated that the site and extent of wall motion abnormalities are closely related to the hemodynamic implications of the infarct and that they carry a prognostic value during ischemia. [25,26] Wall motion abnormalities have been shown to occur much earlier than ST-segment changes on the ECG, and, after prolonged ischemia, continued hypocontractility of the ischemic segments has been demonstrated even after the ECG changes had subsided. Although the wall motion abnormalities often seem to exceed the extent of the electrocardiographic changes, it is assumed that these abnormalities reflect jeopardized myocardium surrounding the infarct zone.

After intubation, the left ventricle can readily be visualized by a two-dimensional short-axis cut at the level of the papillary muscles. The ventricle can then be divided into a number of segments, and for each segment wall motion and systolic wall thickening can be assessed. If during the procedure abnormal motion or thickening is recognized in previously unaffected segments, a restoration of normal function can be attempted by various therapeutic interventions. An additional benefit of 2D-TEE is that global left ventricular function can roughly be estimated.

Induction and Maintenance

The main objectives during the induction will be to maintain hemodynamic stability and to prevent aspiration by rapid control of the airway. To protect the airway, two options can be considered. The first is to perform an intubation with the patient awake. It is unlikely, however, that in this patient an awake intubation could be achieved without some degree of hemodynamic response in the form of tachycardia or hypertension. Either would be deleterious since they could trigger further perioperative ischemia and increase the size of the infarction.[27] Because it is probable that the patient has already been heavily medicated with analgesics such as morphine while in the catheterization laboratory, the administration of additional intravenous sedation to facilitate the awake intubation would be fraught with hazards. The clinician also hesitates to recommend complete topical anesthesia for the posterior pharynx and larynx since it might compromise the patient's ability to reject a foreign body.

The second option would be to perform a rapid-sequence induction combined with a Sellick's maneuver. Under most circumstances, the airway can adequately be protected by this approach and the crucial question then becomes the choice of anesthetic agents. Thiopental, the traditional rapidly acting induction agent, is probably not the best choice for this particular patient. Although the drug is not a pronounced myocardial depressant, it may cause a significant drop in blood pressure due to its vasodilating properties. Furthermore, its action on the central nervous system might be insufficient to totally blunt the response to laryngoscopy and intubation.

Recently a number of investigators have demonstrated that during rapid-sequence induction the hemodynamic response to intubation could be blunted more effectively by the combination of a low-dose barbiturate with a low-dose narcotic.

Cork et al. have described a rapid-sequence induction technique with 2 mg/kg of thiopental and 5 μg/kg of fentanyl, while Kleinman et al. have studied the combined use of thiamylal 2 mg/kg with 1 or 2 μg/kg of sufentanil.[28,29] We, however, hesitate to recommend this approach for the management of our current patient. Indeed, the technique was only investigated in patients with

ASA I and II classification and in a number of instances profound hypotension was noted after the combined administration of sufentanil and thiamylal.

In patients scheduled for elective coronary artery bypass surgery, anesthesia is commonly induced with the highly potent and rapidly acting synthetic narcotics fentanyl and sufentanil. Murkin et al. have demonstrated that these agents can be used for rapid induction.[30] They reported that in nine patients rapid administration of fentanyl 50 μg/kg resulted in satisfactory induction of anesthesia, while in only two patients a moderate drop in blood pressure was noted as the loss of sympathetic tone was accompanied by vasodilation and bradycardia. Our recommended approach then is to administer fentanyl 30 to 50 μg/kg at a fairly rapid rate (two to three minutes) after adequate preoxygenation. Cricoid pressure should be maintained throughout the induction and muscle relaxants should be used judiciously to enhance hemodynamic stability. Rapid paralysis can be achieved with a wide variety of muscle relaxants used alone or in combination with each other. In the presence of bradycardia, pancuronium with its vagolytic and sympathomimetic effects should be of benefit. In tachycardia, succinylcholine might be preferred. Another possible choice is vecuronium that does not appear to disturb hemodynamic stability and acts rapidly provided the priming principle of administration is utilized.[31]

An alternative induction technique would consist of the rapid administration of etomidate and succinylcholine. Etomidate (0.3 mg/kg) has a rapid onset of action (10 to 12 seconds) and a pronounced hypnotic effect. In patients with cardiac disease, remarkable hemodynamic stability was demonstrated after etomidate administration.[32] The side effects of etomidate include pain on injection, thrombophlebitis, and myoclonic movements.

Anesthesia and muscle relaxation can be maintained by intermittent administration of narcotics and muscle relaxants. At the end of cardiopulmonary bypass (CPB), hypoperfusion as a result of inadequate ventricular performance is possible. Weaning from cardiopulmonary bypass might require intra-aortic balloon pumping, inotropes, and vasodilators. If thrombolytic therapy was utilized in combination with angioplasty, coagulation disturbances can also occur after CPB. Even with intracoronary administration of streptokinase, significant fibrinolytic activity has been demonstrated. A case of a patient with severe postbypass coagulopathy who required extensive therapy with fresh frozen plasma, platelets, cryoprecipitate, and ε-amino-caproic acid was recently reported by Goldberg et al.[33]

Summary

In discussing the anesthetic management of this patient, we have discussed a number of options without mentioning others. Every anesthesiologist can undoubtedly recommend alternative regimens that will work in his/her practice. However, little published information is available to substantiate that under circumstances similar to those described in this case any technique is superior to any other. Since in the future more patients will present for surgery following the complicated failure of one of the new therapies for AMI, it is essential that the anesthetic outcome of these patients be documented and published.

REFERENCES

1. Alpert JS, Braunwald E: Acute myocardial infarction: Pathological, pathophysiological and clinical manifestations, in Braunwald E (ed): *Heart Disease.* Philadelphia, WB Saunders Co, 1984, p 1262.
2. Laffel GL, Braunwald E: Thrombolytic therapy: A new strategy for the treatment of acute myocardial infarction. *N Engl J Med* 1984; 311:710(part 1); 311:770(part 2).
3. Reimer KA, Lower JE, Rasmussen MM, et al: The wavefront phenomenon of ischemic cell death. *Circulation* 1977; 56:786.
4. Rentrop KP: Thrombolytic therapy in patients with acute myocardial infarction. *Circulation* 1985; 71:627.
5. Collen D, Topol EJ, Tiefenbrum AJ, et al: Coronary thrombolysis with recombinant human tissue-type plasminogen activator: A prospective, randomized, placebo controlled trial. *Circulation* 1984; 70:1012.
6. Cowley MJ, Hastillo A, Vetrouec GW, et al: Fibrinolytic effects of intracoronary streptokinase administration in patients with acute myocardial infarction and coronary insufficiency. *Circulation* 1983; 67:1031.
7. Anderson JL, Marshall HW, Bray BE, et al: A randomized trial of intracoronary streptokinase in the treatment of acute myocardial infarction. *N Engl J Med* 1983; 308:1312.
8. Topol EJ, Weiss JL, Brinker JA, et al: Regional wall motion improvement after coronary thrombolysis with recombinant tissue plasminogen activator: Importance of coronary angioplasty. *J Am Coll Cardiol* 1985; 6:426.
9. Holmes DR, Smith HC, Vlietstra RE, et al: Percutaneous transluminal coronary angioplasty, alone or in combination with streptokinase therapy, during acute myocardial infarction. *Mayo Clin Proc* 1985; 60:449.
10. DeWood MA, Spores J, Berg R, et al: Acute myocardial infarction: A decade of experience with surgical reperfusion in 701 patients. *Circulation* 1983; 68(suppl 2): II8.
11. Vanhaecke J, Flameng W, Sergeant P, et al: Emergency bypass surgery: Late effects on size of infarction and ventricular function. *Circulation* 1985; 72(suppl 2):II179.
12. Spencer FC: Emergency coronary bypass for acute infarction: An unproved clinical experiment. *Circulation* 1983; 68(suppl 2):II17.
13. Nunley DL, Grunkemeier GL, Teply JF, et al: Coronary bypass operation following acute complicated myocardial infarction. *J Thorac Cardiovasc Surg* 1983; 85:485.

14. Pelletier LC, Pardini A, Renkin J, et al: Myocardial revascularization after failure of percutaneous transluminal coronary angioplasty. *J Thorac Cardiovasc Surg* 1985; 90:265.

15. Brahos GJ, Baker NH, Ewy HG, et al: Aortocoronary bypass following unsuccessful PTCA: Experience in 100 consecutive patients. *Ann Thorac Surg* 1985; 40:7.

16. Sobel BE, Braunwald E: The management of acute myocardial infarction, in Braunwald E (ed): *Heart Disease*. Philadelphia, WB Saunders Co, 1984, p 1317.

17. Gibbs CP, Spohr L, Schmidt D: The effectiveness of sodium citrate as an antacid. *Anesthesiology* 1982; 57:44.

18. Schulze-Delrieu K: Drug therapy: Metoclopramide. *N Engl J Med* 1981; 305:28.

19. Cohen SE, Jasson J, Talafre ML, et al: Does metoclopramide decrease the volume of gastric contents in patients undergoing cesarean section? *Anesthesiology* 1984; 61:604.

20. McGuigan JE: A consideration of the adverse effects of cimetidine. *Gastroenterology* 1981; 80:181.

21. Thys DM: Pulmonary artery catheterization: Past, present, and future. *Mt Sinai J Med* 1984; 51:578.

22. Kaplan JA, Wells PH: Early diagnosis of myocardial ischemia using the pulmonary artery catheter. *Anesth Analg* 1981; 60:789.

23. Lichtenthal PR, Collins JT: Multipurpose pulmonary artery catheter. *Ann Thorac Surg* 1983; 36:493.

24. Morganroth J, Chen CC, David D, et al: Echocardiographic detection of coronary artery disease: Detection of effects of ischemia on regional myocardial wall motion and visualization of left main coronary artery disease. *Am J Cardiol* 1980; 46:1178.

25. Heger J, Weyman AE, Noble RJ, et al: An analysis of the site, extent and hemodynamic consequences of acute myocardial infarction by cross-sectional echocardiography. *Circulation* 1977; 56(suppl 3):III152.

26. Pichler M: Non-invasive assessment of segmental left ventricular wall motion: Its clinical relevance in detection of ischemia. *Clin Cardiol* 1978; 1:173.

27. Slogoff S, Keats AS: Does perioperative myocardial ischemia lead to postoperative myocardial infarction. *Anesthesiology* 1985; 62:107.

28. Cork RC, Weiss JL, Hameroff SR, et al: Fentanyl preloading for rapid-sequence induction of anesthesia. *Anesth Analg* 1984; 63:60.

29. Kleinman J, Marlar K, Silva D, et al: Sufentanil attenuation of the stress response during rapid-sequence induction, abstracted. *Anesthesiology* 1985; 63:SA379.

30. Murkin JM, Moldenhauer CG, Hug CC: High dose fentanyl for rapid induction of anesthesia in patients with coronary artery disease. *Can Anaesth Soc J* 1985; 32:320.

31. Schwarz S, Ilias W, Lackner F, et al: Rapid tracheal intubation with vecuronium: The priming principle. *Anesthesiology* 1985; 62:388.

32. Gooding JM, Weng JT, Smith RA, et al: Cardiovascular and pulmonary responses following etomidate induction of anesthesia in patients with demonstrated cardiac disease. *Anesth Analg* 1979; 58:40.

33. Goldberg M, Colonna-Romano P, Babins NA, et al: Emergency coronary artery bypass surgery following intracoronary streptokinase. *Anesthesiology* 1984; 61:601.

35

Management of Combined Carotid/Coronary Artery Disease

A 65-year-old woman had stable angina pectoris and three-vessel coronary artery disease (CAD). She also had a history of transient ischemic attacks (TIAs) and a 95% occlusion of her right common carotid artery. She was scheduled for a combined carotid endarterectomy (CEA) and coronary artery bypass (CAB) surgery.

Recommendations by Lars R. Newsome, M.D., and C. Craig Moldenhauer, M.D.

ANALYSIS OF THE PROBLEM

Due to the diffuse nature of atherosclerosis, the natural histories of carotid and coronary artery occlusive diseases are clearly intertwined. The incidence of significant internal or carotid bifurcation stenosis in patients scheduled for myocardial revascularization has been reported to be between 6% and 16%.[1, 2] Alternatively, CAD may coexist with carotid obstructive disease in as many as 40% to 60% of patients undergoing CEA.[3-5] Myocardial infarctions are a frequent cause of early death and the most frequent cause (40% to 70%) of late deaths in patients undergoing CEA.[6, 7] Likewise, focal and/or global neurologic injury following CAB surgery remains a significant problem. The optimal management of coexisting carotid artery stenosis in patients requiring coronary artery surgery remains debatable. Some physicians recommend combined or simultaneous operations employing CEA with CAB surgery for patients with coexisting disease, with the anticipation that the risk will be similar to those of coronary or carotid artery procedures done separately.[3, 8] Other physicians, however, have recommended staging the two procedures for certain categories of patients and combining the operations only when definite clinical indications exist.[9] In fact, several studies in patients with asymptomatic cervical bruits indicate that required cardiac or noncardiac surgery can safely be done without a prophylactic CEA.[2, 8, 10, 11]

Cerebrovascular disease refers to any pathologic process that involves the blood vessels supplying the brain. Cerebrovascular insufficiency secondary to atherosclerosis is produced by one of two mechanisms: (1) reduction in cerebral blood flow (CBF) with progressive stenosis (that may even lead to thrombosis), and (2) embolization of platelet, fibrin, or atheromatous debris from an ulcerated plaque. Ischemia occurs when blood flow to a part of the brain becomes insufficient to satisfy metabolic demands. With ischemia and its resultant focal areas of hypoxia, there is loss of neuronal function in the affected area. A TIA is defined as a neurologic deficit that usually resolves completely in minutes, but may last up to 24 hours. Deficits that persist beyond 24 hours are classified as strokes and are the result of brain destruction following profound or prolonged ischemia. Embolic strokes are generally very sudden in onset and may be caused by numerous substances, including blood clots of cardiac origin, fragments of atheromatous debris such as cholesterol released spontaneously or during surgery, or unevacuated (trapped) air introduced at surgery.

In a focal cerebral infarction, similar to myocardial infarction, there is a central area of necrosis that is irreversibly damaged, surrounded by an ischemic penumbra or band of neurons that may be electrically silent due to ischemia but viable and, therefore, salvageable with appropriate therapy.[12] Total arrest of the cerebral circulation leads to complete cessation of neuronal electrical activity, i.e., a flat EEG (synaptic transmission failure) in seconds, followed by deterioration of intracellular ion homeostasis. Depletion of high energy phosphates, $Na^+ - K^+$ transport failure, influx of sodium chloride and water, efflux of intracellular potassium and membrane depolarization (membrane failure) occur next. Under normal conditions, complete cerebral circulatory arrest for more than five or ten minutes results in irreversible cell damage. However, if ischemia is incomplete, the outcome is more difficult to predict and depends upon multiple factors including perfusion pressure, availability of collateral flow, and cerebral metabolic rate. Animal and human studies provide evidence that there is an upper ischemic flow threshold of synaptic failure and a lower ischemic flow threshold of membrane failure. Primate studies suggest that the lowest safe level of CBF lies just above the flow threshold for membrane failure. Membrane failure always precedes structural damage; however, the flow thresholds for each are so closely associated that the critical CBF thresholds for membrane failure and infarction may be considered identical. Also, the development of a cerebral infarction is related both to the severity and duration of the reduction in CBF.[13]

In both human and animal studies the critical threshold of electrical failure of the cerebral cortex varies between 15 and 20 ml/100 gm/minute.[12,14,15] Further primate studies have shown that there is another critical flow threshold of between 10 and 15 ml/100gm/minute below which the extracellular potassium concentration increased massively (and perhaps irreversibly) due to efflux of potassium from the cells.[16] This appears to be the critical threshold to maintain membrane function and cell viability. Thus, the difference in CBF that separates the ischemic thresholds for electrical vs. membrane failure, or viability vs. irreversible damage is relatively small—only about 5 ml/100 gm/minute.

Myocardial infarction is a prominent cause of postoperative morbidity and mortality in patients undergoing CEA. Ennix et al. found that nearly 50% of their patients with carotid artery disease also had significant CAD.[3] These investigators noted the presence of CAD increased operative mortality following CEA from 1.5% to 18.2%. In addition, most series report that myocardial infarction was responsible for up to 70% of all late deaths following CEA.

Coronary artery bypass surgery is also associated with a significant incidence of postoperative neurologic dysfunction, ranging from 1% to 40%.[17,18] In a recent prospective study, the overall incidence of cerebral dysfunction attributable to cardiac surgery and cardiopulmonary bypass (CPB) was 16.2% for transient, and 6.4% for persistent problems (present on the tenth postoperative day).[18] Furthermore, Slogoff et al.[18] found that the incidence of postoperative cerebral dysfunction was more than twice as high in patients undergoing intracardiac vs. extracardiac operations and more than four times as high in patients older than age 60 compared to younger patients. Unlike earlier studies, perfusion pressures less than 50 torr persisting for over 16 minutes were not associated with the development of postoperative cerebral deficits. In fact, even more profound hypotension during CPB has been tolerated without cerebral damage—mean arterial pressures below 30 torr for 30 minutes and below 40 torr for 1 hour.[19] In eight of the nine patients who suffered a focal motor or sensory deficit, the right hemisphere was involved.[18] The laterality of the focal findings and the increased incidence of deficits following valvular and other intracardiac procedures strongly suggests that air or particulate emboli originating within the heart or aorta are the major causes of postbypass neurologic dysfunction.

APPROACH TO THE PROBLEM

Preanesthetic Evaluation

An important aspect of the preanesthetic evaluation of patients with coexisting carotid and coronary artery disease involves deciding which lesion, i.e., carotid or coronary or both, requires the initial surgical repair. Although the majority of neurologic deficits seen after bypass are thought to be embolic in nature, there is concern that coexistent carotid artery diseases may be contributory. Since flow distal to a severe stenosis becomes pressure dependent, CPB, with its occasional periods of hypotension, may further reduce perfusion pressure and CBF, resulting in postoperative neurologic deficits. Unfortunately, the presence of a carotid artery bruit is not a very good indicator of the presence or severity of carotid artery stenosis. Indeed, a silent neck may harbor advanced disease due to extremely low blood flow. For this reason, ultrasound, ocular plethysmography, or intravenous digital subtraction angiography is currently used to evaluate the extent of carotid artery stenosis.

Ivey and colleagues evaluated the risk of perioperative cerebral dysfunction in patients undergoing cardiac procedures.[11] Over a 31-month period, they screened 1,433 consecutive patients scheduled for cardiac surgery. Those with a carotid bruit or a positive neurologic history underwent ultrasonic duplex scanning of the carotid artery. Stenosis greater than 50% was considered hemodynamically significant and, if associated with symptoms and confirmed by angiography, was treated with CEA in combination with the required cardiac procedure. Nine symptomatic patients with bruits and hemodynamically significant lesions underwent angiography and CEA prior to or simultaneous with cardiac surgery. There was one death in this group due to neurologic complications. Of the 82 patients with asymptomatic bruits, 16 had and 66 did not have hemodynamically significant lesions (internal diameter reduction $\geq$ 50%) when evaluated by ultrasonic Doppler scanning. These patients underwent cardiac surgery without further carotid evaluation or treatment and there were no focal postoperative neurologic deficits. While the usual practice of Ivey and colleagues is to maintain perfusion pressure at or above 40 mm Hg during CPB, in the subset of 16 asymptomatic patients with hemodynamically significant lesions, perfusion pressure was kept at 70 mm Hg. The remaining patients without carotid bruits had a 0.7% incidence of focal neurologic deficits postoperatively. They concluded that asymptomatic patients with or without hemodynamically significant stenosis could safely undergo cardiac surgery and CPB without carotid angiography and CEA. The few patients they identified with symptomatic carotid disease received staged or simultaneous procedures, with the physicians' preference being to perform staged procedures if clinically possible.

Controversy continues whether both lesions should be repaired simultaneously or as staged procedures. In most studies, simultaneous procedures have been associated with an increased incidence of stroke and mortality as compared to staged procedures. For example, Hertzer et al. reported a 1.5% perioperative stroke rate in 59 patients having a staged procedure, i.e., with the CEA performed first, followed by CAB surgery a few days to six months later.[9] After the staged CAB surgery, there were no permanent strokes and the early mortality rate was 1.7%. In contrast, a group of 115 patients undergoing combined CEA and CAB surgery had a 4.3% incidence of permanent stroke and a 4.3% operative mortality rate. They concluded that a combined procedure may be associated with a higher risk of intraoperative stroke. In a more recent study by the same investigators, 331 patients received combined operations from 1973 to 1981 and had similar stroke (4.5%) and mortality (5.7%) rates.[20] These results were significantly higher than the 1.8% stroke rate and 1.9% mortality rate for all 22,100 patients who underwent CAB surgery during the same time period. Given these results, Hertzer and his colleagues recommend combined CEA and CAB surgery for only those patients whose coronary and carotid disease is considered too severe to permit staged operations. The 331 patients in their more recent study represent only a minority (1.7%) of the patients having CAB surgery during the same time period. Hertzer et al. recognize that it will require a large, prospectively randomized (probably multicenter) study to resolve the controversy of whether to perform staged vs. combined procedures. Until then they continue to recommend combined procedures for patients with recognized carotid disease who require CAB surgery for (1) severe lesions of the left main coronary artery; (2) diffuse CAD without satisfactory collateral circulation; and (3) severe CAD with unstable angina. Also, the greater incidence of stroke and mortality associated with the combined procedures may only represent a higher risk or sicker group of patients. In general, this group is older, has more extensive CAD including left main coronary artery and left ventricular dysfunction, and a greater percentage of contralateral carotid occlusions.[9]

More recently, Jones et al. reported a lower mortality (3.0% and incidence of perioperative stroke (1.6%) during combined carotid/coronary artery bypass surgery in a series of 132 patients.[8] This perioperative stroke rate was not significantly different from that of a control group having CAB surgery alone. The incidence of postoperative stroke in 5,676 patients undergoing coronary artery bypass surgery alone was 0.9%. The incidence of perioperative stroke in patients with asymptomatic carotid bruits or prior history of stroke or TIA undergoing CAB surgery was 3.3% and 8.6%, respectively. Their indications for simultaneous carotid/coronary operations included *symptomatic* carotid disease (TIA or prior stroke) or bilateral carotid disease and severe or unstable coronary artery disease, left main obstruction, or diffuse multivessel disease.

Staged procedures were recommended for patients with stable angina and symptomatic carotid lesions, especially when difficulty with the CEA was anticipated (for example, a "redo" CEA). They further recommended CAB surgery alone for most patients with asymptomatic cervical bruits, mild-to-moderate carotid artery obstruction, and unstable angina associated with prior stroke, although the latter situation may be accompanied by an increased risk of postoperative neurologic injury.

To return to the patient in the case example, she has severe stenosis of her carotid artery that is symptomatic and requires CEA. The indication for a simultaneous carotid/coronary surgery is debatable since she has stable angina, but it is not an unreasonable approach for this patient, especially given her multivessel coronary disease. One additional benefit from doing both procedures at the same setting is that it will spare the patient the cost and recovery time of a second hospitalization and surgery.

Anesthetic Technique

The problem facing the anesthesiologist involves maintaining a favorable cerebral *and* myocardial oxygen supply/demand ratio in the perioperative period. Ideally, the clinician should maintain an adequate cerebral perfusion pressure, decrease cerebral metabolism, and avoid excessive myocardial depression or ischemia during CEA. A blood pressure about 10% to 20% above normal should be satisfactory. During CPB we would maintain mean arterial pressure between 60 and 80 mm Hg because of the patient's carotid disease. However, there are no hard data to support this practice. Hyperglycemia is avoided if possible and treated aggressively with insulin drips if necessary, as it can exacerbate cerebral ischemia.[21]

Patient monitors include leads II and V_5 of the electrocardiogram (ECG), a radial artery catheter, a pulmonary artery (PA) catheter, and some form of EEG monitoring. The use of a PA catheter is especially useful in combined carotid/coronary procedures. For example, the initial treatment to correct an ischemic EEG during carotid cross-clamping is usually induced hypertension with a phenylephrine drip. In addition to the ECG, the clinician can also use the PA catheter to monitor for early signs of myocardial ischemia that may occur during the hypertensive period. Increases in the pulmonary capillary wedge pressure or the new onset of a V wave on the wedged tracing may reflect myocardial ischemia (papillary muscle dysfunction or a decrease in myocardial compliance) or cardiac failure resulting from the induced hypertension therapy. By monitoring the PA catheter and ECG, the clinician can determine the blood pressure (and heart rate) limit the heart will tolerate. If the EEG still looks ischemic, a shunt should be placed for the CEA. The PA catheter can also be used to detect excessive myocardial depression that can occur with the use of thiopental to decrease cerebral metabolism in the immediate peribypass period and, perhaps, during the CEA as well. Caution should be used when inserting the Swan-Ganz catheter in order to avoid dislodging atherosclerotic plaques that may be present on the contralateral (nonoperated) carotid artery.

There are several monitors and methods for detecting intraoperative cerebral ischemia, including standard multichannel (raw) EEG, various computerized EEG processors, somatosensory evoked potentials, cerebral blood flow measurements, and serial neurologic assessments (only for surgery performed under local or regional anesthesia). Because it is easy to apply and interpret, we routinely monitor the EEG with an automated computer processed EEG (Lifescan or Neurotrac) machine, which eliminates the need for an EEG technician or electroencephalographer in the operating room. Rampil and his colleagues demonstrated the prognostic value of automated EEG analysis during CEA.[22] They found that the majority of abnormal EEG changes during CEA were transient and not associated with any postoperative neurologic deficit. However, all seven patients with ischemic EEG changes lasting longer than ten minutes developed new neurologic deficits postoperatively. Events during the operation were most frequently associated with carotid artery cross-clamping, though several occurred with restoration of carotid flow through either a shunt or the artery itself after closure of the arteriotomy. The use of the EEG for a particular patient will depend somewhat on the surgical technique. Because of the risk of producing emboli, some surgeons will employ a shunt only in selective situations in which there is evidence of cerebral ischemia after carotid artery cross-clamping. In this situation the EEG is used as a diagnostic tool to detect ischemia with carotid artery clamping. If EEG changes occur, a shunt is placed to restore blood flow. The EEG should return to normal if the shunt is working. The EEG is less sensitive in its ability to detect small emboli. Other surgeons routinely shunt all of their patients. In this situation the EEG can tell whether the shunt is functioning properly. The EEG can also be used to guide anesthesia. Moffat et al. demonstrated that while the bolus administration of thiopental (4 mg/kg) prior to carotid artery cross-clamping resulted in EEG burst suppression representing cerebral metabolic depression, this effect was transient and probably inadequate for cerebral protection during carotid artery cross-clamping.[23] However, the use of a barbiturate infusion, titrated to maintain burst suppression throughout carotid cross-clamping would seem to address this problem. Based on earlier work demonstrating that most neurologic injury during CAB surgery and CPB is the result of emboli from the heart or aorta,[19] and the many animal studies demonstrating thiopental's protective effect during focal cerebral ischemia, Nussmeier and Slogoff used a thiopental infusion during CPB to maintain a burst suppression pattern on the EEG during intracardiac procedures.[24] They found a statistically significant reduction in postoperative neurologic deficits in the patients treated with thiopental compared to controls. Additionally, isoflurane may be used as part of the anesthetic technique in patients with good ventricular function, since like barbiturates it seems to provide some cerebral protection by depressing cerebral electric activity and metabolism.[15, 25] Obviously during the CEA, an adequate blood pressure must be maintained without compromising myocardial oxygen supply/demand ratio.

Once cardiopulmonary bypass is initiated, we would maintain perfusion pressure between 60 and 80 mm Hg. This is currently controversial since there are no good studies of neurologic outcome to document any benefit of maintaining high perfusion pressures on CPB. In fact, Govier and colleagues recently evaluated the effects of alterations in perfusion pressure, pump flow, nasopharyngeal temperature, and arterial PCO_2 on regional CBF in patients *without* evidence of carotid disease who were on CPB.[26] They found no relationship between blood pressure or pump flow and CBF. This would tend to imply that normal cerebral autoregulation exists under the nonpulsatile conditions of hypothermic CPB between mean arterial pressures of 30 to 110 mm Hg. The only variables that correlated with CBF were temperature and PCO_2. Specifically, CBF decreased as temperature decreased and increased as PCO_2 increased. It should be emphasized that this study was performed on patients without carotid artery disease. Although the controversy between low pressure, low-flow vs. high pressure, high-flow techniques of CPB continues, if the patient has cerebrovascular disease, we maintain a mean arterial pressure between 60 and 80 mm Hg and a pump flow of 2.5 L/minute/m^2.

Summary

We would use a slow induction with low doses of fentanyl (5 to 30 µg/kg) or sufentanil (1 to 4 µg/kg)/diazepam/O_2/ and pancuronium, vecuronium, or succinylcholine depending upon the heart rate. We would then add low concentrations of isoflurane ($< 1.0\%$), as tolerated, to maintain anesthesia. Isoflurane is titrated to keep the mean arterial pressure in the patient's preoperative range and allow some fast activity on the EEG. The loss of fast EEG activity with carotid clamping can then be used to detect cerebral ischemia. Ventilation is maintained at normocarbia. The head is positioned very carefully since many patients also have lesions of the vertebral arteries that may be totally occluded when the head is turned to the side, flexed, or extended. During the preoperative evaluation, check to see if the patient becomes symptomatic when assuming positions that will be used during surgery. If bradycardia occurs during manipulation of the carotid artery, we ask the surgeon to infiltrate the carotid body with 1% lidocaine.

Even though our surgeons routinely use a shunt prior to carotid cross clamping, we monitor the EEG to assess whether the shunt is functioning. If the EEG does not return to normal immediately after the shunt is opened, the surgeon is notified so that he can check its positioning. If the EEG remained normal or returned to normal after placement of the shunt, the clinician has a choice. An argument can be made to maintain a constant level of anesthesia and continue to monitor the EEG for ischemic changes on the operated side that might occur with decreases in blood pressure or changes in positioning of the shunt. In other words, the EEG can be monitored to detect dangerous decreases in CBF. However, the patient is also at risk for cerebral ischemia secondary to emboli (a risk that may be increased by the use of a shunt). Depending on the size and location of the emboli, they may not be detected by the EEG. For this reason, once the functioning of the shunt is confirmed by the EEG, we administer thiopental for its brain protective effect. A dose of 4 mg/kg of thiopental, given in 50- to 100-mg increments, is administered until there is EEG burst suppression. This EEG pattern is maintained by an infusion of thiopental (usually starting at 0.5 mg/kg/min)[24] during the CEA. A phenylephrine infusion is used as needed to maintain blood pressure during the CEA at preoperative values or at a level 20% greater than preoperative levels. During CPB we maintain mean arterial pressure at 60 to 80 mm Hg and pump flow at 2.5 L/minute/m^2. Because the patient is also at risk for embolic injury during CPB, we may elect to restart the thiopental infusion to produce EEG burst suppression during CPB if, for example, the aorta is very calcified. We try to limit the dose of thiopental to 25 to 40 mg/kg.[24] During hypothermic CPB very little thiopental is required to maintain an isoelectric EEG.

Postoperative hypertension is common after either CEA or CAB surgery and is aggressively treated as it places the patient at greater risk for cerebral and coronary damage. We continue to maintain values for mean arterial pressure (MAP) and heart rate within the patient's preoperative range with the use of β-blockers, calcium entry blockers, or intravenous nitroglycerin, as indicated. When the patient emerges from anesthesia, the physician grossly assesses the patient's condition for postoperative neurologic recovery in the intensive care unit; the patient is then sedated and weaned from the ventilator the next morning.

REFERENCES

1. Barnes RW, Marszalek PB, Rittgers SE: Asymptomatic carotid disease in preoperative patients. *Stroke* 1980; 11:136.
2. Barnes RW, Marszalek PB: Asymptomatic carotid disease in the cardiovascular surgical patient: Is prophylactic endarterectomy necessary? *Stroke* 1981; 12:497–500.
3. Ennix CL Jr, Lawrie GM, Morris GC Jr, et al: Improved results of carotid endarterectomy in patients with symptomatic coronary disease: An analysis of 1,546 consecutive carotid operations. *Stroke* 1979; 10:122–125.

4. Rokey R, Rolak LA, Harati Y, et al: Coronary artery disease in patients with cerebrovascular disease: A prospective study. *Ann Neurol* 1984; 16:50–53.

5. Hertzer NR, Young JR, Beven EG, et al: Coronary angiography in 506 patients with extracranial cerebrovascular disease. *Arch Intern Med* 1985; 145:849–852.

6. Thompson JE, Patman RD, Talkington CM: Asymptomatic carotid bruit: Long-term outcome of patients having endarterectomy compared with unoperated controls. *Ann Surg* 1978; 188:308–316.

7. Hertzer NR, Lees DC: Fatal myocardial infarction following carotid endarterectomy: Three hundred thirty-five patients followed 6–11 years after operation. *Ann Surg* 1981; 194:213–218.

8. Jones EL, Craver JM, Michalik RA, et al: Combined carotid and coronary operations: When are they necessary? *J Thorac Cardiovasc Surg* 1984; 87:7–16.

9. Hertzer NR, Loop FD, Taylor PC, et al: Staged and combined surgical approach to simultaneous carotid and coronary vascular disease. *Surgery* 1978; 84:803–811.

10. Ropper AH, Wechsler LR, Wilson LS: Carotid bruit and the risk of stroke in elective surgery. *N Engl J Med* 1982; 307:1388–1390.

11. Ivey TD, Strandness DE, Williams DB, et al: Management of patients with carotid bruit undergoing cardiopulmonary bypass. *J Thorac Cardiovasc Surg* 1984; 87:183–189.

12. Astrup J, Siesjö BK, Symon L: Thresholds in cerebral ischemia: The ischemic penumbra. *Stroke* 1981; 12:723–725.

13. Jones TH, Morawetz RB, Crowell RM, et al: Thresholds of cerebral ischemia in awake monkeys. *J Neurosurg* 1981; 54:773–782.

14. Sundt TM Jr, Sharbrough FW, Anderson RE, et al: Cerebral blood flow measurements and electroencephalograms during carotid endarterectomy. *J Neurosurg* 1974; 41:310–320.

15. Sundt TM Jr: The ischemic tolerance of neural tissue and the need for monitoring and selective shunting during carotid endarterectomy. *Stroke* 1983; 14:93–98.

16. Astrup J, Symon L, Branston NM, et al: Cortical evoked potential and extracellular K^+ and H^+ at critical levels of brain ischemia. *Stroke* 1977; 8:51–57.

17. Ellis RJ, Wisniewski A, Potts R, et al: Reduction of flow rate and arterial pressure at moderate hypothermia does not result in cerebral dysfunction. *J Thorac Cardiovasc Surg* 1980; 79:173.

18. Slogoff S, Girgis KZ, Keats AS: Etiologic factors in neuropsychiatric complications associated with cardiopulmonary bypass. *Anesth Analg* 1982; 61:903–911.

19. Aren C, Bloomstrand C, Wikkelso C, et al: Hypotension induced by prostacyclin treatment during cardiopulmonary bypass does not increase the risk of cerebral complications. *J Thorac Cardiovasc Surg* 1984; 88:748–753.

20. Hertzer NR, Loop FD, Taylor PC, et al: Combined myocardial revascularization and carotid endarterectomy: Operative and late results in 331 patients. *J Thorac Cardiovasc Surg* 1983; 85:577–589.

21. Welsh FA, Ginsberg MD, Rieder W, et al: Deterioration effect of glucose pretreatment on recovery from diffuse cerebral ischemia in the cat. *Stroke* 1980; 11:355–362.

22. Rampil IJ, Holzer JA, Quest DO, et al: Prognostic value of computerized EEG analysis during carotid endarterectomy. *Anesth Analg* 1983; 62:186–192.

23. Moffat JA, McDougall MJ, Brunet D, et al: Thiopental bolus during carotid endarterectomy—rational drug therapy? *Can Anaesth Soc J* 1983; 30:615–622.
24. Nussmeier NA, Slogoff S: Neuropsychiatric complications after cardiopulmonary bypass: Cerebral protection by a barbiturate. *Anesthesiology* 1985; 63:A387.
25. Newberg LA, Michenfelder JD: Cerebral protection by isoflurane during hypoxemia or ischemia. *Anesthesiology* 1983; 59:29–35.
26. Govier AV, Reves JG, McKay RD, et al: Factors and their influence on regional cerebral blood flow during nonpulsatile cardiopulmonary bypass. *Ann Thorac Surg* 1984; 38:592–600.

36

Thoracic Abdominal Aneurysm Repair With Cardiopulmonary Bypass

A 70-year-old man in otherwise good health presented with back pain. Angiography demonstrated a descending thoracic atherosclerotic aneurysm. It was elected to use cardiopulmonary bypass in this patient to optimize distal aortic perfusion. The proximal aortic cross-clamp was applied just below the left subclavian artery and the distal one above the renal arteries. Cardiopulmonary bypass was established using femoral cannulation, and the systemic pressure decreased from 170/100 to 60/40 mm Hg and pulmonary artery wedge pressure (PAWP) decreased from 12 to 5 mm Hg. There were ST changes in lead V_5 indicative of acute ischemia.

Recommendations by Paolo Flezzani, M.D.

ANALYSIS OF THE PROBLEM

With initiation of partial cardiopulmonary bypass, inadequate myocardial perfusion occurred with resulting myocardial ischemia. Prompt therapy is indicated to avoid myocardial infarction.

APPROACH TO THE PROBLEM

It is likely that our patient became ischemic following a rapid fall in systemic blood pressure (systemic diastolic pressure from 100 to 40 mm Hg) that dropped the coronary perfusion pressure from 88 mm Hg down to 35 mm Hg.

The decrease in pulmonary capillary wedge pressure suggests that the mechanism is a decrease preload, with decrease in both aortic pressure and stroke volume. The most appropriate intervention is to increase preload by tranfusing volume from the bypass pump and by decreasing venous drainage. It is likely that this manipulation will achieve the objective of increasing coronary perfusion pressure and flow (thus O_2 supply) without excessively increasing diastolic wall tension, since the patient's ventricle seems to be on the flat portion of the left ventricular compliance curve. An alternative intervention consists of the infusion of an α-adrenergic agent to further increase arterial impedance (and afterload) and aortic pressure. The drawbacks of this approach are that only coronary perfusion pressure will be increased without probably any increase in coronary blood flow. Second, this ventricle is contracting against a high aortic impedance and any further increase could elevate both afterload and myocardial oxygen consumption, thus limiting or offsetting the gains of the higher coronary perfusion pressure. Also, systemic vasoconstriction could theoretically decrease blood flow to the spinal cord and kidneys. The use of β-adrenergic agents is not advisable because an increase in contractility and possibly heart rate would increase myocardial oxygen demand without probably obtaining any significant increases in O_2 supply since the low preload might prevent significant increases in stroke volume. The use of nitroglycerin could have some beneficial effect in improving collateral myocardial circulation and subendocardial coronary blood flow, but its preload reducing effects will further compromise stroke volume and oxygen supply. Similar considerations hold true for sodium nitroprusside. Both might reduce pressure-dependent flow to the spinal cord and kidneys.[1] Once preload and perfusion pressure are brought back to prebypass levels, both nitroglycerin and sodium nitroprusside could be used to optimize loading of the left ventricle.

DISCUSSION

Background

Aneurysms of the thoracic aorta represent a relatively rare condition, the incidence is approximately 6 cases in 100,000 persons per year.[2] The pathologic process that leads to this disease involves the necrosis and degeneration of both the elastic and muscular layers of the arterial wall secondary to various causes.

Cystic necrosis, atherosclerosis, aortitis of various origins, trauma, and chronic aortic dissection are all possible etiologies. With the loss of the muscular layer and with only the outer fibrous tissue remaining, elasticity (i.e., the ability to deform in response to the systolic wall stress[3] and return to the pre-stress state during diastole) is lost and, over the course of time, dilatation occurs, either localized (saccular) or generalized (fusiform). Since the advent of antibiotic therapy, the incidence of syphilitic aortitis has decreased, while the incidence of atherosclerotic aneurysms has increased.[4] Atherosclerotic aneurysms affect the descending thoracic aorta more than the ascending and are less prone to dissect than other types. Their incidence increases with age and they are more common in males. The pathology associated with this disease includes hypertension (45% to 100%), coronary artery disease, peripheral vascular disease, abdominal aortic aneurysm (13% to 29%).[5, 6]

Diagnosis is difficult since the presenting symptomatology is deceiving.[4] Very often (> 50%) atherosclerotic aneurysms of the descending aorta are totally asymptomatic and represent an incidental finding during routine investigations. When symptoms are present, they result from the compression of adjacent structures, from dissection or free rupture of the aneurysm.

Untreated aneurysms of the aorta have a poor prognosis, although atherosclerotic aneurysms of the descending aorta are generally more amenable to conservative medical treatment than ascending aortic aneurysms. However, the incidence of late rupture (more than a month after diagnosis) is high.[4] Symptoms of pain or the evidence of enlargement are associated with higher morbidity and mortality. Although the perioperative mortality is about 10%, the five-year survival for surgically treated patients is significantly better than that for nontreated patients.[7]

Thoracic aortic aneurysms are classified according to their anatomical position (Fig 36–1).

Perioperative Evaluation

As discussed previously, aortic aneuryms represent a multifactorial disease occurring mainly in the elderly population. Particular care should then be paid to assess the presence of associated pathology through careful history taking, physical examination, and laboratory testing.

The presence of coronary artery disease (angina, dysrhythmia); congestive heart failure (dyspnea on exertion or at rest, peripheral edema, pulmonary congestion); hypertension and hypertensive cardiomyopathy (blood pressure monitoring, chest x-ray film, electrocardiogram); cerebral vascular disease (bruits, transient ischemic attacks, stroke); renal disease (BUN and creatinine determinations); diabetes; pulmonary disease; and coagulation disorders should be carefully investigated. If necessary, additional tests such as stress testing, echocardiograms, or radionuclide scanning should be obtained. Patient medications should be carefully reviewed and an appropriate decision concerning their continuation on the day of surgery should be made.

It is not unusual that a patient will present for surgery with an unremarkable history and that a careful investigation will not reveal any remarkable finding.

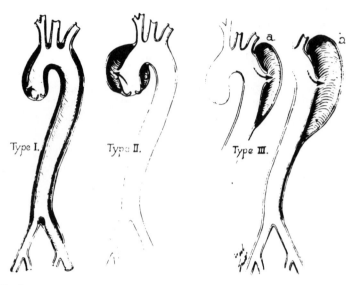

FIG 36–1.
Classification of thoracic aortic aneurysms according to their anatomical positions. Type I and II ➡ type A; Type III ➡ type B. (From DeBakey ME, Henley WS, Cooley DA, et al: Surgical management of dissecting aneurysms of the aorta. *J Thorac Cardiovasc Surg* 1965; 49:130–149. Used by permission.

Two factors should be kept in mind. The first is that the absence of the positive signs or symptoms does not exclude the presence of either coronary artery disease or hypertensive disease. The second is that the surgical procedure causes profound and often sudden changes in loading conditions of the heart, thereby compromising perfusion to critical organs to the extent that subclinical vascular disease becomes of critical importance. This occurred in our patient.

The anesthesiologist must understand the type of repair, its physiologic implication, and devices that might be used to support the circulation during surgery. For example, surgery for the *ascending aorta* and the *arch* is performed through a median sternotomy, and repair of the *descending aorta* is approached through a left lateral thoracotomy. Depending on the type of aneurysm, two different surgical techniques are employed. If the aneurysm is saccular and the diameter of the neck is less than half the circumference of the aorta, a partial aortic cross-clamp can be applied and an aortorrhaphy can be performed. If the aneursym is fusiform (or saccular with large neck), the entire segment of the aorta must be resected and replaced with a graft. This technique requires the application of two cross-clamps, with total obstruction of the aortic flow. This approach changes afterload (addressed later), but there are two problems the anesthesiologist needs to understand. The first problem is that the upper clamp can obstruct the left subclavian artery, so that blood pressure measurements from the left arm are impossible. The second problem (and by far the most critical one) is that perfusion distal to the upper clamp is either stopped or decreased. This situation places the lowest spinal cord and the kidneys at high risk of ischemic complication. Paraplegia (3.7% to 17.7%) and acute renal failure (10% during elective surgery) are two of the most devastating complications of this type of surgery.[8-10] Different approaches have been advocated to prevent these complications. Some groups claim that short (less than one hour) cross-clamping time can be tolerated without complications. The use of heparin-coated shunts or partial cardiopulmonary bypass through femoral route with systemic heparinization have also been advocated. Although there is no evidence that any of these approaches are superior to the others, the use of shunts or cardiopulmonary bypass is preferred when long and difficult repairs are expected. If femoral-femoral cardiopulmonary bypass is used, perfusion pressure and flow distally to the cross-clamp will be determined by the pump. Proximal aortic perfusion will be determined largely by the beating heart, although venous return to the oxygenator will affect preload and therefore cardiac output.

The application of aortic cross-clamp and the institution of cardiopulmonary bypass cause a rapid and relatively complex change in myocardial oxygen balance by means of changes in both oxygen demand and supply.

The cross-clamping of the aorta causes a sharp increase in systemic vascular resistance because of an increase in aortic impedance ($\Delta P/\Delta V$) to left ventricular outflow that thereby increases left ventricular afterload. Afterload is defined either as additional stress (force/cross-sectional area) or tension (force) above the preload developed by the muscle during systole and is linearly related to myocardial oxygen consumption ($M\dot{V}O_2$) (Fig 36-2), so that any increase in afterload will increase oxygen consumption. As is well known, the development of tension represents a major component of myocardial oxygen consumption. At the same time, the increased afterload can cause an increase in left ventricular end systolic volume that, depending on the passive diastolic compliance of the left ventricle, will increase left ventricular end diastolic pressure and tension; this, in turn, will increase resistance to coronary blood flow. Depending on the contractile state of the ventricle, this increase in afterload could lead to a change in the stroke volume; while a normal ventricle will either increase or at least maintain stroke volume by increasing preload and contractility, a failing ventricle will respond by decreasing stroke volume.

Other factors to consider are that any increase in aortic pressure will increase coronary perfusion pressure and that a decrease in stroke volume will decrease coronary blood flow.

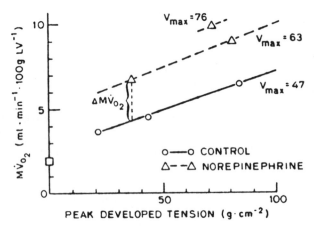

FIG 36–2.
Relationship between myocardial oxygen consumption (MVO₂) and peak developed tension. *LV* = left ventricle; *V$_{max}$* = maximum velocity of myocardial fiber shortening at O load. (From Graham TP Jr, Covell JW, Sonnenblick EH, et al: Control of myocardial oxygen consumption: Relative influence of contractile state and tension development. *J Clin Invest* 1968; 47:375–383. Used by permission.)

On the other side, the initiation of partial cardiopulmonary bypass will affect ventricular mechanics by decreasing preload. The decreasing preload will reduce diastolic wall tension, therefore reducing coronary resistance; but it can also reduce stroke volume, thus reducing coronary blood flow and perfusion pressure, even in the presence of an increase in aortic impedance. It is possible to reach loading conditions that cause a negative myocardial oxygen balance. This will cause acute ischemia in a patient with preexisting coronary artery disease. The severity of the episode and the extent of the damage will depend on the degree of coronary artery disease, the presence of adequate collateral circulation, the maintenance of normal coronary autoregulation and the severity and duration of the ischemic episode.

Summary

The use of cardiopulmonary bypass in thoracic aneurysm repair will facilitate repair and can preserve organ function; however, there can be vastly altered loading conditions of the heart. Reduced preload can reduce cardiac output and jeopardize myocardial perfusion. Proper balance of volume between the patient and perfusion apparatus is essential in maintaining adequate cardiac and systemic perfusion.

REFERENCES

1. Gelman S, Reves JG, Fowler K, et al: Regional blood flow during cross-clamping of the thoracic aorta and infusion of sodium nitroprusside. *J Thorac Cardiovasc Surg* 1983; 85:287.
2. Bickerstaff LK, Pairolero DC, Hollier LH, et al: Thoracic aortic aneurysms: A population-based study. *Surgery* 1982; 92:1103–1108.
3. Prokop EK, Palmer RF, Wheat MW: Hydrodynamic forces in dissecting aneurysms. *Circ Res* 1970; 27:121–127.
4. Pressler V, McNamara JJ: Thoracic aortic aneurysm. *J Thorac Cardiovasc Surg* 1980; 79:489–498.
5. Crawford ES, Cohen ES: Aortic aneurysm: A multifocal disease. *Arch Surg* 1982; 117:1393–1400.
6. Sabawala PB, Strong MJ, Keats AS: Surgery of the aorta and its branches. *Anesthesiology* 1970; 33:229–259.
7. Pressler V, McNamara JJ: Aneurysms of the thoracic aorta. *J Thorac Cardiovasc Surg* 1985; 89:50–54.
8. Wadouh F, Lindemann EM, Arndt CF, et al: The arteria radicularis magna anterior as a decisive factor influencing spinal cord damage during aortic occlusion. *J Thorac Cardiovasc Surg* 1984; 88:1–10.
9. Thompson JE, Mollier LM, Patmanrd, et al: Surgical management of abdominal aortic aneurysms. *Ann Surg* 1975; 181:654.
10. Stokes J, Butcher MR: Abdominal aortic aneurysms: Factors influencing operative mortality and criteria of operability. *Arch Surg* 1973; 107:297.

37

Postoperative Right Ventricular Failure Due to Air in the Coronary Vein Graft

A 60-year-old man underwent coronary artery bypass grafting for severe occlusion of his dominant right coronary artery as well as circumflex and anterior descending coronary arteries. The induction, prebypass, and bypass periods were uneventful and the grafts appeared patent. The patient was weaned from cardiopulmonary bypass without difficulties. Shortly thereafter, a rise in right atrial pressure, decreased cardiac output, and poor right venticular contraction were observed. Air was seen in the coronary vein graft.

Recommendations by Joseph Profeta, M.D., and George Silvay, M.D., Ph.D.

ANALYSIS OF THE PROBLEM

There are two important considerations in this case: the effects of coronary air emboli and the importance of the right ventricle in overall cardiac function.

Air Emboli

The incidence of arterial air or gaseous emboli in coronary artery surgery is not reported but is certainly significant. Systemic arterial air embolus is a well-known complication of open heart surgery. Much has been written on cerebral air emboli following open heart surgery; there is some literature on coronary air emboli following open heart surgery; however, there is very little written on the subject of arterial air emboli following coronary artery bypass graft surgery. The emboli can be either air or oxygen. Air emboli may be introduced through the left ventricular vent site, through interatrial or interventricular defects allowing air to enter the systemic circulation from the venous side, or air trapped in the coronary bypass graft at the time of anastomosis. Gaseous emboli may be introduced via the oxygenator during extracorporeal circulation. Ultrasound has been used to detect gaseous microemboli during cardiopulmonary bypass,[1] and intraoperative echocardiography has also been used to detect gaseous microemboli in the heart and aorta while the patient is on bypass—the quantity of gaseous microemboli being greater with the use of bubble oxygenators than with the use of membrane oxygenators. These microbubbles may, however, coalesce to form larger bubbles. Periods of increased incidence of gaseous microbubbles have been documented—at the onset of extracorporeal circulation, during the induction of hypothermia (as supersaturated cold blood from the oxygenator enters the patient the blood is suddenly warmed and oxygen may come out of solution forming microbubbles), and when the heart starts ejecting blood from its cavities into the systemic circulation.[2] While clinical studies definitely linking gaseous microemboli to significant morbidity during heart surgery are lacking, they are still suspect.

Importance of the Right Ventricle

With the ostium of the right coronary artery at the highest point of the aortic root, the chances of gaseous embolization of this artery are high. Also after aortocoronary bypass grafting the grafts are vulnerable to gaseous or air emboli because of their position on the anterior surface of the aorta. Though the right coronary artery supplies the sinoatrial (SA) node in 55% of instances and the atrioventricular (AV) node in 90% of instances (right dominance) as well as the right ventricle, it is looked upon with less significance than the left coronary artery or either of its two divisions. This is principally due to the historical view of the right ventricle as no more than a conduit moving blood through the lungs to the left side of the heart. Recently, however, the function of the right ventricle has been looked at more carefully and it has been observed that the right ventricle may be the limiting factor governing global cardiac pump function.[3]

APPROACH TO THE PROBLEM

The diagnosis of coronary air embolus is usually made by direct visualization of air in the graft by the surgeon, although the diagnosis must be suspected if on discontinuation of bypass there are ECG changes consistent with ischemia, with or without left ventricular failure, or if there are weak cardiac contractions or ventricular premature contractions. While most air emboli occur immediately after defibrillation and at the termination of extracorporeal circulation, some do not occur until later—when the heart is moved or lifted by the surgeon or even much later when the patient is moved from the operating room table to the intensive care unit bed. This is due to air remaining trapped in the heart and being liberated only by vigorous movement. When the air is released early, it is usually noticed by the surgeon and a 25-gauge needle inserted into the graft to release the air. However, if the embolus is not noticed until after there are signs of failure, three important maneuvers must be performed immediately. The patient should be placed in the Trendelenburg position to avoid cerebral artery embolization by the possible further release of air; as much air as possible must be evacuated from the graft by a 25-gauge needle; the circulation must be supported. If the cannulae are still in place and the lines and oxygenator still primed, the easiest way of supporting the circulation is by going back to extracorporeal circulation. The flow rate should be increased to 1½ to 2 times that of normal for one minute. (Normal is considered to be 2.2 L/minute/m^2 of body surface area).[7] This has been shown to be the most effective means of removing air from the coronary arteries and improving contractility. If the flow rate required exceeds the limit of the pump, isoproterenol should be instituted as a slow drip. Inotropes have been shown to be more effective than vasoconstrictors for the removal of coronary air and the improvement of ventricular contractility. If the combination of high flow and isoproterenol drip do not improve contractility, and if the arterial return cannula is in the ascending aorta, the aorta may be partially constricted distal to the inflow cannula with the surgeon's fingers. If the patient cannot be placed back on extracorporeal circulation, support of the circulation with ephedrine or isoproterenol has been shown to be more effective than with vasoconstrictors. This support should be continued until contractility is good, the myocardium shows no signs of cyanosis, and there are no more premature ventricular contractions.

DISCUSSION

Pathophysiology

Air in the systemic arterial circulation was studied by Chase[4] who found that air acts not only as an obstruction to flow, but can also act as an irritant to the vascular wall and produce segmental spasm followed by vasodilatation of capillaries, collateral arteriolar vessels, and venules. Chase concluded there is probably a neurovascular component to the effects of air in the arterial circulation. This was observed in the arterial supply to the duodenal loop and attached mesentery, but there is little reason to believe the effects would be different in the coronary circulation. Others have studied the effects of coronary air emboli in dogs. Rhodes and McIntosh[5] report a significant decrease in regional blood flow with a redistribution of flow away from the subendocardium, i.e., significantly reduced subendocardial/epicardial blood flow ratio. They also reported a significant increase in mean regional blood flow to the area not infarcted, despite significant decreases in mean arterial pressure and left ventricular contractility and increases in left atrial pressures. Others have shown transmural necrosis following air emboli. Clinically, the signs are those of ischemia: ST-segment depression or elevation, various dysrhythmias, including ventricular fibrillation, wall motion abnormalities from hypokinesia to akinesia, and, if severe enough, acute cardiac failure and myocardial necrosis.[6] The duration of the event will vary depending on the composition of the bubble. Carbon dioxide—being more soluble than oxygen—will be short lived; while air—being composed of mostly less soluble nitrogen—will last much longer. The duration of an oxygen embolus will be between that of air and carbon dioxide.

Prevention of the Problem

Of course, the best method of handling any problem is to prevent its occurrence. This can be accomplished by reducing gaseous microemboli and by performing maneuvers that eliminate gaseous bubbles from the chambers of the heart and the aortic root.

Kurusz[1] has derived seven recommendations for reducing gaseous microemboli:

1. Lower gas-to-blood flow ratios. Most current bubble oxygenators require only a 1:1 flow ratio. This is accomplished by reducing the size of the bubbles, thereby increasing the surface area.

2. Maintenance of high reservoir volumes to allow bubbles more time to dissipate.

3. The extracorporeal circuit should be protected from jarring, which has been shown to release showers of microbubbles.

4. Judicious cooling and rewarming: large gradients between cold blood and warm tissues can cause gas to come out of solution.

5. The circuit should be primed and evacuated of air carefully in the pre-bypass period: use of CO_2 to displace room air can facilitate this because of the greater solubility of CO_2.

6. The use of membrane oxygenators: membrane oxygenators produce fewer gaseous microemboli.

7. Arterial line filtration has been shown to remove gaseous microemboli.

Though these seven steps will significantly reduce the incidence of gaseous microemboli, maneuvers must also be performed to eliminate any gas or air from the chambers of the heart and the root of the aorta. This can be accomplished by filling, venting, and compressing the chambers of the heart prior to discontinuation of cardiopulmonary bypass. This procedure should be repeated.[8] Airway pressure should be increased by either the anesthesia bag or ventilator to force blood and any air bubbles from the pulmonary veins into the left atrium and then into the left ventricle, which is vented. Another maneuver is the slow release of the aortic cross-clamp after three or four beats of the heart, while the clinician is gently pinching the proximal right coronary artery and using an aortic root vent. If more attention is paid to the prevention and removal of air from the heart chambers, aortic root, and vein grafts, there will be less incidence of poor ventricular contractility postbypass, which is usually attributed to a long pump run or diminished myocardial level of adenosine triphosphate (ATP).

Summary

Recent investigation has shown the right ventricle may be the limiting factor governing global cardiac pump function. In light of this, the right coronary artery and right coronary artery bypass graft take on much more significance. Coronary air emboli should be prevented by taking steps to prevent gaseous microemboli from the extracorporeal circuit. In addition, maneuvers should be performed at the time of defibrillation and removal of the aortic cross-clamp to remove any trapped gases from the heart chambers and aortic root. If coronary air embolus still occurs, the patient should be placed back on extracorporeal circulation at 1½ to 2 times that of the normal flow. Vasoconstrictors should be avoided. Inotropes have been shown to be more effective in removing coronary air emboli and improving ventricular contractility.

REFERENCES

1. Kurusz M: Gaseous microemboli: Sources, causes and clinical considerations. *Med Instrum* 1985; 19:73–76.

2. Krebber HJ, Hanrath P, Janzen R, et al: Gas emboli during open heart surgery. *Thorac Cardiovasc Surg* 1982; 30:401–404.
3. Hines R, Biondi J, Barash P: The right ventricle: Master or servant? *Anesthesiology* 1984; 61:A8.
4. Chase WH: Anatomical and experimental observations on air embolism. *Surg Gynecol Obstet* 1934; 59:569.
5. Rhodes GR, McIntosh CL: An experimental evolution of coronary air embolism. *Surg Forum* 1976; 27:275–278.
6. Stegman T, Daniel W, Bellmann L, et al: Experimental coronary air embolism: Assessment of time course of myocardial ischemia and the protective effect of cardiopulmonary bypass. *Thorac Cardiovasc Surg* 1980; 28:141–149.
7. Justice C, Leach J, Edwards WS: The harmful effects and treatment of coronary air embolism during open-heart surgery. *Ann Thorac Surg* 1972; 14:47–53.
8. Lawrence GH, McKay HA, Sherensky RT: Effective measures in the prevention of intraoperative aeroembolus. *J Thorac Cardiovasc Surg* 1971; 62:731–735.

38

Low Cardiac Output and Hypotension

A 67-year-old man underwent coronary artery bypass surgery for five-vessel disease. Weaning from cardiopulmonary bypass was difficult and required dopamine 10 µg/kg/minute, and nitroprusside 1 µg/kg/minute to maintain a cardiac index of 1.8 L/minute/m^2 and a blood pressure (BP) above 100/60 mm Hg. Despite this pharmacologic therapy, the pulmonary artery wedge pressure (PAWP) was 20 mm Hg and he had a persistent metabolic acidosis (pH 7.25) and mixed venous saturation of 55%.

Recommendations by Robert N. Sladen, M.B., M.R.C.P.(U.K.), F.R.C.P.(C.)

ANALYSIS OF THE PROBLEM

It is clear that this patient has a low cardiac output syndrome following cardiopulmonary bypass (CPB). The patient is hypotensive and the cardiac index of 1.8 L/minute/m^2 is somewhat less than the lower limit of normal (2.2 L/minute/m^2). Abnormal left ventricular compliance is indicated by the elevated pulmonary artery wedge pressure (PAWP) of 20 mm Hg (upper limit of normal 12 mm Hg). That perfusion is inadequate for tissue needs is indicated by the marked reduction in mixed venous saturation (S$\bar{v}$O$_2$) to 55%. Under conditions of normal cardiac output, the tissues remove 25% of oxygen delivered. Since normal arterial saturation (SaO$_2$) is close to 100%, S$\bar{v}$O$_2$ is normally about 75%. An S$\bar{v}$O$_2$ of 55% implies that the tissues are being grossly underperfused, so that tissue oxygen extraction is markedly increased. [An alternative explanation could be a dramatic decrease in SaO$_2$ to 80%, equivalent to an arterial oxygen tension (PaO_2) of 50 mm Hg.] The evidence for tissue ischemia or hypoxia is reinforced by the presence of a metabolic acidosis. Indeed, this patient's condition qualifies for the term cardiogenic shock.

APPROACH TO THE PROBLEM

1. Normalize heart rate and rhythm. Treat bradycardia or block with atrial or atrioventricular (AV) sequential pacing. Treat tachyarrhythmias with direct current (DC) cardioversion.

2. Optimize preload by fluid challenge with red blood cells (RBCs), fresh frozen plasma (FFP), or normal saline, as appropriate. Push PAWP in steps of 2 to 4 mm Hg and assess effect on cardiac output, stroke volume, SvO_2, and pH.

3. Normalize pH with judicious hyperventilation or bicarbonate. Enhance contractility by adding epinephrine 0.02 to 0.10 µg/kg/minute. Decrease dopamine to 2 to 3 µg/kg/minute to promote renal perfusion. Give calcium chloride 10 to 20 mg/kg over 10 to 15 minutes intravenously (IV) if blood is being rapidly transfused. Restrict or curtail these maneuvers if myocardial ischemia is present and worsens; consider early insertion of intra-aortic balloon pump.

4. Decrease afterload by judicious use of nitroprusside, limited by effect on blood pressure—do not reduce mean arterial pressure (MAP) < 60 mm Hg. Restore preload to former levels with repeated fluid challenges to achieve full benefit of afterload reduction. Curtail this maneuver if myocardial ischemia is present: start nitroglycerin 0.25 to 0.5 µg/kg/minute and consider early insertion of intra-aortic balloon pump.

5. If low cardiac output state (and/or myocardial ischemia) persists despite the above interventions, insert intra-aortic balloon pump and support on 1:1 basis.

6. Continue above approach into the postoperative period. Sedate heavily and plan to ventilate overnight or until there is hemodynamic improvement.

DISCUSSION

Causes

Causes of low cardiac output after cardiopulmonary bypass (CPB) are summarized in Table 38–1. The most likely causes of severe myocardial dysfunction are persistence of previously poor left ventricular function, acute myocardial depression, or acute myocardial ischemia. These will be discussed further. Anaphylactic reactions to protamine or blood products (e.g., fresh frozen plasma) are uncommon but dramatic events. Certainly all the manifestations of low cardiac output presented in this case may be present, except that hypotension is related to a combination of myocardial depression and vasodilation, so that nitroprusside would not be tolerated or indicated. Additional clues to an anaphylactic event include the temporal relationship to the administration of the offending agent, tachycardia, urticaria, hematuria, and pulmonary edema. Low cardiac output can result from profound arterial hypoxemia due to pulmonary edema, pneumothorax, or a misplaced endotracheal tube, which should be excluded. These entities will not be further discussed.

Persistence of Poor Left Ventricular Function

Primary myocardial failure could be due to the fact that the patient had poor ventricular function to begin with that was exacerbated by the stress of aortic cross-clamping and cardiopulmonary bypass and not corrected by the surgical procedure. My evaluation would depend on the history, examination, and special investigations performed on the patient before surgery. Suggestive findings include a history of effort dyspnea or congestive heart failure and evidence of left ventricular failure on preoperative examination (cardiomegaly, gallop, pulmonary edema).

TABLE 38–1.

Causes of Low Cardiac Output After Cardiopulmonary Bypass

Persistence of abnormal ventricular function
  (not corrected by surgery)
Acute myocardial depression
  Drug effects (nadolol, atenolol);
  Acidosis
  Hyperkalemia
  Hypocalcemia
Acute myocardial ischemia
  Intraoperative myocardial infarction
  Prolonged aortic cross-clamp
  Inadequate revascularization
  Kinked or clotted grafts
  Coronary air embolism
  Coronary artery spasm
  Left ventricular distension
Anaphylaxis
  (protamine, blood products)
Severe hypoxemia

On cardiac catheterization the clinician would have expected to have seen an enlarged, poorly contracting ventricle with regional or diffuse abnormalities of wall movement. The most useful quantitative index of *systolic* pump function of the left ventricle is the ejection fraction (EF), which represents that fraction of end diastolic volume ejected as stroke volume. An EF of less than 0.5 suggests clinically significant myocardial dysfunction, and EF of less than 0.25 usually denotes cardiomyopathy. However, if a discrete left ventricular aneurysm is present, it may induce a low total EF even if the residual myocardium has good contractility. In this case the EF may misrepresent the potential improvement in ventricular function possible with resection of a large discrete aneurysm.

Indices of left ventricular filling pressure such as left ventricular end diastolic pressure (LVEDP), pulmonary artery wedge pressure (PAWP), and pulmonary artery diastolic pressure (PAD) provide a guide to ventricular *diastolic* function and ventricular compliance. Elevated resting filling pressures indicate poor compliance due to fibrosis or necrosis of the myocardium and are usually associated with poor systolic pump function. However, in many instances, filling pressures are normal at rest (<12 mm Hg) but become sharply abnormal (>20 mm Hg) after dye injection. This indicates diffuse coronary artery disease; ventricular stiffness increases due to the ischemic and volume stress of the injected dye.[1] In this situation, systolic function (EF, cardiac output) is frequently normal or even hyperdynamic.

Further evidence of poor left ventricular reserve would be obtained by noting hypotension, tachycardia, or tachyarrhythmias in response to stressful events, notably anesthetic induction and cardiac cannulation. During anesthetic induction there is a decrease in sympathetic tone and decrease in venous return (muscle relaxation, positive pressure ventilation). Once the chest is open, an impression of myocardial function can be obtained by direct observation of poor global or regional wall motion in the left ventricle. Cannulation of the great veins and right atrium interferes with venous return, decreases atrial filling, and often precipitates supraventricular arrhythmias. Patients with limited cardiac reserve do not tolerate loss of the atrial "kick" or preload and hypotension often results.

Myocardial Depression

The duration of aortic cross-clamping is an important determinant of postbypass ventricular function. While the aorta is cross-clamped, the myocardium is subject to ischemia. The use of cold potassium cardioplegia with mannitol mitigates the degree of ischemia and interstitial edema, but even so there is a marked deterioration in myocardial function when cross-clamping is prolonged beyond 90 minutes. In addition, although cold is protective, it decreases ventricular compliance and increases the incidence of conduction defects in the early postbypass period. Even in patients with previously normal ventricular function, it may take up to 24 hours before myocardial function returns to preoperative levels.[2]

Postbypass myocardial depression can be induced by drugs, electrolyte, and acid-base abnormalities. Preoperative administration of short-acting β-blockers such as propranolol does not cause problems, but long-acting agents such as nadolol or atenolol can contribute to myocardial depression and bradyarrhythmias after CPB. Calcium blockers with negative inotropic action such as verapamil or diltiazem have a short duration of action and are unlikely to pose problems.

Hyperkalemia can cause profound depression of myocardial contractility and conduction. It may be due to excessive administration or inadequate clearing of potassium cardioplegia. I have seen it in one case in which oliguria was induced by excessive use of vasoconstrictors to maintain coronary perfusion pressure after release of the aortic cross-clamp. Myocardial depression improved once potassium was decreased from 6.5 to 5.0 mEq/L by furosemide-induced diuresis. Ionized calcium levels are frequently low in the early postbypass period. Calcium is sequestered by extracorporeal circulation and chelated by citrated blood products (blood, fresh frozen plasma) and human albumin. Hypocalcemia can contribute to myocardial depression and impair the response to endogenous and exogenous catecholamines. Acidosis (pH<7.25) has similar effects.

Acute Myocardial Ischemia

Low cardiac output after CPB induced by acute myocardial ischemia may have one of several precipitating factors. The patient may have suffered acute myocardial ischemia or infarction in the immediate preoperative period, during anesthetic induction or in the prebypass period. Revascularization may have been inadequate or inappropriate. A graft may have become kinked or thrombosed. Coronary air embolism is an insidious and ever-present threat. Rarely, unexplained coronary artery spasm may precipitate acute ischemia after CPB.

The most important single determinant of perioperative myocardial infarction is the presence of unstable angina in the preoperative period.[3] Unstable angina implies new onset angina, angina that is worsening in severity, rest pain, or angina that is poorly responsive to medication. Other clues to the severity of preoperative myocardial ischemia exist. Chest pain, arrhythmias, or systolic hypotension during exercise testing implies diffuse ischemia. Thallium scanning can quantitate the amount of myocardium involved by ischemia.

Early detection of myocardial ischemia during anesthesia requires appropriate lead placement. With a five-lead system (chest lead at V_5, episodes of lateral (>50% of cases) or inferior ischemia (15% of cases) may be detected. If a three-lead system is used, the left arm lead should be placed at the V_5 position. Lead I will detect anterior ischemia, and lead II inferior ischemia. [4] Subendocardial ischemia is implied by ST depression; ST elevation above 1 mm implies transmural ischemia or coronary artery spasm.

An important sign of myocardial ischemia is a decrease in ventricular compliance, manifested by a sudden increase in filling pressure (PAD or PAWP). This in itself may justify the use of pulmonary artery catheters in patients with unstable angina. Blood pressure may increase (a reflex response to ischemia) or decrease (if output is impaired). Transesophageal echocardiography, if available, can demonstrate regional wall motion abnormalities, even in the absence of ECG or PAWP changes.

Using the above monitoring, ischemia may have been detected during periods of sympathetic stress: the preinduction period (especially if lines were placed before anesthesia), anesthetic induction, skin incision, sternal split, and aortic root dissection. Hypotension and tachyarrhythmias may have induced ischemia during caval cannulation. Acute ischemia could have occurred independently of these events due to coronary artery spasm. Signs of ischemia before CPB should have alerted the clinician to the possibility of ischemia-induced low cardiac output after CPB.

Prolonged aortic cross-clamping provides an ischemic insult that increases exponentially with duration greater than 90 minutes. This will be greatly increased if there has been inadequate venting of blood return to the left ventricle from thebesian vessels, bronchial, and noncoronary collaterals. Ventricular distention during cross-clamping induces subendocardial ischemia, impairs myocardial cooling, and overstretches myocardial fibers. Clues to acute ischemia may be given by the observation of elevated ST segments or ventricular irritability after aortic cross-clamp release that do not improve with connection of the proximal bypass grafts.

Coronary air embolism is a constant threat, despite efforts to vent the heart after aortic cross-clamp release. It is an important cause of sudden, otherwise unexplained, myocardial depression. Not infrequently, entrapped air is dislodged into the coronary arteries when the patient is moved from the operating table to the gurney. The diagnosis is usually made by direct visualization of the heart, which may actually reveal air in the coronaries or areas of inadequate perfusion (pallor, duskiness, hypokinesis).

Management Options

Poor Ventricular Function

The fundamental approach to the hemodynamic management of poor ventricular function is summarized in Table 38–2.

TABLE 38–2.

Hemodynamic Management of Low Cardiac Output Syndrome

1. Correct acid-base and electrolyte abnormalities; ensure adequate oxygenation
2. Optimize preload (serial fluid challenges)
3. Enhance contractility with inotropic agents
4. Reduce afterload with vasodilator drugs
   (steps 3 and 4 are additive)
5. Restore preload to former level if decreased by vasodilator
6. Intra-aortic balloon counterpulsation if low output persists
   (use early if myocardial ischemia present)

Normalize Rate and Rhythm.—The primary goal is to achieve an appropriate heart rate (90 to 100 beats per minute) with an intact atrial kick.

Bradycardia and Atrioventricular (AV) Conduction Defects.—The most direct and successful intervention is for the surgeon to place atrial and ventricular epicardial pacing wires. Sinus or junctional bradycardias can usually be overcome by atrial pacing. However, if AV block exists, sequential atrioventricular pacing is required. Ventricular pacing alone is never as effective—the more depressed and stiff the myocardium, the more dependent it is on atrial contraction for optimal ventricular filling. Indeed, the ability to provide atrial (or sequential AV) pacing often greatly influences the success of weaning from CPB. To attain the equivalent output with ventricular pacing, rates of 110 to 120 beats per minute are required, which shortens diastolic coronary filling time. Placement of a multipurpose pulmonary artery catheter (''pacing Swan'') may be helpful in patients with conduction problems in the prebypass period, but it should not be relied upon in favor of epicardial wires. A slow infusion of isoproterenol (1 to 2 μg/minute) can be helpful in speeding up a sinus bradycardia but is less predictable than direct pacing and can potentially cause unwanted ischemia and vasodilation.

Tachyarrhythmias.—Sinus tachycardia (ST) (120 to 160/beats per minute) is generally a symptom of inadequate anesthesia, intravascular hypovolemia, or a poor stroke volume. The underlying cause—not the tachycardia itself—should be treated. A very useful clinical sign that ventricular function is improving is the gradual slowing of heart rate with the same BP and cardiac output, i.e., stroke volume has increased. Supraventricular arrhythmias (atrial tachycardia, atrial flutter, atrial fibrillation) should immediately be treated with cardioversion (10 to 15 joules applied with sterile paddles directly to the heart if the chest is open). In the early postbypass period, calcium blockers such as verapamil should be used only when concomitant myocardial ischemia is suspected and β-blockers should be avoided altogether. Ventricular tachycardia or fibrillation obviously require emergent cardioversion.

At the same time, predisposing factors such as hypokalemia, hypoxemia, and acidosis should be sought and eliminated. We use a "K Scale" to guide potassium replacement: for every 0.1 mEq less than 4.5 mEq/L, 1 mEq KCL is given in dilute infusion over two minutes (e.g., if the level of serum potassium were 3.0 mEq/L, 15 mEq of diluted KCl is given over 30 minutes). Myocardial hypothermia is a common cause of ventricular irritability when attempts are made to wean from CPB before the heart has warmed sufficiently. Persistent ventricular irritability is an indication for lidocaine (1mg/kg IV bolus, followed by IV infusion at 2 mg/minute), or magnesium sulfate (8 to 16 mEq, or 1 to 2 ml of a 50% solution).

Optimize Preload.—The optimum preload is that filling pressure that is associated with maximal efficiency of cardiac function. Although this patient has a PAWP of 20 mm Hg, it may not yet be adequate in the presence of depressed myocardial function or compliance. Optimum preload is found by sequential fluid challenges with hemodynamic evaluation; although while the chest is open, an astute estimate of intravascular volume can be achieved by direct observation of the heart—whether the chambers appear full or tend to "collapse." The type of fluid to be administered depends on the circumstance. If the patient's hematocrit (Hct) reading was less than 30%, I would use packed red blood cells (RBCs) because this would enhance oxygen-carrying capacity. If the patient was bleeding and had a prolonged prothrombin time, I would use fresh frozen plasma (FFP). If Hct reading and coagulation status were normal, I would use normal saline in aliquots of 250 to 500 ml (there is no intrinsic advantage in using colloids such as human albumin or hetastarch). A favorable response to fluid challenges is assessed by an increased BP in the face of decreased inotropic drug requirement, increased stroke volume (increased cardiac output at the same heart rate or decreased heart rate with the same cardiac output), and improvement in tissue oxygenation (i.e., increased SvO_2 above 65%, increased pH above 7.3).

In this case optimal preload may be a PAWP of 24, 28, or even 30 mm Hg. However, lack of favorable response to increased preload suggests that the limit of preload reserve has been reached (i.e., the "flat portion" of the Frank-Starling curve). In particular, if fluid challenges cause increased lung stiffness (increased peak inspiratory pressure, or PIP), increased alveolar-arterial O_2 gradient ($AaDO_2$) or frank pulmonary edema, then alternative approaches should be applied. In the face of already severely compromised tissue oxygenation (SvO_2 55%), it would be essential to maintain PaO_2 greater than 100 mm Hg to ensure 100% arterial saturation.

Enhance Contractility.—The metabolic acidosis (pH 7.25) must be normalized to allow appropriate catecholamine effects on the heart. If cardiac output increases in response to control of heart rate and preload augmentation, the acidosis should resolve. Moderate hyperventilation (to a $PaCO_2$ of 25 to 30 mm Hg) can compensate to improve pH. If not, sodium bicarbonate 25 to 50 mEq IV should be given with the goal to improve pH to greater than 7.30. Excessive bicarbonate administration may induce metabolic alkalosis, hypokalemia, hypocalcemia, and increase CO_2 production.

If the low cardiac output syndrome persists at a dose of dopamine of 10µg/kg/minute, I would add epinephrine. At doses of above 10 µg/kg/minute, dopamine has a progressively greater α- adrenergic, chronotropic, and bathmotropic effect. This results in cutaneous, renal, and splanchnic vasoconstriction, increased systemic vascular resistance, tachycardia, and ventricular irritability. In addition, about 50% of dopamine's action is indirect, via the release of myocardial norepinephrine, which may be depleted in long-standing cardiomyopathy. Epinephrine is a much more potent, direct-acting inotropic agent. The dose of epinephrine (1 mg in 250 ml 5% dextrose = 4 µg/ml or 4,000 ng/ml) ranges from 20 to 100 ng/kg/minute. At doses greater than 100 ng/kg/minute, effects identical to those described with dopamine become increasingly prominent. The addition of epinephrine facilitates successful weaning from CPB in many cases in which dopamine has failed.

Once epinephrine is started, dopamine should be weaned to the 2 to 3 µg/kg/minute range, rather than discontinued. The rationale is to attempt to promote renal and splanchnic blood flow with low-dose dopamine, and possibly even to counteract the effects of epinephrine on renal blood flow. There is some animal evidence that this maneuver may protect the kidney against potent vasopressors.[5] At Stanford University, calcium chloride has traditionally been added to the epinephrine infusion (1 gm in 250 ml 5% dextrose: epical). On a pharmacokinetic basis, it would seem logical to first give a loading bolus of calcium chloride (10 to 20 mg/kg over 10 to 15 minutes).

Isoproterenol is a very potent inotropic agent, but it causes unacceptable tachycardia and tachyarrhythmias. Dobutamine is far less chronotropic than isoproterenol and is a potent direct-acting inotropic drug. However, its peripheral (β$_2$-adrenergic) vasodilator effect can cause disconcerting hypotension, particularly in patients who already have low blood pressure. Norepinephrine is also a potent inotropic agent, but its profound vasoconstrictor effect increases SVR and afterload, and may worsen cardiac output and tissue perfusion. Amrinone is a nonadrenergic inotropic agent with vasodilator activity that has been released but its clinical efficacy has not yet been established in this situation. It has side effects (thrombocytopenia, ventricular arrhythmias) that may limit its acceptance.

Reduce Afterload.—As myocardial function deteriorates, it becomes less responsive to inotropic support and more dependent on afterload reduction. Drugs that dilate the arterial bed decrease systemic vascular resistance (SVR) and the impedance to ventricular outflow. The ventricle is able to perform less pressure work and more volume work, which increases stroke volume and decreases oxygen consumption. It is important to recognize that pharmacologic afterload reducers all have the potential to drop aortic diastolic (and therefore coronary perfusion) pressures and worsen myocardial ischemia.

Sodium nitroprusside has the distinct advantage that it is extremely rapid-acting, so that it may be exquisitely titrated to effect. However, because nitroprusside has a balanced vasodilator effect on arteries and veins, it tends to decrease preload at the same time as it decreases afterload. If preload drops below optimal levels, hypotension and decreased cardiac output result. In fact, hypotension is the limiting factor in achieving afterload reduction with nitroprusside. In order to achieve the full benefit of afterload reduction with nitroprusside, preload must be restored to its former level[6] (Fig 38–1). This requires frequent fluid challenges.

Clinically, nitroprusside [50 mg in 250 ml 5% dextrose = 200 μg/ml] is titrated against the mean arterial pressure (MAP), which is used as an indirect index of afterload. In the present case the MAP is already 73 mm Hg on 1

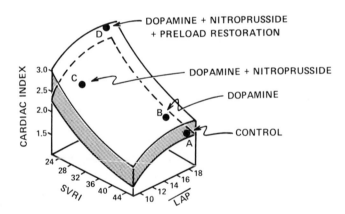

FIG 38–1.
Hemodynamic management. Three-dimensional schematic diagram integrating preload, afterload, and contractility effects. *LAP* = mean left atrial pressure. *SVRI* = systemic vascular resistance index. At *point A*, preload (LAP) is elevated at 16 mm Hg, afterload (SVRI) is elevated at 44 Wood Units (= 3,520 dyne/sec/cm^{-5}), and cardiac index is decreased at 1.75 L/min/m^2. At *point B*, dopamine has been added. Inotropic effect increases cardiac index with slight improvement in preload and afterload. At *point C*, nitroprusside has been added. Afterload reduction is striking: SVRI decreases to 26 Wood Units (= 2,080 dyne/sec/cm^{-5}) and cardiac index increases to 2.7. However, preload is simultaneously decreased to 12 mm Hg. At *point D*, after preload restoration to an LAP of 16 mm Hg with a fluid challenge, the full benefit of afterload reduction is realized, and cardiac index increases above 3 L/min/m^2. (From Miller DC, et al: *Surgery* 1980; 88:108–117. Used by permission.)

μg/kg/minute of nitroprusside, so that there is not a great deal of BP reserve for further afterload reduction. However, I would carefully increase the dose of nitroprusside to titrate the MAP to about 65 mm Hg, below which I would become concerned about coronary perfusion pressure. Cardiac output should then again be measured, in the hope that it has increased as SVR has decreased. If acute myocardial ischemia is present, nitroprusside should be used with great care because it decreases aortic diastolic pressure and shunts blood away from ischemic areas of the myocardium.

Hydralazine is a pure arterial dilator, and so has the potential to decrease afterload without affecting preload. It is particularly useful in low cardiac output syndromes in which the combination of afterload reduction with the maintenance of a high preload is required. However, it has a half life of between 1.5 and 8 hours and cannot easily be titrated to effect. It is therefore not useful in the operating room or in the early postoperative period when vasodilator requirements rapidly fluctuate. However, once the patient has warmed up in the intensive care unit, hydralazine can be extremely useful in providing specific afterload reduction while preserving preload and allowing nitroprusside and inotropic agents to be weaned. [7]

Prostaglandin E1 is an investigational drug currently undergoing evaluation. It promotes coronary and pulmonary dilatation and has been lifesaving in cases of low cardiac output syndrome associated with right ventricular decompensation and severe pulmonary hypertension. However, because it is a balanced vasodilator, hypotension results, and the systemic circulation may have to be supported with a concurrent infusion of norepinephrine via the left atrium to maintain blood pressure. [8]

Acute Myocardial Ischemia.—Fundamentally, the approach to the low cardiac output syndrome caused by acute myocardial ischemia is the same as that discussed above, except that the effect of these maneuvers on myocardial oxygen balance must be taken into primary consideration. In certain situations, such as left ventricular distention or suspected coronary air embolism, the most expeditious approach is to have the patient go back on to CPB. This allows time for the ventricle to be properly vented or for coronary air to be flushed (occasionally induced hypertension on CPB is helpful in this regard) and for the ventricle to recover. Kinked or clotted grafts may have to be replaced.

The major clinical determinants of *myocardial oxygen demand* are heart rate, contractility, afterload, and preload. Increasing heart rate is the most oxygen-expensive means of increasing cardiac output. Tachycardia increases cardiac work per unit time, at the expense of diastolic time and myocardial oxygen supply. In addition, tachycardia causes a reflex increase in contractility. In contrast, preload augmentation is the most efficient and least oxygen-expensive means of increasing cardiac output. However, if the heart is overdistended, afterload increases (because it is related to intracavitary ventricular radius) and negates this benefit. Myocardial oxygen balance is adversely affected by excessive use of inotropic drugs that increase heart rate and contractility, or overzealous volume challenges that distend the heart.

Myocardial oxygen supply depends on oxygen transport and coronary perfusion. During diastole 70% to 90% of coronary perfusion to the left ventricle occurs. In the presence of acute ischemia the coronary arteries are maximally dilated, so that flow is very dependent on the pressure gradient across them. The coronary perfusion pressure (CPP) is the gradient between the aortic diastolic pressure (ADP)—the pressure head—and the left ventricular diastolic pressure (LVDP), which compresses the subendocardial vessels.

$$CPP = ADP - LVDP$$

Therefore, interventions that decrease ADP out of proportion to LVDP can worsen acute ischemia. This applies to the use of any arterial vasodilator: nitroprusside, hydralazine, and even calcium blockers such as nifedipine.

In contrast, nitroglycerin, which has a predominantly venodilator effect at lower doses, can decrease LVDP without affecting ADP. In addition, it has been demonstrated that nitroglycerin increases blood flow into ischemic areas by dilating conductance (epicardial) rather than resistance (intramuscular) coronary vessels. However, it is not a very effective afterload reducer except inasmuch as it decreases overdistended ventricular radius.

If the low cardiac output syndrome were due to acute myocardial ischemia, I would still try nitroprusside initially to provide afterload reduction, but I would add nitroglycerin. If there were acute ST changes, I would titrate the nitroglycerin to relieve them as long as BP was maintained and would continue the infusion at between 0.25 and 1.0 µg/kg/minute as a "background" to facilitate coronary perfusion. If BP decreased when the nitroglycerin was started, nitroprusside should be weaned or discontinued. Myocardial ischemia not responsive to nitroglycerin may be due to coronary artery spasm. If this is suspected, verapamil 2.5 to 5.0 mg IV can be given. However, this may adversely affect contractility and precipitate hypotension.

Intra-aortic Balloon Counterpulsation.—Intra-aortic balloon counterpulsation (IABC) is the only method available that provides afterload reduction while simultaneously maintaining coronary perfusion pressure. A serious limitation of all pharmacologic maneuvers to decrease afterload is that these arterial vasodilator drugs all decrease ADP as well. Afterload reduction is gained at the expense of impaired myocardial oxygen supply.

The principle of IABC is that balloon inflation creates a positive pressure wave just after the aortic valve closes that markedly increases ADP and coronary filling (diastolic augmentation). In mid-diastole the balloon deflates, creating a negative pressure wave that reaches its nadir at the end of diastole (end diastolic dip). Impedance to ventricular outflow at the next systole is thereby reduced, decreasing peak systolic pressure (afterload reduction) (Fig 38–2).

The IABC improves pump function and increases cardiac output an average of 0.5 to 0.8/L/minute. Myocardial oxygen balance is markedly improved because of decreased afterload and systolic pressure work (decreased demand) and improved diastolic perfusion pressure (increased supply). Because left ventricular ejection is enhanced, the required filling pressure is decreased and the reduced heart size further decreases myocardial oxygen demand.

The important decision in this case is to determine when to place the intra-aortic balloon. If a low cardiac output syndrome (hypotension, tachycardia, low SvO_2, metabolic acidosis) persists despite adequate heart rate, preload augmentation and maximal inotropic support (dopamine 10 μg/kg/minute +

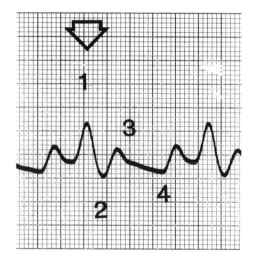

FIG 38–2.

Intra-aortic balloon counterpulsation (IABC). Peripheral arterial waveform illustrating desired effects of IABC. For the sake of clarity, assist is at 1:2 and the balloon wave is indicated by the arrow. At *point 1* inflation proceeds, *after* the dichrotic notch (aortic valve closure); this is important to avoid ejection against an inflated balloon. For maximal coronary perfusion, the diastolic pressure wave should exceed the preceding systolic pressure (diastolic augmentation). At *point 2* the balloon has been deflated and a negative pressure wave has been created—end diastolic pressure (EDP). Impedance to outflow from the next beat is decreased (afterload reduction), and the peak systolic pressure is correspondingly reduced (*point 3*). Note that the EDP after an unassisted beat (*point 4*) is higher than that after an assisted beat (*point 2*), illustrating the effect of afterload reduction. The IABC decreases afterload while improving coronary perfusion pressure.

epinephrine 100 ng/kg/minute), IABC must be considered. In this situation the major function of the balloon would be to support cardiac pump function; blood pressure should *increase*. However, if there is acute myocardial ischemia, the balloon should be placed at an earlier stage, before maximal inotropic support is considered. In this situation the major function of IABC is to improve myocardial oxygen balance; systolic blood pressure might even *decrease*.

In about 12% of cases, insertion fails, most often because of severe atheromatous disease of the femoral and iliac vessels and the descending aorta. The IABC is started at 1:1, i.e., every beat is assisted. However, with irregular arrhythmias and with tachyarrhythmias of greater than 130 beats per minute, the balloon, which usually triggers off the R wave of the ECG, cannot track accurately and support becomes erratic. The IABC can be triggered by a pacing spike, if necessary.

Postoperative Management.—The hemodynamic management[9] outlined above should be continued into the postoperative period without interruption. In order to facilitate a smooth transition and to reduce variables, the patient should be kept heavily sedated and paralyzed, and controlled mechanical ventilation should be continued overnight. Hypokalemia should be diligently managed because it is the commonest cause of ventricular irritability in the early postoperative period. Oliguria should be anticipated but the primary treatment remains efforts to improve cardiac output, although diuretic therapy with low-dose dopamine (1 to 3 μg/kg/minute), mannitol and furosemide may protect against acute tubular necrosis. Bleeding is more likely to occur because CPB times have usually been protracted and low flow and acidosis promote the development of disseminated intravascular coagulation (DIC).

REFERENCES

1. Forfang K, Anderson A, Simonen S, et al: Relation between intraventricular filling pressure and angiographic findings in coronary heart disease: Ventriculography used as a stress test. *Br Heart J* 1977; 39:67–72.
2. Berger RL, Weisel RD, Vito L, et al: Cardiac output measurement by thermodilution during cardiac operations. *Ann Thorac Surg* 1976; 21:43–47.
3. Fennell WH, Chua KG, Cohen L, et al: Detection, prediction, and significance of perioperative myocardial infarction following aortocoronary bypass. *J Thorac Cardiovasc Surg* 1979; 78:244–253.
4. Bazaral M, Norfleet E: Comparison of V5 and CB5 leads for intraoperative monitoring. *Anesth Analg* 1981; 60:849–853.
5. Shaer GL, Fink MP, Parillo JE: Norepinephrine alone versus norepinephrine plus low-dose dopamine: Enhanced renal blood flow with combination pressor therapy. *Crit Care Med* 1985; 13:492–496.

6. Miller DC, Stinson EB, Oyer PE, et al: Postoperative enhancement of left ventricular performance by combined inotropic-vasodilator therapy with preload control. *Surgery* 1980; 88:108–117.

7. Sladen RN, Rosenthal MH: Specific afterload reduction with parenteral hydralazine following cardiac surgery. *J Thorac Cardiovasc Surg* 1979; 78:195–202.

8. D'Ambra MN, LaRaia PJ, Philbin DM, et al: Prostaglandin E1: A new therapy for refractory right heart failure and pulmonary hypertension after mitral valve replacement. *J Thorac Cardiovasc Surg* 1985; 89:567–572.

9. Sladen RN: Management of the postoperative cardiac surgery patient, in Ream AK, Fogdall RP (eds): *Acute Cardiovascvular Management: Anesthesia and Intensive Care*. Philadelphia, JB Lippincott Co, 1982, pp 481–548.

39

Mitral Insufficiency With Coronary Artery Disease

A 65-year-old man with severe three-vessel coronary artery disease and unstable angina was scheduled to have bypass surgery. The patient was anesthetized with fentanyl, enflurane, pancuronium, and oxygen. During sternotomy the heart rate increased from 75 to 85 beats per minute and the blood pressure (BP) went from 140/90 to 100/50mm Hg. The pulmonary artery wedge pressure (PAWP) increased from 10 to 22 mm pressure Hg and there were prominent V waves.

Recommendations by Steven N. Konstadt, M.D., Mark Trager, M.D., and Joel A. Kaplan, M.D.

ANALYSIS OF THE PROBLEM

This case presents deterioration in hemodynamic status and evidence of mitral valve incompetence. Therapy is indicated since a patient with ischemic heart disease requires adequate perfusion or myocardial injury will occur. The presumed cause of this problem is myocardial ischemia.

APPROACH TO THE PROBLEM

Monitoring for signs of ischemia and mitral valve competency should be carefully implemented. Therapy is designed to ensure adequate cardiac and systemic perfusion. Nitroglycerin administered intravenously (IV), starting at 0.5 μg/kg/minute, is the treatment of choice. Other possible drug interventions include β-adrenergic and calcium entry blockers (see discussion below).

DISCUSSION

Background

Median sternotomy and spreading of the chest can cause a massive sympathetic discharge. In patients with normal left ventricular function, this often results in hypertension and tachycardia. However, in patients with poor left ventricular function and coronary artery disease (CAD), the increase in afterload may not be tolerated, and they may respond to sternotomy by developing myocardial ischemia and/or congestive heart failure.

Three significant hemodynamic alterations occurred during sternotomy in this patient. First, there was an increase in heart rate from 75 to 85 beats per minute. Though a heart rate of 85 beats per minute is not usually considered a tachycardia, in a patient with CAD under anesthesia, a 15% increase in heart rate can be significant. The differential diagnosis of this increase in heart rate includes inadequate depth of anesthesia, hypovolemia, anemia, vasodilation, hypoxia, hypercarbia, fever, dysrhythmia, myocardial ischemia, and/or valvular dysfunction.

Second, the patient's blood pressure dropped from a mean arterial pressure (MAP) of 107 to 67 mm Hg, i.e., approximately a 40% decrease. This decrement could be caused by a dysrhythmia, hypovolemia, vasodilation, valvular dysfunction, decreased myocardial contractility, ischemia, various drugs, or manual compression.

Third, the pulmonary capillary wedge pressure (PCWP) increased over 100% and prominent "V" waves appeared. In the normal PCWP tracing, two waves may be seen. The A wave, which occurs after the P wave on the electrocardiogram (ECG), is produced by left atrial contraction. The V wave of the left atrial or PCWP tracing reflects atrial filling and is normally produced by the flow of blood into the left atrium against a closed mitral valve. The V wave occurs at the time of the T wave on the ECG. In pathologic situations the PCWP tracing may be altered. The A wave will be absent in the presence of atrial fibrillation. Conversely, large A waves will be seen when there is an increased resistance to left atrial emptying, (e.g., mitral stenosis). Giant A waves, or cannon A waves, can be seen when the left atrium contracts against a closed mitral valve. This is frequently seen during anesthesia when a nodal rhythm occurs. In the past, it was believed that large V waves were diagnostic of mitral regurgitation. However, recently, Pichard et al. studied 237 patients undergoing catheterization; in those cases 27 patients had large V waves.[1]

Ventriculograms were used to diagnose mitral regurgitation, and 17 patients were found to have mitral regurgitation, while 10 had no significant regurgitant flow. The only significant difference found between patients with and without mitral regurgitation was that the slope of the ascent of the V wave was steeper in patients without regurgitation. In a similar study, Fuchs et al. came to identical conclusions looking at 1,021 cardiac catheterizations.[2] Fifty patients with large V waves (10 or more mm Hg greater than the mean PCWP) were studied; 36% of the patients had no mitral regurgitation. Therefore, caution is called for in diagnosing mitral regurgitation by PCWP tracings alone. The differential diagnosis of the "V" wave in this patient includes (1) acute mitral regurgitation, (2) ventricular distention, or (3) reduced myocardial compliance.

There are two groups of papillary muscles in the left ventricle, called the posteromedial and the anterolateral muscles. The blood supply to the anterolateral papillary muscle is usually from branches of the left circumflex coronary artery. The blood supply to the posteromedial muscle is more variable, reflecting the variability of supply of the posterior septal attachment. In hearts with a left dominant circulation, the left circumflex coronary artery may supply the posterior muscle. In hearts with a right dominant circulation, the muscle is supplied by posterior descending branches of the right coronary artery.[3] Mitral regurgitation can be a relatively common finding in either acute or chronic ischemia, since the papillary muscles are subendocardial structures and are particularly vulnerable to ischemia. Papillary muscle dysfunction is much more likely to occur than a ruptured muscle. If papillary muscle ischemia is treated, the mitral regurgitation should resolve. However, if the ischemia is untreated, an infarct may occur with subsequent papillary muscle rupture. In the event of an infarct, rupture most often occurs between the second and third days after the myocardial infarction. Another potential etiology of acute mitral regurgitation is rupture of a chorda tendineae. However, this is unlikely in the present case since there is no prior history of rheumatic fever or bacterial endocarditis.

Acute ventricular dilatation may also produce mitral regurgitation. In this situation, the papillary muscles are stretched and mitral valve opposition is prevented, creating valvular incompetence. Volume loading, left ventricular dysfunction, and an increase in left ventricular afterload are the common etiologies of acute dilatation.

Myocardial ischemia is a common cause of altered myocardial compliance. This was demonstrated by Mann et al. in 12 patients atrially paced during cardiac catheterization.[4] All patients developed segmental contraction abnormalities and demonstrated decreased left ventricular compliance prior to developing angina. Gausch et al. also studied ventricular compliance changes and found that the elevated filling pressure was not always a result of transient left ventricular failure with increased left ventricular volumes.[5] It appeared that during ischemia there was an impairment of ventricular relaxation and the left ventricular diastolic pressure/volume curve was shifted upward. For any given diastolic volume, left ventricular pressure is, therefore, higher and an increased PCWP with a prominent "V" wave can be seen.

As a result of these and other studies, Kaplan and Wells advocated use of the pulmonary artery catheter to detect V waves as a means of diagnosing early myocardial ischemia.[6] They demonstrated that 55% of patients in their study developed myocardial ischemia, i.e. a mean PCWP of greater than 15 mm Hg or a V wave greater than 20 mm Hg, without concurrent ECG changes. It is recognized that other factors such as changes in airway pressure, anesthetic depth, or afterload may also affect the PCWP tracing.[7]

Since it will alter the management of this patient, it is important to answer the following questions:

1. Is mitral regurgitation present?

2. Is there associated myocardial ischemia?

Intraoperatively, there are two ways to determine if mitral regurgitation is present. Since the chest is open, the surgeon can palpate the left atrium. If mitral regurgitation is present, a thrill will be felt in this area. Alternatively, the diagnosis can be made by the use of intraoperative echocardiography or color-flow Doppler. Goldman et al. have reported the use of intraoperative contrast (microbubbles) injection into the left ventricle to test for the presence of mitral regurgitation.[8] If mitral regurgitation is present, contrast will appear in the left atrium during systole. Without contrast injection, mitral regurgitation can be diagnosed by using pulse-wave Doppler or color-flow Doppler across the mitral valve.[9] These echocardiographic techniques can be performed using either a sterile probe placed directly on the heart or by a transesophageal approach (Fig 39–1).[10]

The presence of myocardial ischemia can be confirmed by several techniques. The method most commonly in use is the electrocardiogram. Blackburn et al. first showed that 89% of ST-segment information can be found in precordial lead V_5 from the twelve-lead exercise-stress ECG.[11] Kaplan and King first applied this information to the operating room in 1976, and lead V_5 or a modification, such as CM_5, is now monitored for diagnosing anterolateral ischemia; while lead II is monitored for inferior ischemia.[12] To detect posterior ischemia, Kates and coworkers advocate use of the esophageal electrocardiographic probe.[13] Despite these improvements in electrocardiographic monitoring, it still has severe limitations. Electrocautery interferes with the signal, temperature and electrolyte changes alter ST-segment repolarization, and positional changes alter the lead configuration. Most importantly, electrocardiographic changes are not early indicators of myocardial ischemia.

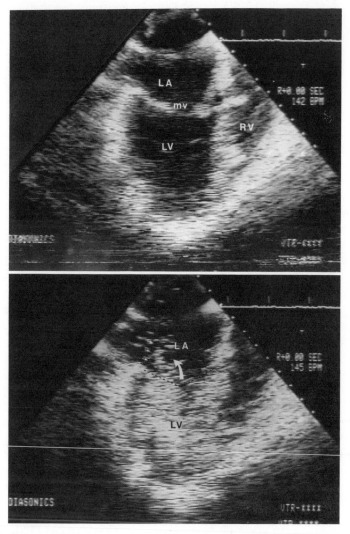

FIG 39–1.
A, preinjection four-chamber transesophageal echocardiographic view. *LA* = left atrium;
LV = left ventricle; *RV* = right ventricle; *MV* = mitral valve. **B,** identical view during agitated saline injection into the left ventricle. The large white arrow indicates the direction of regurgitant flow from the LV into the LA. The small white arrows point to the contrast that appeared in the LA that demonstrates mitral regurgitation.

In 1935, Tennant and Wiggers first demonstrated that left ventricular contractile function was impaired shortly after coronary artery ligation. [14] Since then the correlation of myocardial blood flow and ventricular function has become clearer. Forrester et al. studied the effects of graded coronary perfusion and ventricular function as measured by pressure-length relationships and showed that stepwise reductions in perfusion pressure produced a predictable progression of segmental contractile abnormalities. [15] Vatner correlated actual blood flow with ventricular function and obtained similar results. [16] In dogs anesthetized with halothane, Lowenstein et al. showed that regional wall motion abnormalities were limited to areas of myocardium supplied by narrowed coronary arteries. [17] Further, they noted that the epicardial ECG was insensitive to ischemia. Based on these studies, regional wall motion is now considered to be a reliable indicator of myocardial blood flow. [18-20]

Numerous studies have shown that, in response to decreased myocardial blood flow, changes in regional wall motion consistently occur prior to ECG changes. In anesthetized dogs, Miller et al. placed intramural ultrasonic elements and ECG electrodes at the same depth of myocardium. [21] When the left anterior descending coronary artery was constricted, changes in segmental shortening of the myocardium were noted prior to changes in the ECG. Similar results were obtained by Butler et al. [22] and Smith et al. [23] In man, Upton et al. studied ventricular function by radionuclide angiocardiography during exercise in 25 patients. [24] At a low level of exercise, no patients developed angina or ST-segment depression, but 14 of the 25 patients had segmental contractile abnormalities. Sugishita et al., also using radionuclide scanning, found that regional wall motion abnormalities occurred on the average 30 seconds after the onset of exercise, whereas ECG changes took 90 seconds to occur in patients with coronary artery disease. [25] Thus, regional wall motion abnormalities often appear prior to ECG changes in response to ischemia.

Clinically, regional wall motion abnormalities can be detected using echocardiography. In myocardial infarction, two-dimensional echocardiography is more sensitive in detecting and localizing segmental pathologic lesions than either postmortem study [26] or technetium pyrophosphate scanning. [27] Kisslo et al. correlated echocardiographically diagnosed wall motion abnormalities with those obtained by left ventricular cineangiography. [28] They found a close correlation between the two techniques.

Intraoperatively, echocardiography has been reported to aid in the diagnosis of ischemia. Using transthoracic M-mode echocardiography, Elliot and coworkers detected significant changes in wall motion in 10 of 24 patients studied during the induction of anesthesia for coronary artery bypass surgery. [29] Only one patient developed corresponding ECG changes. Beaupre et al. reported two cases where two-dimensional transesophageal echocardiography revealed imporant clinical information. [30] In one case, only 1 mm of ST-segment depression was evident in leads I, AVL and V_5 at the time of diagnosis despite "pronounced anterior septal akinesis." The patient later developed ECG changes consistent with those of a transmural anteroseptal myocardial infarction, and levels of creatine phosphokinase (CPK) were noted to be greater than 3,000 IU/L, postoperatively. In the second case, improved segmental wall motion was documented after cardiopulmonary bypass and aortocoronary grafting without any improvement in the ECG signs of ischemia. Another case in which transesophageal echocardiography aided in the diagnosis of myocardial ischemia in the absence of ST-segment changes was reported by Konstadt et al.[31] In that report, good correlation was shown between the appearance of wall motion abnormalities and the presence of pathologic "V" waves. In addition, nitroglycerin resulted in normalization of the segmental wall motion abnormality and a reduction in the PCWP and "V" waves. These clinical observations have recently been confirmed by a prospective study reported by Smith et al.[32] Using transesophageal echocardiography to detect segmental wall motion abnormalities, they found that 24 of 50 patients developed intraoperative myocardial ischemia. During this period, ECG monitoring detected only six episodes of myocardial ischemia, and no patient had ST-segment changes without corresponding segmental wall motion abnormalities.

Management Options

Assuming that one process is responsible for the three observed hemodynamic alterations, the diagnosis of myocardial ischemia, mitral regurgitation, or dysrhythmia must be considered. The presence of sinus rhythm on the ECG can easily rule out a dysrhythmia as the primary cause of the hemodynamic alterations. Thus, in the discussion of the management of this patient, it will be assumed that the patient's diagnosis is acute myocardial ischemia with papillary muscle dysfunction leading to mitral regurgitation and moderate left ventricular dysfunction.

There are three main therapeutic goals: (1) Increase myocardial oxygen supply; (2) decrease myocardial oxygen demand; and (3) ensure adequate systemic perfusion. Myocardial oxygen supply is dependent on an adequate coronary perfusion pressure and diastolic time interval. Therefore, the objectives are to maintain diastolic blood pressure, lower left ventricular end diastolic pressure, dilate coronary arteries, and slow the heart rate. To decrease myocardial oxygen demand, a slow heart rate and decreased myocardial wall tension are needed. Since there is moderate left ventricular dysfunction in this patient, it is necessary to assess the adequacy of the systemic circulation and, if necessary, to intervene. To maintain cerebral and renal blood flow, a MAP of at least 50 mm Hg and a cardiac index (CI) of 1.5–2.5 L/minute/m^2 is necessary.

Given these objectives, nitroglycerin (NTG) is the drug of choice in this patient. Nitroglycerin has been shown to relieve the symptoms of angina and prevent its occurrence during both atrial pacing and exercise. Its effects on the peripheral circulation including dilatation of both the arterial and venous systems are most important. As a result, there is a reduction in preload, afterload, and cardiac size. A reduction in myocardial wall tension occurs with subsequent reduced demand for myocardial oxygen. In the setting of elevated left ventricular pressures, nitroglycerin rarely causes a significant increase in heart rate and usually results in an increased cardiac output. Improved coronary blood flow may occur due to a direct dilator action on the larger conducting arteries or due to a decrease in the left ventricular end diastolic pressure with a resultant increase in the coronary perfusion pressure. [33]

The dose of NTG should be started at 0.5 μg/kg/minute, and increased until the ECG changes resolve; regional wall motion abnormalities disappear; the V wave is reduced; and the PCWP falls to baseline, i.e. 10 mm Hg; or until the MAP falls below 55 mm Hg. The blood pressure will most likely not decrease, but rather increase when the ischemia and mitral regurgitation are resolved.

If the ischemia persists in the presence of a rapid heart rate and the MAP is greater than 55 mm Hg, it may be useful to add a β-adrenergic blocker or a slow calcium-channel blocker to the treatment regimen.

Since a decrease in heart rate will improve coronary blood flow and decrease myocardial oxygen consumption, the administration of a β-blocker is indicated. In chronic stable left ventricular failure, the use of a β-blocker is relatively contraindicated. However, in the case of acute left ventricular dysfunction secondary to ischemia, the beneficial effects of β-blockade in treating ischemia and improving ventricular performance outweigh its deleterious direct negative inotropic effects.

Currently there are three β-blockers available for intravenous use: propranolol, metoprolol, and labetalol. In the future, esmolol, a new $β_1$ selective antagonist may prove to be the drug of choice in this setting, due to its short duration of action, (β half-life is 9 minutes). [34] It is administered by intravenous infusion and can be easily titrated. In the event of an overdose, the duration of the untoward effects will be short-term. In this patient, a β-blocker should be carefully titrated to reduce the heart rate to 60 to 70 beats per minute while monitoring for hypotension or worsening left ventricular function.

Verapamil is the only calcium-entry blocking drug now approved for intravenous use and it has been effective in the intraoperative treatment of coronary artery spasm. [35] It has been used successfully for the treatment of angina pectoris and is effective in reducing myocardial oxygen demand. Verapamil's mechanism of action includes peripheral vasodilatation [36] as well as direct coronary vasodilatation. [37] While its coronary vasodilating potency is less than nifedipine's, effective blood levels can be achieved rapidly and easily via the intravenous route.

Nifedipine has been extensively used for the treatment of chronic stable angina, and its use has recently been extended to patients in the operating room on an experimental basis. Its mechanisms of action include systemic vasodilatation with a decrease in myocardial oxygen requirements and a direct coronary vasodilating effect with increased coronary blood flow. Sublingual,[38] intravenous, intracoronary,[39] and nasogastric[40] administration of nifedipine have been shown to result in prompt recovery of myocardial function when used alone or in combination with intravenous nitroglycerin.

Since the patient is undergoing coronary artery surgery, if the ischemia is refractory to therapy or worsens and systemic hypotension results, cardiopulmonary bypass should be immediately instituted.

In the setting of noncardiac surgery with severe ischemia and left ventricular dysfunction and/or mitral regurgitation, the intra-aortic balloon pump (IABP) could be used to salvage ischemic myocardium and prevent further damage. The IABP is inflated during diastole to displace a volume of blood proximally and increase coronary blood flow, and then is deflated prior to the next systole. Arterial impedance to ejection of blood from the left ventricle is decreased, and cardiac output and coronary blood flow are augmented. By decreasing preload and afterload and increasing coronary blood flow, the myocardial oxygen balance, as well as ventricular function, are improved.

SUMMARY

In summary, a case of myocardial ischemia with acute mitral regurgitation and left ventricular dysfunction has been discussed. Through the integration of several monitoring modalities, the diagnosis was reached and a therapeutic plan was outlined. As a recent study has shown, myocardial ischemia occurring prior to cardiopulmonary bypass correlates with perioperatiave myocardial infarctions.[41] Therefore, it is important to prevent myocardial ischemia, and, if it occurs, early diagnosis and appropriate treatment will help to reduce operative morbidity and mortality.

REFERENCES

1. Pichard AD, Kay R, Smith H, et al: Large V waves in the pulmonary wedge pressure tracing in the absence of mitral regurgitation. *Am J Cardiol* 1982; 50:1044–1049.
2. Fuchs RM, et al: Limitations of pulmonary wedge "V" waves in diagnosing mitral regurgitation. *Am J Cardiol* 1982; 49:849–854.

3. Estes EH, Daltum FM, Entman ML, et al: The anatomy and blood supply of the papillary muscles of the left ventricle. *Am Heart J* 1966; 21:356–362.

4. Mann T, Brodie B, Grossman W, et al: Effect of angina on the left ventricle diastolic pressure-volume relationship. *Circulation* 1977; 55:761–766.

5. Gausch WH, Levine HJ, Zuinones MA: Left ventricular compliance: Mechanisms and clinical implications. *Am J Cardiol* 1976; 38:645–653.

6. Kaplan JA, Wells PH: Early diagnosis of myocardial ischemia using the pulmonary artery catheter. *Anesth Analg* 1981; 60:789–793.

7. Lieberman RW, Orkin FO, Jobes DR, et al: Hemodynamic predictors of myocardial ischemia during halothane anesthesia for coronary artery revascularization. *Anesthesiology* 1983; 59:36–41.

8. Goldman M, Mindich B, Teichholz L, et al: Intraoperative contrast echocardiography to evaluate mitral valve operations. *J Am Coll Cardiol* 1984; 4:1035–1040.

9. Maurer G, Czer L, DeRobertis M, et al: Intraoperative Doppler color-flow mapping in valvular and congenital heart disease, abstracted. *Circulation* 1985; 72:III-206.

10. Kremer P, Rodewald G, Aschenberg W, et al: Mitral valvuloplasty: Assessment of functional result by intraoperative transesophageal 2-D echocardiography, abstracted. *Circulation* 1985; 72:III-396.

11. Blackburn H, Taylor HL, Okamoto N, et al: The exercise electrocardiogram: A systemic comparison of chest lead configuration employed for monitoring during exercise, in Karloman M (ed); *Physical Activity and the Heart*. Springfield, Ill, Charles C Thomas Publisher, 1966.

12. Kaplan JA, King SD: The precordial electrocardiographic lead (V_5) in patients who have coronary artery disease. *Anesthesiology* 1976, 45:570–574.

13. Kates RM, Zaidan JR, Kaplan JA: Esophageal lead for intraoperative electrocardiographic monitoring. *Anesth Analg* 1982; 61:781–785.

14. Tennant R, Wiggers CJ: Effects of coronary occlusion on myocardial contraction. *Am J Physiol* 1935; 112: 351–361.

15. Forrester JS, Wyatt, HL, Pa Luz PL, et al: Functional significance of regional ischemic contraction abnormalities. *Circulation* 1976; 54:64–70.

16. Vatner SF: Correlation between acute reductions in myocardial blood flow and function in conscious dogs. *Circ Res* 1980; 47:201–207.

17. Lowenstein E, Foex P, Philbin D, et al: Regional ischemic ventricular dysfunction in myocardium supplied by a narrowed coronary artery with increasing halothane concentration in the dog. *Anesthesioogy* 1981; 55:349–359.

18. Komer RR, Edalzi A, Hood WB: Effects of nitroglycerin on echocardiographic measurements of left ventricular wall thickness and regional myocardial performance during acute coronary ischemia. *Circulation* 1979; 59:926–937.

19. Pandian NG, Kieso RA, Kerber RE: Two dimensional echocardiography in experimental coronary stenosis. *Circulation* 1982; 66:603–611.

20. Kerber RE, Martins JB, Marcus ML: Effect of acute ischemia, nitroglycerin and nitroprusside on regional myocardial thickening, stress and perfusion. *Circulation* 1979, 60:121–129.

21. Miller MM, Thorvaldson J, Ilebekk A, et al: Myocardial ischemia: Relationship between local flow, function and ST- segment elevation. *Eur J Cardiol* 1979; 10:7–18.

22. Battler A, Froelicher VF, Gallagher KP, et al: Dissociation between regional myocardial dysfunction and ECG changes during ischemia in the conscious dog. *Circulation* 1980; 62:735–744.
23. Smith HJ, Kent KM, Epstein SE: Relationship between regional contractile function and ST segment elevation after experimental coronary artery occlusion in the dog. *Cardiovasc Res* 1978; 12:444–448.
24. Upton MT, Resych SK, Newman GE, et al: Detecting abnormalities in left ventricular function during exercise before angina and ST segment depression. *Circulation* 1980; 62:341–439.
25. Sugishita Y, Susumu K, Matsuda M, et al: Dissociation between regional myocardial dysfunction and ECG patients with angina pectoris. *Am Heart J* 1983; 106:1–8.
26. Weiss JL, Bulkley BH, Hutchins GM, et al: Two-dimensional echocardiographic recognition of myocardial injury in man: Comparison with postmortem studies. *Circulation* 1981; 63:401–408.
27. Meltzer RS, Woythaler JN, Buda AJ, et al: Two-dimensional echocardiographic quantification of infarct size alteration by pharmocologic agents. *Am J Cardiol* 1979; 44:257–262.
28. Kisslo J, Ideker R, Harrison L, et al: Serial wall changes after acute myocardial infarction by two-dimensional echo, abstracted. *Circulation* 1979; 60(suppl 11): 11–151.
29. Elliot PL, Schauble JF, Weiss J, et al: Echocardiography and LV function during anesthesia, abstracted. *Anesthesiology* 1980; 53:S105.
30. Beaupre P, Kremer P, Cahalan M, et al: Intraoperative detection of changes in left ventricular segmental wall motion by transesophageal two-dimensional echocardiography. *Am Heart J* 1984; 107:1021–1023.
31. Konstadt S, Goldman M, Thys D, et al: Intraoperative diagnosis of myocardial ischemia. *Mt Sinai J Med* 1985; 52:521–525.
32. Smith J, Cahalan M, Benefiel D, et al: Intraoperative detection of myocardial ischemia in high risk patients: Electrocardiography versus two-dimensional transesophageal echocardiography. *Circulation* 1985; 72:1015–1021.
33. Najmi M, Griggs D, Kasparian H, et al: Effects of nitroglycerin on hemodynamics during rest and exercise in patients with coronary insufficiency. *Circulation* 1967; 35:46–53.
34. Girard D, Shulman B, Thys D, et al: The safety and efficacy of esmolol during myocardial revascularization. *Anesthesiology* 1986; 65:157–165.
35. Nussmeier N, Slogoff S: Verapamil treatment of intraoperative coronary artery spasm. *Anesthesiology* 1985; 62:539–541.
36. Ferlinz J, Tuobow M: Antianginal and myocardial metabolic properties of verapamil in coronary artery disease. *Am J Cardiol* 1980; 46:1019–1026.
37. Singh B, Chew C, Josephson M, et al: Pharmacology and hemodynamic mechanisms underlying the antianginal actions of verapamil. *Am J Cardiol* 1982; 50:886–893.
38. Kopf, G, Ribg A, Zito R: Intraoperative use of nifedipine for hemodynamic collapse due to coronary artery spasm following myocardial revascularization. *Ann Thorac Surg* 1982; 34:457–460.

39. Kaltenbach M, Schultz W, Kober G: Effects of nifedipine after intravenous and intracoronary administration. *Am J Cardiol* 1979; 44:832–837.
40. Cohen D, Foley R, Ryan J: Intraoperative coronary artery spasm successfully treated with nitroglycerin and nifedipine. *Ann Thorac Surg* 1983; 36:97–100.
41. Slogoff S, Keats A: Does perioperative myocardial ischemia lead to postoperative myocardial infarction? *Anesthesiology* 1985; 62:107–114.

40

Reoperation for Coronary Artery Bypass

A 60-year-old patient had two-vessel coronary artery bypass grafting five years prior to developing unstable angina. At catheterization, a graft to the left anterior descending (LAD) was patent, but the right graft was occluded and there was 95% stenosis in the circumflex artery and 50% stenosis in the left main coronary artery. The patient was scheduled for reoperation because of increasing anginal symptoms. With sternotomy, the right ventricle was cut with massive blood loss and loss of perfusion pressure.

Recommendations by Narda Croughwell, C.R.N.A. and J. G. Reves, M.D.

ANALYSIS OF THE PROBLEM

Atherosclerosis is a progressive disease. Even patients with patent grafts continue to develop ischemic heart disease as other major vessels suffer occlusive disease, therefore, it is common that patients are presenting for anesthesia and operation for a second time for the treatment of ischemic heart disease. This case represents such a patient as well as a relatively common complication, massive hemorrhage with cutting of the right ventricle. The proper treatment of such a patient is based on two principles: (1) preparation for the catastrophe and (2) swift action if a hemorrhagic disaster occurs.

APPROACH TO THE PROBLEM

Preparation

In preparing for a patient having a reoperation, there are certain principles that must be observed in anticipation of hemorrage.

1. Two 14-gauge venous cannula catheters should be placed for volume expansion. One catheter should be placed in the patient's right arm because left innominate vein tears are common in patients presenting for reoperation.

2. Intravenous fluid (1,000-ml) bags (for example, lactated ringer's) should be placed in blood pump bags and connected to the 14-gauge catheters.

3. The lungs should be kept deflated during sternotomy.

4. The heparin dose should be calculated and ready to administer immediately.

Treatment of This Problem

1. The crystalloid should be administered as rapidly as possible by inflating the blood administration bags.

2. If the blood pressure is significantly reduced, a vasoconstrictor (for example phenylephrine 100 to 200 µg) should be administered.

3. Surgical repair of the right ventricle tear should be made expeditiously but without panic.

4. The heparin dose should be administered through the distal part of a pulmonary artery catheter (if available) if surgical repair without cardiopulmonary bypass is impossible.

5. Perfusionists should administer half the heparin dose to their prime.

6. After heparinization, blood may be scavenged to the pump (this is an option even if cardiopulmonary bypass is not instituted).

7. If a surgical repair cannot be completed prior to cardiopulmonary bypass, the groin should be incised and the arterial perfusion line placed in the femoral artery; the right ventriculotomy may be used as venous return for cardiopulmonary bypass.

DISCUSSION

In most cardiovascular hospitals, the percentage of patients with coronary artery disease having secondary operations averages approximately 5% to 10% of the practice; therefore, it is common to have patients present for reoperation. Patients who have reoperation for coronary disease present multiple problems to the anesthesiologists.[1] These include longer operating times, greater blood use, and higher morbidity and mortality. The anesthesiologist needs to be prepared for these complications by anticipating the need for greater blood and blood product utilization, use of inotropic drugs, and a planned procedure longer than that of the primary operation.

Indications for reoperation include progression of disease and/or graft occlusion. There are a number of reports of the results of reoperation for coronary artery bypass graft operations.[1-12] Some of these reports suggest an increased risk with a second operation, while others report similar risks to the first operation. Two reports show the development of left ventricular dysfunction, myocardial damage, and high blood utilization in coronary reoperation patients.[1,2]

In the preoperative evaluation of reoperative patients there may be an important history of congestive heart failure, unstable angina, and arrhythmias.[1] During the operative course there is a greater need for intraoperative and postoperative use of dopamine, nitroglycerin, and the intra-aortic balloon pump to treat low cardiac output than that seen in patients undergoing a first procedure.[1] Myocardial damage is increased in patients having reoperation as detected by CKMB isoenzyme release, a sensitive and specific index of myocardial damage. The myocardial damage can occur at any time during the perioperative period secondary to inadequate anesthetic or surgical management or inadequate myocardial preservation during cardiopulmonary bypass. Severe hypotension would obviously compromise coronary blood flow in the prebypass period, whereas noncoronary collateral flow through the adhesions can rewarm the heart and wash out cardioplegia during the period of cross-clamp during cardiopulmonary bypass. It is essential that supplemental measures to improve myocardial protection in these patients include periodic reinfusions of cardioplegic solutions and a reduction in the systemic perfusate temperature, flow, and pressure. Cold saline irrigation of the pericardial cavity or other topical hypothermic techniques are additionally important in keeping the heart cold, but these methods may be technically difficult in reoperation patients.

SUMMARY

There are an increasing number of patients having reoperation for coronary artery surgery. In addition to the usual anesthetic management designed to optimize the oxygen supply-to-demand ratio, the management plan should include anticipation of needs for high volume infusion as well as special attention to myocardial protection during cardiopulmonary bypass.

REFERENCES

1. Brummet C, Reves JG, Lell WA, et al: Patient care problems in patients undergoing reoperation for coronary artery grafting surgery. *Can Anaesth Soc J* 1984; 31:213–220.
2. Estafanous FG: Anaesthesia and heart reoperations. *Cleve Clin Q* 1981; 48:93–6.
3. Qazi A, Garcia JM, Mispireta LA, et al: Reoperation for coronary artery disease *Ann Thorac Surg* 1981; 32:16–18.
4. Adam M, Geisler GF, Lambert CJ, et al: Reoperation following clinical failure of aorta-to-coronary artery bypass vein grafts. *Ann Thorac Surg* 1972; 14:272–281.
5. Kobayashi T, Mendez AM, Zubiate P, et al: Repeat aortocoronary bypass grafting. *Chest* 1978; 73:446–449.
6. Benedict JS, Buhl TL, Henney RP: Re-vascularization of the ischemic myocardium. *Arch Surg* 1974; 108:40–2.
7. Winkle RA, Alderman EL, Shumway NE, et al: Results of reoperation for unsuccessful coronary artery bypass surgery. *Circulation* 1975; 51(suppl 1):161–165.
8. Oglietti J, Angeline P, Leachman RD, et al: Myocardial revascularization: Early and late results after reoperation. *J Thorac Cardiovasc Surg* 1976; 71:736–740.
9. Stiles QR, Lindesmith GG, Tucker BL, et al: Experience with fifty repeat procedures for myocardial revascularization. *J Thorac Cardiovasc Surg* 1976; 72:849–851.
10. Irarrazaval MJ, Cosgrove DM, Loop RD, et al: Reoperations for myocardial revascularization. *J Thorac Cardiovasc Surg* 1977; 73:181–188.
11. Norwood WI, Cohn LH, Collins JJ: Results of reoperation for recurrent angina pectoris. *Ann Thorac Surg* 1977; 23:9–13.
12. Schaff HV, Orxzulak TA, Gersh BJ, et al: The morbidity and mortality of reoperation for coronary artery disease and analysis of late results with use of actuarial estimate of event-free interval. *J Thorac Cardiovasc Surg* 1983; 85:508–515.

PART SIX

Pharmacology

41

Digitalis Toxicity

A 50-year-old woman with mitral regurgitation and heart failure was brought to the operating room for a mitral valve replacement. She had been receiving 0.25 mg of digoxin daily, was in atrial fibrillation, and her ventricular rate averaged 50 to 60 beats per minute. She also was taking furosemide (Lasix) and a potassium supplement, but her serum potassium level on the morning of surgery was 3.5 mEq/L. She received her morning dose of digoxin. She underwent a relatively uneventful induction with diazepam, fentanyl, oxygen and 50% nitrous oxide, except that her ventricular rate slowed to 45 beats per minute and she began having premature ventricular contractions. At the time of the arrhythmia, her pH was 7.50 with a $PaCO_2$ of 28 mm Hg.

Recommendations by R. William McIntyre, M.D.

"The foxglove, when given in very large and quickly repeated doses occasions . . . A slow pulse, even as low as 35 in a minute . . ."[1]

ANALYSIS OF THE PROBLEM

In this case of mitral regurgitation, heart failure, and atrial fibrillation, the preoperative ventricular rate of 50 to 60 beats per minute would indicate the possibility of early digoxin toxicity. This slow ventricular response was possibly exacerbated by the decision to administer the daily digoxin dose on the day of surgery. Further slowing of the ventricular rate to 45 beats per minute was due to the effects of premedication and anesthesia on adrenergic regulation of atrioventricular (AV) nodal conduction. In addition, acute hypocapnic depression of extracellular K^+ from hyperventilation was evidenced by the blood gas data that demonstrated a respiratory alkalosis. For every 10 torr decrease in $PaCO_2$ a concomitant 0.5 mEq/L decrease in K^+ has been demonstrated.[2] Therefore a further reduction in K^+, to approximately 3.0 mEq/L or less, may have occurred. The normal compensatory mechanisms in mitral regurgitation involve an increase in sympathetic tone with tachycardia, increased contractility, and compensatory use of the Frank-Starling reserve. Critical slowing of the ventricular rate in mitral regurgitation in addition to a reduction in the inotropic state of the heart secondary to general anesthesia may combine in a situation such as this to cause an increase in the regurgitant fraction and acute hemodynamic deterioration. The severity of these changes and the urgency for intervention would depend on the degree and rapidity of changes in monitored parameters: blood pressure, pulmonary artery wedge pressure, cardiac output and mixed venous oxygen saturation.

APPROACH TO THE PROBLEM

Treatment should be directed at the underlying cause of dysrhythmias. First, correction of the $PaCO_2$ and pH should be accomplished by normalization of ventilation. This maneuver would result in an increase in K^+, perhaps to the extent of eliminating the premature ventricular contractions (PVCs). In addition, the potassium effect may improve AV conduction and accelerate ventricular response. However, it is likely, because of the potential urgency of this problem, that an immediate increase in the fraction of atrial impulses being propagated through the AV node would be desirable by the use of intravenous (IV) atropine, 0.4 mg initially, and up to 2.0 mg in divided doses. An infusion of K^+ (20 mEq in 100 ml of D5W) should be started and administered at 0.5 to 1 ml/minute through a central venous catheter. It would be impractical to consider decreasing the anesthetic level as an intervention, although an increase in central adrenergic tone would hypothetically increase AV conduction. In the event of persistent bradycardia and hemodynamic deterioration, an adrenergic agonist such as ephedrine (5 to 10 mg IV) should be administered. An acute increase in lung water, evidenced by a decrease in PaO_2 and possibly an increase in airway pressure, should be treated by furosemide (5 to 20 mg IV). This has the immediate effect of reducing left ventricular filling pressure, independent of its renal properties.[3]

If the ventricular arrhythmia were to progress in severity, lidocaine 1 mg/kg should be administered. This is a type IB antiarrhythmic. In addition to suppressing PVCs, it can enhance AV conduction and therefore increase ventricular rate.[4] Cautious use is advised in the presence of rapid atrial tachycardia, because a catastrophic ventricular rate response can occur.[5]

Should pharmacologic intervention fail to achieve a satisfactory increase in

AV conduction, application of epicardial pacing wires and ventricular pacing to a rate of 80 to 90 beats per minute should be considered.

Cardioversion can increase manifestations of digitalis toxicity. However, in the presence of life-threatening ventricular arrhythmia such as ventricular tachycardia or fibrillation, low-energy direct current (DC) cardioversion would necessarily be undertaken.

DISCUSSION

Digitalis toxicity is common, occurring in approximately 25% of hospitalized patients who are receiving digitalis therapy.[6] Toxicity is usually a manifestation of the drug's effect on the electrophysiologic properties of the heart. In addition to ionic effects due to inhibition of membrane-bound Na^+, K^+-adenosine triphosphase (Na^+, K^+-ATPase), digoxin effects are a reflection of its pharmacology and pharmacokinetics. Drug and metabolic interactions, particularly those involving potassium-regulating processes, account for the most significant exacerbating factors in digitalis toxicity.

Intraoperatively the inotropic, chronotropic, and dromotropic effects of digoxin occur in the pathophysiologic context of changes in the underlying cardiac disease and the autonomic consequences of anesthesia.

Digoxin is 50% to 70% absorbed from the gastrointestinal tract. The small volume of coadministered fluid given preoperatively with digoxin does not affect bioavailability.[7] The therapeutic end point for control of ventricular rate by digoxin in patients with atrial fibrillation is approximately 65 to 95 beats per minute at rest and 90 to 110 beats per minute after exercise. This usually requires more digoxin than that required to exert an inotropic effect in the failing heart. However, the therapeutic index for digoxin is low and the relationship between "therapeutic" serum levels and the efficacy of controlling ventricular response to atrial fibrillation is variable and unpredictable.[8] For example, satisfactory slowing of the ventricular rate in patients with chronic stable atrial fibrillation is accomplished in only 60% of patients when digoxin levels are therapeutic or subtherapeutic (< 2 ng/ml). Slowing of ventricular rate frequently requires "toxic" concentrations of digoxin (2.5 to 6.0 ng/ml). The temporal relationship of the last dose of digoxin is a determinant of the serum level. In patients with atrial fibrillation with a ventricular response of < 70 beats per minute, elimination of the digoxin dose on the day of anesthesia should be considered.

Digoxin is the most frequently employed cardiac glycoside. Given by the oral route, it has a half-life for distribution and binding (T1/2α) of 50 minutes.[9] Following intravenous administration the T1/2α is 30 minutes. The half-life of digoxin for metabolism and elimination (T1/2β) is 30 to 40 hours for both the oral and intravenous routes of administration. Protein binding of digoxin is approximately 20% to 25%. The pharmacokinetics of digoxin is based on a two-compartment model and there is preferential uptake in the heart and kidney. The ratio of heart muscle to serum digoxin concentration (43:1) is relatively constant, a classic example of the Ferguson principle. However, because of other factors such as the influence of sympathoadrenal and parasympathetic function on AV nodal conduction, there is a frequent lack of correlation between blood levels of digoxin and drug effect. This has important anesthetic implications in that changing sympathoadrenal activity may occur because of mismatching of the depth of anesthesia and the degree of surgical stress so that toxic manifestations of digoxin may occur at therapeutic serum levels.

Cardiac anesthesia for patients receiving digoxin includes a consideration of the effects of cardiopulmonary bypass on the pharmacokinetics of the drug. In view of the small degree of protein binding, the effects of hemodilution secondary to bypass on the free fraction and volume of distribution of digoxin are small. Serum concentration of digoxin decreases on bypass but reequilibration with tissue stores occurs during the postoperative period because of the relatively long elimination half-life. This, however, is influenced by the hypothermic reduction in perfusion of skeletal muscle, the major depot for body digoxin stores. Postoperatively, digoxin clearance is reduced in parallel with any reduction in creatinine clearance. Current evidence suggests a rebound peak in the concentration of serum digoxin following cardiopulmonary bypass and the possibility of associated dysrhythmia. [10] Consideration should therefore be given to reducing the dose of digoxin administered after cardiopulmonary bypass.

The effect of digoxin on inotropy is due to inhibition of the Na^+, K^+-ATPase within the transverse tubular system. [11] Active extrusion of Na^+ is diminished so that more intracellular Na^+ is available for exchange with extracellular Ca^{++}. Toxic manifestations of digoxin are commonly due to its effects on AV-nodal conduction and specialized ventricular conducting tissue. [12] There is direct depression of conduction of impulses through the AV node that results in an increase in the effective refractory period. With increasing digoxin effect and toxicity, AV block ultimately occurs. The indirect effects of digoxin on the AV node result from enhanced vagal activity and a decreased sensitivity to catecholamines (antiadrenergic effect). There is evidence for central nervous system adrenergic-receptor mediation for the cardiotoxic action of digoxin. [13] These direct and indirect effects combine to decrease the rate at which atrial impulses can be transmitted to the ventricle and to increase the fraction of blocked atrial impulses in the presence of atrial fibrillation. The random reentry of atrial impulses during atrial fibrillation results in impulses arriving at the AV node at approximately 500 per minute. Most impulses fail to enter the AV node because of refractoriness; some enter but do not propagate (concealed conduction), and some are propagated to the His bundle. The ventricular response is determined by the effective refractory period of the AV node. Digoxin toxicity at the AV node is therefore manifest as a result of the summation of the indirect vagal effect, direct digoxin effect, and adrenergic influence, which is modified by general anesthesia.

Ectopic ventricular pacemaker activity, manifest as premature ventricular contractions (PVCs), can occur as a result of bradycardia secondary to AV nodal toxicity. The PVCs also result from the effect of digoxin on phase 4 (diastolic depolarization) of the action potential (Fig 41–1). This effect varies with the concentration of extracellular potassium (K^+). At low K^+ concentration, the slope of phase 4 is increased, with resulting augmented automaticity. At higher concentrations of K^+, delayed after-depolarizations appear (Fig 41–2). The after-depolarizations are initially subthreshold but as toxicity progresses their amplitude increases and extra-action potentials can be initiated. Therefore, digoxin can initiate ectopic impulses by two different mechanisms, enhancement of normal phase 4 depolarization or the development of delayed after-depolarization.

The effects of potassium on the action potential in ventricular conducting fibers is shown in Fig 41–3. Hypokalemia increases the slope of phase 4 and in this way can augment the toxic effects of digoxin.[14] The mechanism for this is probably like digoxin, an inhibition of Na^+, K^+-ATPase. If the level of extracellular potassium (K^+) is low or normal, an increase will usually suppress ectopic ventricular beats and improve AV conduction. This is due to the immediate decrease in the binding of digoxin to heart tissue and also direct antagonism of its cardiotoxic effects. If K^+ is high, potassium administration may increase the degree of AV block. Magnesium changes have similar effects to those of potassium. Acidosis and hypercalcemia both depress the Na^+-K^+ pump and therefore exacerbate digoxin toxicity. Intraoperative sympathoadrenal activity

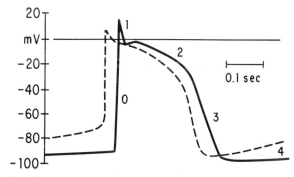

FIG 41–1.
Digoxin effect on the action potential in Purkinje's fibers (– – –).

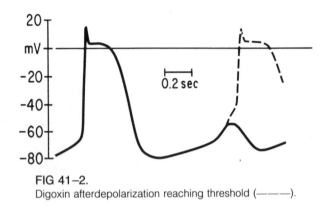

FIG 41–2.
Digoxin afterdepolarization reaching threshold (———).

reflects the balance between the depth of anesthesia and surgical stress and may influence extrarenal potassium regulation and digitalis toxicity. [15] Adrenergic extrarenal potassium regulation involves both α- and β_2-receptor mechanisms. The β_2-stimulation can cause hypokalemia. [16] Toxicity is increased following electrical cardioversion, probably as a consequence of catecholamine release and potassium changes.

In chronic mitral regurgitation, digoxin normalizes intracellular ionic concentrations while increasing myocardial contractility. [17] The development of significant hemodynamic disturbances and heart failure frequently requires the use of diuretic therapy. Potassium-losing diuretics such as furosemide can result in a substantial reduction in both total body and extracellular K^+. Therefore, it is widespread practice to administer K^+ supplements to patients in this group. However, the end points of potassium therapy are unclear and controversial. Perioperatively, it has been suggested that patients who are not at serious cardiac risk during surgery and anesthesia who have a modest reduction in

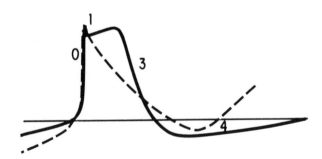

FIG 41–3.
Hypokalemia: effect on action potential (———) and slope of phase 4.

level of K$^+$ (3.0 to 3.50 mEq/L) should not have their surgery postponed.[18] Recent evidence in patients with ischemic heart disease suggests that even minor changes in K$^+$ are associated with increased ventricular electrical instability.[19] However, there are no data to base definitive criteria for postponement of cardiac surgery in order to correct potassium deficits. Long-term diuretic therapy can be associated with total body potassium depletion of up to several hundred milliequivalents and replacement is unpredictable and time-consuming.

REFERENCES

1. Withering WM: An account of foxglove and same of its medical uses. Birmingham, England, Robinson Publishers, 1785.
2. Edwards R, Winnie AP, Ramamurthy S: Acute hypocapnic hypokalemia: An iatrogenic anesthetic complication. *Anesth Analg* 1977; 56:786–792.
3. Dikshit K, Vyden JK, Forrester JS, et al: Renal and extrarenal hemodynamic effects of furosemide in congestive heart failure after acute myocardial infarction. *N Engl J Med* 1973; 288:1087–1090.
4. Vaughan-Williams EM: A classification of antiarrhythmic action reassessed after a decade of new drugs. *J Clin Pharmacol* 1984; 24:129.
5. Marriott HJL, Bieza CF: Alarming ventricular acceleration after lidocaine administration. *Chest* 1972; 61:682–683.
6. Bellor GA, Smith TW, Abglman WH, et al: Digitalis intoxication: A prospective clinical study with serum level correlations. *N Engl J Med* 1971; 284:989–997.
7. Bustrack JA, Katz JD, Hull JH, et al: Bioavailability of digoxin capsules and tablets: Effect of coadministered fluid volume. *J Pharm Sci* 1984; 73:1397–1400.
8. Goldman S, Probst P, Selzer A, et al: Inefficacy of "therapeutic" serum levels of digoxin in controlling the ventricular rate in atrial fibrillation. *Am J Cardiol* 1975; 35:651–655.
9. Doherty JE, de Soyza N, Kane JJ, et al: Clinical pharmacokinetics of digitalis glycosides. *Prog Cardiovasc Dis* 1978; 21:141–158.
10. Holley FO, Ponganis KV, Stanski DR: Effect of cardiopulmonary bypass on the pharmacokinetics of drugs. *Clin Pharm* 1982; 7:234–251.
11. Smith TW, Wagner H, Markis JE, et al: Studies on the localization of the cardiac glycoside receptor. *J Clin Invest* 1972; 51:1777–1789.
12. Hoffman BF, Bigger JT: Cardiovascular drugs, in *The Pharmacological Basis of Therapeutics*, ed 6. New York, Macmillan Publishing Co, 1980, pp 729–760.
13. Plunkett LM, Tackett RL: Central α-receptors and their role in digoxin cardiotoxicity. *J Pharmacol Exp Ther* 1983; 227:683–686.
14. Lloyd EA, Surawicz B: Tachycardia related to electrolyte imbalance, in Surawicz B (ed): *Tachycardias*. Boston, Martinus Nijhoff, 1984, pp 407–412.
15. McIntyre RW, Knopes KD, Ossey KD: The relationship between sympathoadrenal activity and extrarenal potassium regulation. *Anesthesiology* 1985; 63:230–231.

16. Brown MJ, Brown DC, Murphy MB: Hypokalemia from β_2-receptor stimulation by circulating epinephrine. *N Engl J Med* 1983; 309:1414–1419.
17. Prasad K, O'Neil CL, Bharadwaj B: Effects of chronic digoxin treatment on cardiac function, electrolytes, and sarcolemmal ATPase in the canine failing heart due to chronic mitral regurgitation. *Am Heart J* 1984; 108:1487–1493.
18. McGovern B: Hypokalemia and cardiac arrhythmias. *Anesthesiology* 1985; 63:127–129.
19. Stewart DE, Ikram H, Espiner EA, et al: Arrhythmiogenic potential of diuretic induced hypokalaemia in patients with mild hypertension and ischaemic heart disease. *Br Heart J* 1985; 54:290–297.

42

Procainamide Toxicity

A 74-year-old man with left main coronary artery disease and history of ventricular tachycardia underwent coronary artery bypass grafting without complications. Postoperatively, the creatinine and BUN levels began to climb despite satisfactory urine output. He was given procainamide (Pronestyl) for premature ventricular beats (500 mg orally four times a day) beginning on the first postoperative day and on the third postoperative day nurses reported widened QRS, inability to pace the atrium, and multiple ventricular tachyarrhythmias. The procainamide level was 20 μg/ml before administration of the last dose, which just preceded the conduction disturbance and ventricular arrhythmias.

Recommendations by Roger L. Royster, M.D.

ANALYSIS OF THE PROBLEM

This case illustrates the development of toxic side effects from accumulation of a drug during renal insufficiency and underscores the necessity of understanding the pharmacokinetics and pharmacodynamics of each drug. Oral administration of procainamide is 250 to 500 mg every three to four hours. Sustained released procainamide is available and is given at intervals of six hours or longer. Oral procainamide is well absorbed with the bioavailability being 80% to 90%; however, in patients with an acute myocardial infarction, the oral absorption is reduced.[1] This possibly occurs in the immediate postoperative period as well. The therapeutic plasma concentration is usually between 4 and 10 μg/ml. In patients with congestive heart failure, due to a reduction in the volume of distribution, the plasma concentration usually rises. In contrast, the volume of distribution increases during cardiopulmonary bypass, but probably has returned to normal values in this patient by the third postoperative day.

Due to unpredictable absorption and distribution during the immediate post-operative period, intravenous administration is preferable to the oral route.

Patients may develop toxic symptoms at plasma concentrations as low as 8 μg/ml and toxic symptoms usually are present at plasma concentrations greater than 16 μg/ml. The toxic level of 20 μg/ml in our patient is primarily the result of problems with elimination and not absorption or distribution. Approximately 50% of procainamide is eliminated unchanged in the urine and 50% is metabolized by the liver. When renal function decreases, the fraction metabolized in the liver by acetylation to N-acetylprocainamide (NAPA) increases. The NAPA is almost entirely eliminated by renal excretion and in acute renal failure, procainamide and NAPA levels usually rise. The NAPA has cardiac electrophysiologic effects and adds to the cardiac toxicity of procainamide. The measurement of NAPA plasma levels is helpful in patients requiring higher dosages, in patients with renal failure or congestive heart failure, and in patients who acetylate the drug rapidly.

Adverse effects of procainamide include gastrointestinal symptoms such as nausea, vomiting, and diarrhea. Fever, myalgias, skin rashes, and arthralgias may occur, producing a syndrome common during chronic oral therapy that resembles systemic lupus erythematosus. However, symptoms of the lupus-like syndrome associated with positive serology have been reported after only seven days of therapy. Depression, anxiety, leukopenia, and agranulocytosis are rare side effects.

Procainamide has electrophysiologic effects similar to those of quinidine. The PR, QRS, and QT intervals may become prolonged but not of the magnitude associated with quinidine. Like quinidine, procainamide may have a proarrhythmic effect, especially when the QRS and QT intervals are prolonged, creating heterogenous areas of depolarization and repolarization predisposing to reentry. Multiple ventricular arrhythmias including polymorphic ventricular tachycardia (torsade de pointes) may occur.[2] Rapid intravenous infusion of procainamide causes hypotension secondary to vasodilatation, and/or direct myocardial depression. Toxic levels from oral administration also may cause these hemodynamic problems.

APPROACH TO THE PROBLEM

The development of nonoliguric renal failure in this case is probably secondary to preexisting renal insufficiency, poor renal blood flow, and reduced cardiac output. The volume of distribution of procainamide is reduced due to poor peripheral perfusion and combined with a reduction in elimination in renal failure; an increase in the patient's procainamide level results. The plasma level of 20 μg/ml is certainly in the toxic range and explains the widened QRS complex and ventricular arrhythmias. Failure to pace the atrium in this case may be secondary to an elevated pacing threshold. Changes in pacing threshold are caused by a multitude of factors including electrolyte abnormalities, hypoxemia, acidosis, and drugs.[3] Pronestyl may elevate the pacing threshold at toxic levels and has been reported to cause various other pacing abnormalities.[4] The atrial effective refractory period is usually prolonged more than the ventricular effective refractory period. A pacemaker operating during the effective refractory period of the atria or ventricle will not capture the rhythm. As the QT interval lengthens, the T waves usually widen and increase in amplitude. A pacemaker in the inhibited (sensing) mode may oversense the T waves, and failure to pace or pacing at a decreased rate results.

The patient's procainamide should be discontinued and electrolyte abnormalities, arterial blood gas abnormalities, and hemodynamic problems should be treated. Hypokalemia causes membrane destabilization and increases the slope of phase 4 of the action potential and increases QT prolongation, leading to a propensity for arrhythmias. Extracellular alkalosis will shift potassium intracellularly, reversing these arrhythmogenic effects. Metabolic alkalosis created by the administration of sodium bicarbonate or sodium lactate has been shown to be protective in procainamide cardiotoxicity.[5] The administered sodium ions may play a role in reversing the depressed phase 0 of the action potential caused by procainamide. Gay and Brown reported sodium bicarbonate or sodium lactate given intravenously narrowed the QRS, shortened the QT interval, and reversed pacemaker failure.[4] In contrast, hyperkalemia may intensify the procainamide effect, especially worsening the conduction system abnormalities. Pacing the patient at a faster heart rate will shorten the QT interval and may be effective in treating ventricular arrhythmias by creating a more homogenous repolarization pattern and preventing the development of reentry pathways. In addition, isoproterenol has been used in patients with prolonged QT intervals having ventricular arrhythmias that are not responsive to other means of therapy. The β-receptor stimulation increases the heart rate, shortens the QT interval, and reverses myocardial depression. If arrhythmias persist and intravenous xylocaine is not effective, oral quinidine may be used since its elimination is not dependent on renal clearance.

DISCUSSION

Procainamide, the amide analogue of procaine hydrochloride, is a Class I antiarrhythmic agent with local anesthetic properties. Procainamide, like quinidine, depresses phase 0 of the action potential, prolongs the action potential duration, prolongs the effective refractory period of the atrium and ventricle, and depresses phase 4 of the action potential. Decreasing the slope of phase 4 reduces automatic rhythms and by prolonging the refractoriness of conducting tissue prevents reentry. A mild vagolytic effect increases heart rate and atrioventricular conduction. Clinically, procainamide appears less effective in treating atrial arrhythmias but more effective in treating ventricular arrhythmias when compared to quinidine. Procainamide is usually a second-line drug after lidocaine in treating patients with ventricular arrhythmias. Frequently, procainamide may be effective in patients that have ventricular arrhythmias refractory to lidocaine. Cautious administration is necessary in patients with bundle-branch blocks and atrioventricular conduction defects because complete heart block may result.[6]

It is generally recommended that procainamide be given intravenously during the perioperative period because of changes in bioavailability. An intravenous loading dose is required and is usually given 100 mg every five minutes while blood pressure and heart rate are noted, until the ventricular arrhythmia is suppressed or until a loading dose of 15 mg/kg or 1 gm is given. The continuous infusion dosage of procainamide is 2 to 6 mg/minute. Intravenous procainamide is generally well tolerated with hypotension being a limiting factor; however, severe hypotension may result if intravenous loading is given more frequently than every five minutes. In patients with renal failure or congestive heart failure, adverse side effects are more likely to occur and plasma levels are helpful in determining adequate therapeutic concentrations. Myerburg et al. showed that the mean plasma level required to suppress 85% of premature ventricular contractions in patients with ischemic heart disease was 9.3 µg/ml.[7] Achieving adequate NAPA levels with higher dosages of procainamide aids in the treatment of some refractory ventricular arrhythmias. N-acetylprocainamide produces less prolongation of conduction times, causes similar changes in refractory periods and electrocardiographic intervals, and is less potent as compared to procainamide. The efficacy of NAPA as a sole antiarrhythmic agent is controversial.[8]

REFERENCES

1. Koch-Weser J: Pharmokinetics of procainamide in man. *Ann. NY Acad Sci* 1971; 179:370–382.
2. Strasberg B, Sclarovsky S, Erdberg A, et al: Procainamide-induced polymorphous ventricular tachycardia. *Am J Cardiol* 1981; 47:1309–1314.
3. Preston TA, Fletcher RD, Lucchesi BR, et al: Changes in myocardial threshold: Physiologic and pharmacologic factors in patients with implanted pacemakers. *Am Heart J* 1967; 74:235–242.
4. Gay RJ, Brown DF: Pacemaker failure due to procainamide toxicity. *Am J Cardiol* 1974; 34:728–732.

5. Bellet S, Hamden G, Somlyo A, et al: A reversal of the cardiotoxic effects of procaine amide by molar sodium lactate. *Am J Med Sci* 1959; 237:177–188.
6. Josephson ME, Caracta AR, Ricciutti MA: Electrophysiologic properties of procainamide in man. *Am J Cardiol* 1974; 33:596–603.
7. Myerburg RJ, Kessler KM, Kiem I, et al: Relationship between plasma levels of procainamide, suppression of premature ventricular complexes and prevention of ventricular tachycardia. *Circulation* 1981; 64:280–290.
8. Kluger J, Drayer D, Reidenberg M, et al: The clinical pharmacology and antiarrhythmic efficacy of acetyl procainamide in patients with arrhythmias. *Am J Cardiol* 1980; 45:1250–1257.

43

Valium-Fentanyl Interaction

A 65-year-old man with coronary artery disease was given 75 µg/kg of fentanyl but remained conscious, so 10 mg of diazepam was given over 5 minutes to complete the anesthesia induction. The arterial blood pressure, which had been stable, decreased over the next minute from 130/70 to 80/60 mm Hg.

Recommendations by J. G. Reves, M.D., and
Narda Croughwell, C.R.N.A.

ANALYSIS OF THE PROBLEM

Hypotension during induction of general anesthesia in a patient with ischemic heart disease may jeopardize oxygen delivery to the heart, resulting in ischemia and possibly myocardial necrosis. Although moderate to high-dose fentanyl anesthesia is frequently used in these patients without hemodynamic disturbances, opioids are not complete anesthetics when used for cardiac surgery. Indeed, Lowenstein states: "Every narcotic anesthetic requires administration of a neuromuscular blocking drug and an anesthetic adjuvant."[1] Adjuvant anesthetics like benzodiazepines, most commonly diazepam, are used as supplement anesthetics to produce sleep (hypnosis) and amnesia. Unfortunately, the combination of opioids and benzodiazepines may produce hypotension as in this case.

When used alone benzodiazepines[2, 3] and opioids[4-7] produce remarkably few hemodynamic changes, even in large doses. However, when used together, a variety of hemodynamic interactions have been reported.[4, 8-12] The principal hemodynamic interaction is supra-additive hypotension. Supra-additive hypotension is defined as greater hypotension from the drug combination than that which would be predicted from the effect of each drug alone.[13] Thus, benzodiazepines and opioids given together can and frequently do produce hypotension as seen in this case. Diazepam (10 mg) given to patients who have mi-

356

tral valvular disease anesthetized with fentanyl (up to 50 μg/kg) produced mild, but statistically significant, depression of the cardiac output (21%), mean arterial blood pressure (BP) (10%), and stroke volume (17%), while the heart rate was unchanged.[4] When fentanyl (50 μg/kg) was infused after doses of diazepam, either 0.125, 0.25, or 0.5 mg/kg, hypotension secondary to a decrease in systemic vascular resistance (SVR) occurs[8] (Fig 43–1). There appears to be no dose-effect relationship, that is, the lowest dose (0.125 mg/kg) of

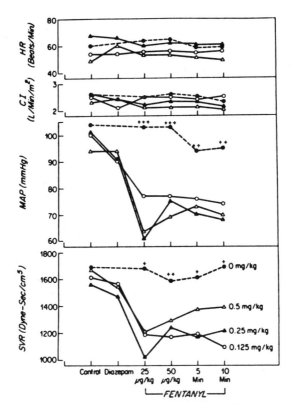

FIG 43–1.

Hemodynamic data for four groups of patients: Group 1, (control)—no diazepam; Group 2, 0.125 mg/kg diazepam; Group 3, 0.25 mg/kg diazepam; and Group 4, 0.5 mg/kg. Significant intergroup difference designated by + (*P*<0.05), ++(*P*<0.01), or +++(*P*<0.001). Note that there is a significant reduction in SVR and MAP when fentanyl and diazepam are combined. The diazepam effect is not dose related. *HR* = heart rate, *MAP* = mean arterial pressure, *CI* = cardiac index, and *SVR* = systemic vascular resistance. (From Tomicheck RC, Rosow CE, Philbin DM, et al: Diazepam-fentanyl interaction: Hemodynamic and hormonal effects in coronary artery surgery. Anesth Analg 1983; 62:881–884. Used by permission.)

drug produced decreases in BP and SVR similar to those of the highest dose (0.5 mg/kg). The administration of fentanyl with midazolam (0.075 mg or 0.15 mg/kg) also produces marked hypotension that is not dose related.[10] Thus, the combination of fentanyl with two commonly used benzodiazepines, diazepam and midazolam, will produce hypotension despite low doses of the benzodiazepines. Diazepam (0.125 mg/kg) given with alfentanil (100 or 200 μg/kg) produces hypotension when alfentanil alone does not.[13] Finally, sufentanil also produces significant decreases in BP and SVR when given after diazepam.[12] The degree of hypotension is similar to that seen with fentanyl.

The apparent reason for the hypotension with combined fentanyl and diazepam is a decrease in systemic vascular resistance (SVR).[8] There is also a possibility that venous pooling occurs with the combination of benzodiazepines and opioids, resulting in a slight decrease in cardiac output secondary to reduced left-sided heart filling.[10] A partial explanation for the decreased SVR is that diazepam given with fentanyl is associated with a decreased serum level of catecholamines;[8] thus, sympathetic reflexes are apparently obtunded and compensatory vasoconstriction is attenuated during induction. There may be other factors that cause this drug interaction, perhaps a synergistic direct effect on vascular smooth muscle. It is not a direct myocardial depressant effect, since ventricular function (as reflected by cardiac output at a given filling pressure) is not altered in man,[8] and the doses required to produce additive negative inotropic effects in vitro[15] are far beyond those in clinical use. The recent findings by Flacke et al. that dogs, rendered devoid of autonomic function by vagotomy and pharmacologic sympathectomy (subarachnoid block), do not exhibit the typical fentanyl-diazepam hemodynamic interaction argue for a central interaction.[16] It then appears that benzodiazepines block the normal sympathetic tone and thereby produce hypotension when given to patients anesthetized with opioids.

APPROACH TO THE PROBLEM

The management of hypotension that occurs in a patient with ischemic heart disease during induction with fentanyl and diazepam is designed to correct the underlying cause of the hypotension: systemic vasodilation with resultant hypovolemia. Appropriate treatment is administration of an α-adrenergic agonist as a bolus (e.g., phenylephrine 50 to 200 μg IV) as well as the administration of fluid (either crystalloid or colloid) to increase ventricular filling pressures to normal. These two simultaneous interventions should restore the hemodynamics to acceptable limits.

DISCUSSION

The induction of general anesthesia is always accompanied by direct hemodynamic effects of the particular compounds. These direct effects are counteracted by compensatory responses, usually mediated by the baroreflex and the sympathetic nervous system[17] (Fig 43–2). An example of the sympathetic response to induction of anesthesia may be seen with the induction of morphine anesthesia (3 mg/kg IV) that produces a significant decrease in systemic arterial pressure (from 98 to 84 mm Hg, $P<0.01$) and twofold increase in plasma norepinephrine (from 246 to 488 pg/ml, $P<0.01$) and fourfold increase in plasma epinephrine (from 129 to 570 pg/ml, $P<0.01$).[9] Presumably the increase in catecholamines is mediated by the baroreflexes as a compensatory response to morphine-induced hypotension (Fig 43–2). Thus, a functioning sympathetic response is necessary to maintain stable hemodynamics during induction of anesthesia, and, if this response is absent, hypotension will occur. Diazepam attenuates the increase in catecholamines in patients given 75 μg/kg of fentanyl[8] and the resultant hypotension illustrates the importance of an intact sympathetic nervous system during induction of anesthesia. When there is an attenuated catecholamine response to anesthesia induction, vasodilation and hypotension result (as in this case).

Since the mechanism of hypotension caused by the drug interaction of fen-

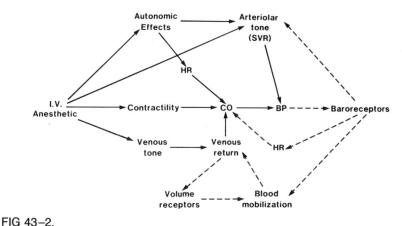

FIG 43–2.
Direct (*solid arrows*) and indirect (*broken arrows*) effects of intravenous anesthetics on cardiovascular function. CO indicates cardiac output; HR, heart rate; BP, blood pressure; SVR, systemic vascular resistance. (From Reves JG, Gelman S: Cardiovascular effects of intravenous anesthetic drugs, in *Effects of Anesthesia.* American Physiological Society, 1985, pp 179–193. Used by permission.)

tanyl with diazepam is systemic arterial and venous vasodilation, the appropriate therapy is an α-adrenergic agonist (vasoconstrictor). An α$_1$-agonist is the first-choice drug along with volume replacement to maintain central blood volume and therefore cardiac filling. It is not appropriate to give positive inotropic drugs, since there is no evidence that myocardial depression is responsible for the hypotension. If a bradycardia occurs with fentanyl,[18] administration of atropine (0.4 to 0.8 mg IV) and/or a mixed α- and β-agonist drug (e.g., ephedrine 5 to 10 mg IV) may be indicated. However, drugs that increase heart rate are contraindicated in hypotensive patients with ischemic heart disease, since this therapy could increase an imbalance of the oxygen supply/demand ratio. Increases in heart rate when the perfusion pressure is reduced increase the chance of ischemia.[19, 20] Positive chronotropic drugs are indicated if the cardiac output is reduced because of a profound bradycardia (heart rate <40 beats per minute). The indication for positive inotropic drugs is evidence of ventricular failure (e.g., reduced cardiac output with elevated pulmonary capillary wedge pressure). If the pulmonary artery wedge pressure is elevated, despite hypotension, nitroglycerin should be considered. Positive chronotropic and inotropic drugs will increase myocardial oxygen consumption and are only indicated if cardiac output is reduced secondary to reduced heart rate or contractility, respectively.

SUMMARY

Although opioids and benzodiazepines when used alone are accompanied by hemodynamic stability, their combination can be associated with serious hypotension. Treatment is directed toward correction of a decreased systemic vascular resistance and maintenance of adequate intravascular volume.

REFERENCES

1. Lowenstein E: Narcotics in anesthesia: Past, present, and future, in Estafanous FG (ed): *Opioids in Anesthesia*. Stoneham, Mass, Butterworth, 1984, pp 3–6.
2. Samuelson PN, Lell WA, Kouchoukos NT, et al: Hemodynamics during diazepam induction of anesthesia for coronary artery bypass grafting. *South Med J* 1980; 73:332–334.
3. Samuelson PN, Reves JG, Kouchoukos NT, et al: Hemodynamic responses to anesthetic induction with midazolam or diazepam in patients with ischemic heart disease. *Anesth Analg* 1981; 60:802–809.
4. Stanley TH, Webster LR: Anesthetic requirements and cardiovascular effects of fentanyl-oxygen and fentanyl-diazepam-oxygen anesthesia in man. *Anesth Analg* 1978; 57:411–416.

5. Lunn JK, Stanley TH, Eisele J, et al: High dose fentanyl anesthesia for coronary artery surgery: Plasma fentanyl concentrations and influence of nitrous oxide on cardiovascular responses. *Anesth Analg* 1979; 58:390–395.

6. Waller JL, Hug CC Jr, Nagle DM, et al: Hemodynamic changes during fentanyl-oxygen anesthesia for aortocoronary bypass operation. *Anesthesiology* 1981; 55:212–217.

7. Sebel PS, Bovill JG, Boekhorst RAA, et al: Cardiovascular effects of high-dose fentanyl anaesthesia. *Acta Anaesthesiol Scand* 1982; 26:308–315.

8. Tomicheck RC, Rosow CE, Philbin DM, et al: Diazepam-fentanyl interaction: Hemodynamic and hormonal effects in coronary artery surgery. *Anesth Analg* 1983; 62:881–884.

9. Hoar P, Nelson N, Mangano D, et al: Adrenergic response to morphine-diazepam anesthesia for myocardial revascularization. *Anesth Analg* 1981; 60:406–411.

10. Heikkilä H, Jalonen J, Arola M, et al: Midazolam as adjunct to high-dose fentanyl anaesthesia for coronary artery bypass grafting operation. *Acta Anaesthesiol Scand* 1984; 28:683–689.

11. Heikkilä H, Jalonen J, Laaksonen V, et al: Lorazepam and high-dose fentanyl anaesthesia: Effects on hemodynamics and oxygen transportation in patients undergoing coronary revascularization. *Acta Anaesthesiol Scand* 1984; 28:357–361.

12. George J, Samuelson PN, Lell WA, et al: Hemodynamic effects of diazepam-sufentanil compared to diazepam-fentanyl. Personal communication.

13. Silbert BS, Rosow CE, Keegan CR, et al: The effect of diazepam on induction of anesthesia with alfentanil. *Anesth Analg* 1986; 65:71–77.

14. Reves JG: Interaction of benaodiazepines and narcotics, in Estafanous F.G. (ed): *Opioids in Anesthesia*. Stoneham, Mass, Butterworth 1984, pp 249–252.

15. Reves JG, Kissin I, Fournier S, et al: Additive negative inotropic effect of a combination of diazepam and fentanyl. *Anesth Analg* 1984; 63:97–100.

16. Flacke JW, Davis LJ, Flacke WE, et al: Effects of fentanyl and diazepam in dogs deprived of autonomic tone. *Anesth Analg* 1985; 64:1053–1059.

17. Reves JG, Gelman S: Cardiovascular effects of intravenous anesthetic drugs, in *Effects of Anesthesia*. American Physiological Society, 1985, pp 179–193.

18. Reitan JA, Stengert KB, Wymore ML, et al: Central vagal control of fentanyl-induced bradycardia during halothane anesthesia. *Anesth Analg* 1978; 57:31–36.

19. Reves JG, Kissin I, Mardis M: Is the rate-pressure product a misleading guide? *Anesthesiology* 1980; 52:373–374.

20. Buffington CW: Hemodynamic determinants of ischemic myocardial dysfunction in the presence of coronary stenosis in dogs. *Anesthesiology* 1985; 63:651–662.

44

Protamine Hypotension

A 56-year-old, 50-kg woman with mitral valve disease had previously undergone a mitral commissurotomy and was scheduled to have a mitral valve replacement. The anesthetic course was uneventful and cardiopulmonary bypass was discontinued without difficulty. At this time, a protamine infusion was begun (calculated dose 3 mg/kg). But after 50 mg had been given, the blood pressure dropped from 120/80 to 50/35 mm Hg, with an increase in pulmonary artery pressure from 30/15 to 50/20 mm Hg, while the left atrial pressure was 5 mm Hg.

Recommendations by Denis R. Morel, M.D., and Edward Lowenstein, M.D.,

ANALYSIS OF THE PROBLEM

The neutralization of heparin by protamine is usually devoid of important adverse effects. On occasion, however, it may be followed by major cardiocirculatory and pulmonary reactions requiring early recognition and prompt intervention. The reaction described consists of acute systemic hypotension associated with pulmonary hypertension and a low left atrial pressure.

APPROACH TO THE PROBLEM

The primary aim in treating pulmonary hypertensive protamine reactions is to support the blood pressure until the pulmonary vasculature relaxes. In the presence of right ventricular distention or elevated venous pressure, we have administered drugs with pulmonary vasodilating properties into the right side of the circulation, while administering vasoconstrictors or inotropic drugs via a left atrial cannula (if in place). If the aortic perfusion cannula is still in place, a modest infusion may maintain systemic pressure. In contrast, right-sided volume infusion may further distend the right ventricle and compromise circulatory integrity.

Abrupt relief of pulmonary vasoconstriction may lead to sudden transfer of blood through the pulmonary vasculature, left ventricular hypervolemia and dramatic systemic hypertension until the circulation is again "balanced," (Fig 44–1). Systemic vasodilation with isoproterenol or a pure vasodilator has proved effective. Since pulmonary vasoconstriction appears to be due to a single burst of mediator release and is therefore short-lived, it is important to avoid iatrogenic complications.

Rarely, the systemic hypotension will persist despite supportive therapy. In that case, it is necessary to reheparinize the patient and reinstitute cardiopulmonary bypass. We have been able to reverse heparin by slow administration of protamine whenever pulmonary vasoconstriction has been the principal manifestation of the adverse response.

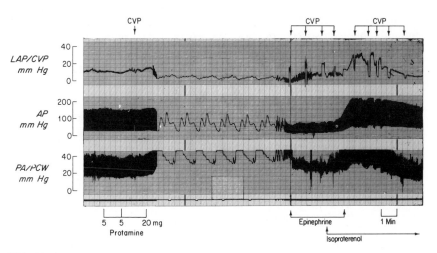

FIG 44–1.
Adverse response to protamine reversal of heparin following myocardial revascularization in a patient receiving intra-aortic balloon counterpulsation for refractory preinfarction angina pectoris.

The right atrial pressure (CVP) is measured intermittently by the same transducer used to measure left atrial pressure (LAP). Note the abrupt increase in pulmonary artery pressure (PA), the precipitous decline of LAP and systemic blood pressure (AP), the reversal of the normal relationship between the LAP and CVP, and the persistent hypotension despite counterpulsation. When the pulmonary vasculature dilates, there is rapid transfer of blood from the right side to the left side of the circulation, LAP and AP increase to abnormally high levels and CVP declines, reflecting relief of right ventricular volume and pressure overload. (From Lowenstein E, Johnston WE, Lappas DG, et al: Catastrophic pulmonary vasoconstriction associated with protamine reversal of heparin. *Anesthesiology* 1983; 59:470–473. Used by permission.)

DISCUSSION

This case represents one of a number of types of adverse responses to protamine neutralization of heparin. We shall provide an overview of the pathophysiology, clinical course, and treatment of the different types of responses, but emphasize the syndrome described in this case report. Understanding of this area remains incomplete. It is likely that concepts will change as further research is performed.

The incidence of adverse reactions to the administration of protamine has not yet been well established. No published prospective studies address this particular point. The reactions occur sporadically and, to date, unpredictably. The incidence undoubtedly varies with different underlying pathophysiologic mechanisms.

Moderate systemic hypotension and vasodilation may occur more frequently than recognized, especially when protamine is administered by rapid intravenous injection. More severe hemodynamic reactions associated with important pulmonary vasoconstriction and bronchospasm probably occur considerably less frequently than in 5% of cases. Prior exposure to protamines, especially in the form of protamine-zinc insulin or neutral protamine Hagedorn (NPH) insulin, has been suspected to be associated with an increased risk of a major protamine reaction.[1] However, the syndrome has also been reported in patients with no history of prior exposure to protamine. Furthermore, some protamine reactions seem to be independent of the dosage and rate of administration, since even minimal doses of protamine (20 mg) have produced this syndrome.[2] Neither underlying pulmonary vascular disease nor general anesthesia and prior extracorporeal circulation appear to be prerequisites for a reaction.[1]

Pathophysiology

Nonimmunological, Complement-Dependent Mechanism

That the complement system can be activated by a nonimmunologic mechanism was first described in vitro by Rent and colleages in 1975.[3] Their studies demonstrated that, similar to antibody-antigen complexing, the interaction of polyanions (e.g., heparin) and polycations (e.g., protamine) activate the complement system via the classic pathway, through which C3a, C4a, and C5a anaphylatoxin generation may occur. Recent prospective clinical studies have documented that plasma levels of C3a and C4a are increased immediately after protamine administration for heparin neutralization in patients undergoing cardiopulmonary bypass surgery,[4-6] thereby confirming in humans the occurence of nonimmunologic complement activation by heparin-protamine interaction.

Several studies have investigated the effects produced by intravenous complement activation, especially the effects of C5a anaphylatoxin. A common stimulus is the intravenous infusion of autologous plasma previously incubated with zymosan particles, which induces complement activation. Infusion of zymosan activated plasma into experimental animals causes an acute profound peripheral leukopenia with pulmonary white blood cell sequestration and the release of the potent prostaglandin vasoconstrictor thromboxane by cells within the lung, resulting in transient pulmonary hypertension and hypoxemia.[7] Since these symptoms are similar to the syndrome observed in patients sustaining an acute reaction to protamine in the form of pulmonary hypertension and bronchospasm, it has been postulated that this nonimmunologic, complement-dependent pathway could explain some of the acute adverse effects to protamine administration.

However, complement activation resulting in increased plasma concentrations of C3a and C4a fragments as well as transient leukopenia are common during protamine reversal of heparin, whereas pulmonary vasoconstriction is rare. The reason for this discrepancy is not clear, but it is most probably due to insufficient production of activated complement anaphylatoxins in vivo. Individual variations in factors inhibiting the complement cascade (e.g., carboxypeptidase B) or a C3a receptor desensitization during multiple activations that occur during cardiopulmonary bypass may account for differences in reactivity among patients. Furthermore, sufficient complement activation is strongly dependent on an optimal heparin-protamine ratio,[3, 8] which is probably rarely realized in vivo.

Interaction of the anionic polyelectrolyte heparin with the cationic protamine depends on their relative "free" plasma concentration. Heparin's plasma half-life measured by its metachromatic activity, which reflects its complexing rather than its anticoagulant propriety, is 13.6 minutes,[9] whereas its anticoagulant activity remains effective for more than 2 hours with a single intravenous dose. Therefore, at the usual time of protamine administration, heparin has probably lost most of its ability to form heparin-protamine complexes. This hypothesis is supported by experimental studies in pigs, which have shown that protamine injected only five minutes after heparinization elicits a reproducible pulmonary hypertensive response, whereas injection of protamine alone has no effect.[10, 11] Similarly, Fehr and Rohr reported an acute granulocytopenic response induced by protamine injection two minutes after intravenous heparin administration.[8] Maximal response was related to an optimal protamine-to-heparin ratio. Complete abolition of this reaction was observed when the animals had been complement depleted.

In a follow-up study to the case reports described previously,[2] in which even minimal doses of protamine induced catastrophic pulmonary vasoconstriction with low left atrial pressure and systemic hypotension, we have recently conducted a prospective study to investigate the mediators responsible for adverse reactions to protamine reversal of heparin anticoagulation.[6] Activation of the complement system by classic pathway mechanism was demonstrated by elevated plasma concentration of both C3a and C4a, which was associated with transient leukopenia proportional to the quantity of neutralized heparin as well as to the increased plasma C3a and C4a levels. Two of 48 patients undergoing cardiopulmonary bypass grafting or mitral valve replacement demonstrated a sudden increase of airway pressure, acute pulmonary hypertension, and systemic hypotension one to three minutes after an intravenous bolus injection of protamine. A marked increase in levels of plasma thromboxane B_2 and C5a occurred in these two subjects, whereas levels were unchanged in the others measured. Plasma histamine was not involved in this reaction. These results strongly suggest that pulmonary vasoconstriction and bronchoconstriction associated with protamine reversal of heparin in humans is mediated through the generation of high levels of C5a anaphylatoxins and thromboxane.

The clinical time course of this type of adverse protamine reaction appears short, starting within one minute of protamine administration (if injected by bolus), and lasting less than ten minutes. A characteristic hemodynamic pattern is presented in Figure 44–1. If carefully monitored, the increase in airway pressure is usually the first sign observed. This time course is similar to that observed in experimental animal studies. The latter are usually performed in young and healthy animals that recover spontaneously without treatment or further sequelae. In particular, no effect on pulmonary vascular permeability has been reported to isolated C5a infusion in rabbits[12] or heparin neutralization with protamine in sheep.[13] However, when combining complement activation with another stimulus such as transient hypoxia, lung vascular permeability was increased in rabbits.[14] Therefore, in a clinical situation, such as after cardiopulmonary bypass, which by itself can lead to some degree of lung injury,[15] the clinician might expect occasional more persistent consequences. Importantly, though the described reaction is usually evanescent, the associated systemic hypotension may acutely compromise coronary blood flow sufficiently to induce irreversible cardiovascular collapse unless it is promptly treated. Occasionally, reestablishment of cardiopulmonary bypass has been necessary.[2]

True Anaphylactic Reaction to Protamine Sulfate

Since commercially prepared protamine is a protein derived from salmon sperm, it is not surprising that it may trigger antibody production by the immune system. Indeed, circulating IgG antibodies to salmon protamine have been measured in patients receiving protamine-containing insulins[16, 17] and in vasectomized men, in whom an immunologic cross-reaction between human and salmon protamines has been documented.[18] Others have reported a prevalence of antiprotamine IgE antibody.[19, 20] A history of fish allergy has also been shown to be associated with IgE-mediated anaphylactic reactions to protamine injection.[21] Several case reports as well as prospective clinical studies have emphasized the increased risk of adverse protamine reaction in diabetic patients receiving protamine-insulins.[2, 20, 22]

However, despite previous sensitization to protamine, immediate type I allergic reactions are very rare. The dozen published case reports are not always sufficiently documented to establish true anaphylaxis. No cases of adverse reactions to protamine have been reported in vasectomized patients, despite the documentation of cross-reacting antibodies to protamine. Though positive immediate skin tests have been observed in some patients who had adverse protamine reactions, other investigators failed to demonstrate them.

Insulin-dependent diabetics may have other reasons to be particularly susceptible to adverse protamine reactions. In our prospective study (see above[6]) one of four diabetics receiving NPH insulin demonstrated acute pulmonary vasoconstriction and bronchoconstriction, but he did not have a plasma histamine level compatible with that of an immediate type I allergic reaction.

Protamine-Induced Isolated Histamine Release

A third pathophysiologic mechanism of protamine reaction has been postulated, supported by the fact that protamine in vitro is able to bind and degranulate mast cells causing histamine release.[23, 24] This nonimmunologic, noncomplement-mediated mechanism may be another explanation for acute decreases in systemic vascular resistance and/or urticaria, facial flushing, skin edema, or bronchospasm that are occasionally observed after protamine administration. In our prospective study, one patient developed acute hypotension due to a decreased systemic vascular resistance. This was associated with a fifteen-fold increase in histamine concentration to 10 ng/ml. Histamine level declined to the preadministration level of protamine by ten minutes after drug injection, and the hypotensive episode was successfully treated with vasopressors without further recognizable sequelae.

Suspected Protamine-Associated Fulminant Noncardiogenic Pulmonary Edema

Recently, a newly recognized syndrome that consists of fulminating noncardiogenic pulmonary edema occurring within two hours after cardiopulmonary bypass has been described.[25–27] Its mechanism remains unknown, but some investigators have suspected its cause to be an adverse reaction to protamine by exclusion of other possible factors, despite its occurrence more than 30 minutes after protamine administration. It is possible that some instances of this type of reaction represent a rare dramatic example of the mechanisms described above.

Anesthetic Evaluation and Management

Candidates for heparin and protamine should be questioned for a history of prior protamine administration. This should include adverse reactions to intravenous protamine during previous vascular surgery, cardiac catheterization, or dialysis and leukapheresis. Diabetic patients with chronic administration of protamine zinc or NPH insulin, and patients with a history of allergic reactions to ingestion of fish[21] are probably at increased risk of presenting an acute anaphylactic reaction to protamine injection. In case of a suspected hypersensitivity reaction, immediate sensitivity skin testing (intradermal or prick test) should be performed. If the patient reacts to a low concentration of protamine (< mg/ml), we advise that protamine be avoided. Alternatives to protamine administration include heparin neutralization by hexadimethrine bromide (Polybrene), a synthetic heparin antagonist,[28] and spontaneous reversal of the heparin anticoagulant activity.[29] Postoperative blood loss due to residual anticoagulation can be reduced by withdrawal of autologous blood prior to heparinization and by reinfusing it in the postoperative period.[30] Infusion of platelet concentrates has also been reported to be effective.[31]

Since the incidence of adverse protamine reaction is low even in high-risk patients, routine prophylactic measures are probably not warranted. The clinician may consider antihistaminic and corticosteroid pretreatment. Since most of the reactions are unpredictable, however, the major point when administering protamine for reversal of heparin anticoagulation is to be aware of the risk of inducing an anaphylactic or anaphylactoid reaction. Continuous monitoring of systemic and pulmonary arterial pressure, if available, just before and during infusion is advisable. In awake, spontaneously breathing patients, respiratory symptoms (such as coughing, sensation of retrosternal oppression, sudden tachypnea, or dyspnea with or without bronchospasm) may indicate the onset of an adverse reaction; cutaneous signs of facial flushing, periorbital or perioral swelling, and angioedema are possible. Under anesthesia with controlled ventilation the first sign may be an increase in airway pressure detected on the manometer of the breathing circuit. Systemic blood pressure usually decreases after approximately one minute with bolus injection, but the decrease may be delayed with a slow protamine infusion rate. Pulmonary vasoconstriction may impede transfer of blood across the lungs, resulting in right atrial and ventricular distention, decreased blood volume and pressures in the left side of the heart, and systemic hypotension.

It is our clinical impression that it is safer to administer protamine as a slow continuous infusion (i.e., maximum 5 mg/minute) rather than by bolus. However, adverse responses have been observed with doses as low as 0.5 mg/kg delivered in divided doses and very low infusion rates. At least acute nonspecific mast cell degranulation and histamine release will probably be minimized by this mode of drug administration.[32] A small test dose (e.g., 5 mg) before starting the planned infusion may also reduce the risk of excessive adverse reaction.

REFERENCES

1. Stewart WJ, McSweeney SM, Kellett MA, et al: Increased risk of severe protamine reactions in NPH insulin-dependent diabetics undergoing cardiac catheterization. *Circulation* 1984; 70:788–792.
2. Lowenstein E, Johnston WE, Lappas DG, et al: Catastrophic pulmonary vasoconstriction associated with protamine reversal of heparin. *Anesthesiology* 1983; 59:470–473.
3. Rent R, Ertel N, Eisenstein R, Gewurz H: Complement activation by interaction of polyanions and polycations: I. Heparin-protamine induced consumption of complement. *J Immunol* 1975; 114:120–124.
4. Cavarocchi NC, Schaff HV, Orszulak TA, et al: Evidence for complement activation by protamine-heparin interaction after cardiopulmonary bypass. *Surgery* 1985; 98:525–530.
5. Kirklin JK, Chenoweth DE, Naftel DC, et al: Effects of protamine administration after cardiopulmonary bypass on complement, blood elements, and the hemodynamic state. *Ann Surg* (in press).
6. Morel DR, Zapol WM, Thomas SJ, et al: C5a generation and thromboxane release associated with pulmonary vaso- and broncho-constriction during protamine reversal of heparin. (Submitted)
7. Cooper JD, McDonald JWD, Ali M, et al: Prostaglandin production associated with the pulmonary vascular response to complement activation. *Surgery* 1980; 88:215–221.
8. Fehr J, Rohr H: In vivo complement activation by polyanion-polycation complexes: Evidence that C5a is generated intravascularly during heparin-protamine interaction. *Clin Immunol Immunopathol* 1983; 29:7–14.
9. Zollner N, Kaiser W: Uber Verteilungsraum und Halbweitszeit von intravenos injiziertem Heparin. *Res Exp Med* 1972; 158:89–94.
10. Stefaniszyn HJ, Novick RJ, Salerno TA: Toward a better understanding of the hemodynamic effects of protamine and heparin interaction. *J Thorac Cardiovasc Surg* 1984; 87:678–686.
11. Fiser WP, Fewell JE, Hill DE, et al: Cardiovascular effects of protamine sulfate are dependent on the presence and type of circulating heparin. *J Thorac Cardiovasc Surg* 1985; 89:63–70.
12. Webster RO, Larsen GL, Mitchell BC, et al: Absence of inflammatory lung injury in rabbits challenged intravascularly with complement-derived chemotactic factors. *Am Rev Respir Dis* 1982; 125:335–340.
13. Morel DR, Nguyenduy T, Collee G, et al: Thromboxane mediates acute pulmonary vasoconstriction during heparin reversal by protamine in sheep. *Fed Proc* 1985; 44:625.

14. Larsen GL, Webster RO, Worthen GS, et al: Additive effect of intravascular complement activation and brief episodes of hypoxia in producing increased permeability in the rabbit lung. *J Clin Invest* 1985; 75:902–910.
15. Anyanwu E, Dittrich H, Gieseking R, et al: Ultrastructural changes in the human lung following cardiopulmonary bypass. *Basic Res Cardiol* 1982; 77:309–322.
16. Kurtz AB, Gray RS, Markanday S, et al: Circulating IgG antibody to protamine in patients treated with protamine-insulins. *Diabetologia* 1983; 25:322–324.
17. Lakin JD, Blocker TJ, Strong DM, et al: Anaphylaxis to protamine sulfate mediated by a complement-dependent IgG antibody. *J Allergy Clin Immunol* 1978; 61:102–107.
18. Samuel T, Kolk AHJ, Rumke P, et al: Autoimmunity to sperm antigens in vasectomized men. *Clin Exp Immunol* 1975; 21:65–74.
19. Sharath MD, Metzger WJ, Richerson HB, et al: Protamine-induced fatal anaphylaxis: Prevalence of antiprotamine immunoglobulin E antibody. *J Thorac Cardiovasc Surg* 1985; 90:86-90.
20. Moorthy SS, Pond W, Rowland RG: Severe circulatory shock following protamine (an anaphylactic reaction). *Anesth Analg* 1980; 59:77–78.
21. Knape JTA, Schuller JL, De Haan P, et al: An anaphylactic reaction to protamine in a patient allergic to fish. *Anesthesiology* 1981; 55:324–325.
22. Weiler JM, Freiman P, Sharath MD, et al: Serious adverse reactions to protamine sulfate: Are alternatives needed? *J Allergy Clin Immunol* 1985; 75:297–303.
23. Keller R: Interrelations between different types of cells: II. Histamine release from the mast cells of various species by cationic polypeptide of polymorphonuclear leukocyte lysosomes and other cationic compounds. *Int Arch Allergy Appl Immunol* 1968; 34:139–144.
24. Schnitzler S, Renner H, Pfuller U: Histamine release from rat mast cells induced by protamine sulfate and polyethylenimine. *Agents Actions* 1981; 11:73–74.
25. Olinger GN, Becker RM, Bonchek LI: Noncardiogenic pulmonary edema and peripheral vascular collapse following cardiopulmonary bypass: Rare protamine reaction? *Ann Thorac Surg* 1980; 29:20–25.
26. Culliford AT, Thomas S, Spencer FC: Fulminating noncardiogenic pulmonary edema: A newly recognized hazard during cardiac operations. *J Thorac Cardiovasc Surg* 1980; 80:868–875.
27. Just-Viera JO, Fischer CR, Gago O, et al: Acute reaction to protamine: Its importance to surgeons. *Am Surg* 1984; 50:52–60.
28. Godal HC: A comparison of two heparin-neutralizing agents: Protamine and polybrene. *Scand J Clin Lab Invest* 1960; 12:446–452.
29. Castaneda AR: Must heparin be neutralized following open-heart operations? *J Thorac Cardiovasc Surg* 1966; 52:716–724.
30. Campbell FW, Goldstein MF, Atkins PC: Management of the patient with protamine hypersensitivity for cardiac surgery. *Anesthesiology* 1984; 61:761–764.
31. Walker WS, Reid KG, Hider CF, et al: Successful cardiopulmonary bypass in diabetics with anaphylactoid reactions to protamine. *Br Heart J* 1984; 52:112–114.
32. Stoelting RK, Henry DP, Verburg KM, et al: Haemodynamic changes and circulating histamine concentrations following protamine administration to patients and dogs. *Can Anaesth Soc J* 1984; 31:534–540.

45

Hyperkalemia During Bypass

A 65-year-old man with ischemic heart disease and a long-standing history of hypertension was treated with diuretics, antihypertensives, propranolol, and nifedipine. The preinduction serum potassium level was 3.5 mEq/L, and a slow potassium infusion containing 25 mEq/L was started. The potassium was maintained in the 3.8 to 4.2 mEq/L range through cardiopulmonary bypass. During aortic cross-clamping, 50 mEq of potassium was administered in the cardioplegic fluid. After cardiopulmonary bypass the patient started diuresing, and the potassium infusion rate was increased. After ten minutes a widened QRS and a high peaked T wave were noted. The level of serum potassium drawn at this time was 6.0 mEq/L.

Recommendations by Carol L. Lake, M.D.

ANALYSIS OF THE PROBLEM

The ECG changes in this patient are the result of hyperkalemia. Although a serum potassium level of 6.0 mEq/L is not life threatening, it is clearly abnormal and has changed the ECG.

APPROACH TO THE PROBLEM

Since there is diuresis to remove potassium and a presumed cause, iatrogenic potassium administration, therapy is:

1. Discontinue the administration of potassium.

2. Monitor diuresis and ECG.

Should there be continued rise in serum potassium level or cardiac complications, therapy for moderate or severe hyperkalemia (see discussion below) should be instituted.

DISCUSSION

Potassium Physiology

Only 2% of the potassium in the human body is extracellular (a usual serum concentration of 3.5 to 4.5 mEq/L), while the remaining 98% is intracellular (an intracellular concentration of 150 mEq/L). This balance is maintained by the cell-membrane adenosinetriphosphatase (ATPase) pump that actively extrudes sodium from the cell. Inhibition of this pump (digitalis overdose) prevents cellular maintenance of intracellular potassium with resultant hyperkalemia.

For ease of measurement, extracellular potassium is customarily estimated. Either arterial, peripheral venous, or central venous sampling sites may be used since there is no significant difference between their plasma concentrations.[1] Plasma levels are usually 0.1 to 0.7 mEq/L lower than those of serum samples since potassium is released by ruptured platelets during the coagulation process.[2] Despite the usual measurement of extracellular concentrations, clinicians must recognize the factors involved in total body potassium homeostasis.

Determinants of Extracellular Potassium Concentration

Acid-base balance, insulin, adrenergic activity, and aldosterone are important determinants of extracellular potassium concentration.

Acid-Base Effects.—Although recent studies question the role of acidosis in cellular potassium distribution, acidosis is believed to cause outward potassium movement; and alkalosis, intracellular movement. An intracellular shift of hydrogen ion in exchange for potassium and sodium ions induces hyperkalemia in acidosis. The outward shift of potassium from the cell occurs only in acidosis mediated by mineral acids such as hydrochloric acid, not organic acids such as lactic or acetoacetic acid.[3] Generally for each 0.1 unit decrease in blood pH, plasma potassium level increases 0.5 to 1.0 mEq/L[4] with a greater increase with metabolic than with respiratory acidosis. The value of plasma potassium also increases with a decreased bicarbonate concentration, even when blood pH is unchanged.[4] Acute hypercapnia increases serum potassium values in a linear fashion.[5]

Potassium secretion in the distal tubule is also affected by acid-base changes. Acute metabolic and respiratory alkalosis increases and acidosis decreases potassium secretion.[6] These effects may be secondary to changes in potassium uptake across the peritubular membrane that are modulated by intracellular pH.[7]

Neuroendocrine Effects.—α-Adrenergic stimulation causes outward movement of potassium while β-adrenergic activity produces an intracellular shift.[3] Catecholamines initially release potassium from hepatocytes, followed by its uptake into hepatic and skeletal muscle cells.[8]

Hyperkalemia stimulates aldosterone production. The role of aldosterone in the distribution of potassium is controversial, but it does affect renal potassium excretion.[3] Aldosterone controls sodium reabsorption and, thus, transtubular potential. Sodium reabsorption in the distal tubule creates a potential difference across the epithelial cell, causing the lumen to be more electronegative. Aldosterone also increases the permeability of the luminal membrane to potassium and stimulates active transfer of potassium into cells at the peritubular membrane, thus enhancing potassium secretion.[9]

Renal Excretion of Potassium.—The kidney excretes about 90% of daily ingested potassium (Fig 45–1). Potassium is freely filtered at the glomerulus and its concentration in the proximal tubule is similar to that in the glomerular

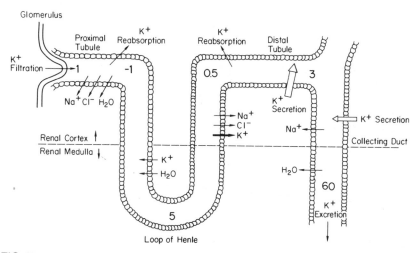

FIG 45–1.
Renal excretion of potassium. The major site of potassium secretion is in the distal convoluted tubule, although small amounts are secreted into the ascending loop of Henle and the collecting duct. Intraluminal numbers represent the tubular fluid/plasma potassium concentration ratios. (Redrawn from Barrett LJ: Potassium handling by the kidney: Hyperkalemia. *Aust NZ J Med* 1981; 2(suppl 1):16–22.

filtrate. At the tip of the loop of Henle, the potassium concentration is higher than in the proximal tubule because of water reabsorption along the descending limb and potassium diffusion inward from the medullary interstitium. [10] There is net potassium reabsorption in the ascending loop of Henle, although a small amount is secreted into tubular fluid. The potassium concentration in the beginning of the distal tubule is lower than that in plasma. Renal potassium excretion is regulated in the distal tubule and collecting duct of the kidney by the following factors: (1) the magnitude of the negative transtubular potential difference; (2) the concentration gradient across the luminal membrane of the tubular cell; (3) distal tubular flow rate; and (4) aldosterone. Thus, the potassium concentration in the distal tubule cells determines secretion of potassium ion into the tubular lumen. If cellular potassium concentration is high and lumen potassium concentration low, secretion is facilitated and vice versa. The electronegativity of tubular fluid anions and the sodium reabsorptive mechanism determines transtubular potential. The concentration gradient is also influenced by peritubular potassium transport, which is a function of membrane ATPase activity, serum potassium, and acid-base balance.

More significant than sodium concentration in controlling potassium secretion may be the flow rate in the distal tubule. An increased flow rate increases potassium secretion even when sodium concentration remains constant. [11] The net result is an increase in tubular fluid potassium from 2 to 3 mmole/L in the beginning of the distal tubule to 12 to 20 mmole/L at the end of the tubule. [10] The concentration of potassium in tubular fluid also increases as it passes through the collecting duct because of water reabsorption. [10]

Etiology of Perioperative Hyperkalemia in Cardiac Patients

Numerous situations occurring in the context of cardiovascular surgery can increase the level of serum potassium. Among these are: (1) pseudohyperkalemia; (2) decreased renal excretion of potassium; (3) a change in transcellular potassium gradient, and (4) increased potassium intake or load (Table 45–1).

Pseudohyperkalemia

Pseudohyperkalemia, release of potassium by cells during the clotting or separation process, occurs with leukocytosis (leukemia); with samples obtained by heel stick or from a transiently ischemic extremity from a tourniquet that is too tight—hemolysis during sampling; and in the presence of hemolysis, as occurs during cardiopulmonary bypass with bubble oxygenators. The presence of potassium release by hemolysis can be determined by comparing plasma and serum concentration since normally the serum level should be no more than 0.5 mEq/L higher than the plasma.

TABLE 45–1.

Causes of Hyperkalemia

Decreased renal potassium excretion
  Inadequate distal tubular sodium delivery and decreased urine
    flow (examples: acute renal failure, acute pulmonary edema in patients with
    chronic renal insufficiency)
  Defective renin-angiotensin-aldosterone axis (examples: Addison's, 1°
    hypoaldosteronism, drugs such as β-blockers and captopril)
  Renal tubular secretory defect (examples: obstructive uropathy, lupus)
  Inhibition of tubular secretion (examples: acidosis, toxins, drugs such as
    spironolactone, digitalis)
Abnormal distribution of potassium
  Insulin deficiency and hyperglycemia
  Tissue damage
  Acidosis
  Exercise
  Drugs (digitalis, succinylcholine, β-blockers, arginine hydrochloride)
Factitious
  Pseudohyperkalemia
  Laboratory error

Decreased Renal Potassium Excretion

Inadequate Distal Sodium Delivery and Decreased Distal Tubular Urine Flow.—Acute or chronic renal failure obviously decrease renal potassium excretion. The normal human excretes between 40 and 90 mEq of potassium in the urine every 24 hours with a normal oral intake of 40 to 100 mEq. Nevertheless, patients with chronic renal disease increase the fractional excretion of potassium as glomerular filtration rate decreases. Thus, potassium excretion is maintained in chronic renal failure due to increased ATPase activity in the cells of the collecting duct in the presence of aldosterone[12] until very low levels of renal clearance occur. There is also more rapid transfer of potassium into cells of patients with renal failure, a process probably mediated by aldosterone.[13] However, other investigators have demonstrated a defect in cellular uptake of potassium[14] and decreased intracellular potassium concentrations in muscle, erythrocytes, and leukocytes in uremia.[4]

In acute renal failure, hyperkalemia is more common since: (1) glomerular filtration rate, distal sodium delivery, and urine flow are often more severely reduced; (2) there is insufficient time for renal and extrarenal adaptive mechanisms to occur; (3) acute insults are often associated with increased tissue breakdown causing hyperkalemia; and (4) acute renal diseases are associated with widespread damage to portions of kidney responsible for potassium secretion.

Defective Renin-Angiotensin-Aldosterone Axis.—Many patients with hypoaldosteronism (Addison's disease, adrenogenital syndrome, or diabetes) will have hyperkalemia due to diminished urinary, intestinal, and sweat potassium excretion. The combination of hyperglycemia, insulin deficiency, and hypoaldosteronism may be required for hyperkalemia to develop in the diabetic state. Hyperglycemia in the diabetic patient can also produce hyperkalemia by an increase in serum osmolarity that results in movement of potassium-containing fluid from cells.[15] The lack of insulin also impairs the movement of potassium from extracellular to intracellular locations.

Drugs such as propranolol, captopril, and the prostaglandin inhibitors can induce a state of functional hypoaldosteronism. Propranolol inhibits renin secretion and, secondarily, conversion of angiotensin II and aldosterone secretion. Hyperkalemia has been noted in patients with chronic renal failure or diabetes during propranolol therapy as potassium shifts from the intracellular to extracellular compartment.[4]

Inhibition of Tubular Secretion or Tubular Secretory Defect.—Some patients even with normal glomerular filtration, aldosterone, and cortisol have defective renal potassium excretion, requiring thiazide or loop diuretic therapy. Patients on potassium-sparing diuretics (triamterene, spironolactone) may become hyperkalemic because of interference with the distal tubule sodium reabsorptive-potassium secretory exchange mechanism. Obstructive uropathy with distal renal tubular acidosis or renal tubular insensitivity to aldosterone can cause defective renal potassium secretion. Chronic heparin anticoagulation decreases aldosterone secretion leading to hyperkalemia.[3] The mechanism is unclear but may involve either a specific enzyme in the synthetic pathway for production of aldosterone or nonspecific inhibition of zona glomerulosa function.[3]

Abnormal Distribution of Potassium

Metabolic acidosis, shock, or rhabdomyolysis can occur during or after cardiopulmonary bypass. Rhabdomyolysis would be most likely as a complication of accidental cannulation of an aortic arch vessel or after prolonged hypothermia with circulatory arrest. Metabolic acidosis and shock commonly occur with low cardiac output states after cardiopulmonary bypass. However, inadequate extracorporeal perfusion causes metabolic acidosis, and extracorporeal circulation at low to moderate flow rates is essentially a state of "controlled shock." The mechanism for hyperkalemia in these disease states has been described earlier.

Increased Intake of Potassium

Massive blood transfusions, systemic absorption of potassium cardioplegia solution, and intravenous administration of potassium are possible sources of an increased potassium intake in the perioperative period. Another less common iatrogenic cause of hyperkalemia is the administration of arginine hydrochloride for the treatment of metabolic alkalosis. Arginine is exchanged for potassium in the cells. [11]

Potassium Flux During Cardiac Surgery

Potassium Homeostasis.—Although most patients undergoing cardiac surgery have normal total body potassium concentrations, [16] during cardiopulmonary bypass extracellular potassium usually decreases to 2 to 3 mEq/L due to urinary excretion, hypokalemic perfusate, hypocarbia, and preoperative diuretics. [17, 18] Potassium increases during the rewarming phase after hypothermic cardiopulmonary bypass, possibly as a result of washout from underperfused regions or a change in transmembrane potassium ion distribution. [19] Williams and colleagues noted the development of hyperkalemia in 17 of 150 adult cardiac surgical patients within 24 hours of surgery. [20]

Potassium Cardioplegia.—With the use of potassium cardioplegia, no change or an increase in potassium may be seen during cardiac surgery. [21] Cardioplegia solutions containing potassium result in three problems upon myocardial reperfusion: (1) systemic hyperkalemia; (2) complete atrioventricular (AV) block; and (3) flaccid, asystolic hearts. Systemic hyperkalemia, a consequence of systemic absorption of cardioplegia solution, [22] is usually self-limiting if renal function is adequate; but, occasionally, therapy may be required. Complete AV block may also be related to the potassium content of the cardioplegia solution and generally responds to AV sequential pacing. However, the pacing threshold will be increased at potassium concentrations greater than 8 mEq/L. [23] Asystole usually responds to pacing or to additional reperfusion time to wash out metabolites and potassium. [24]

Hyperkalemia during the reperfusion phase after aortic clamping can be beneficial as Lake and colleagues [25] reported more rapid resumption of cardiac electrical activity at a lower myocardial temperature when plasma potassium was greater than 5.0 mEq/L as a result of cardioplegia solution. The defibrillation threshold is also decreased. [26] The increased catecholamine concentrations seen during cardiac surgery promote myocardial potassium loss by activation of the sodium-potassium ATPase, [27] predisposing to arrhythmias. [28] Ischemia also causes an efflux of potassium from myocardial cells. [29] Hypokalemia increases the likelihood of dysrhythmias during acute myocardial ischemia and infarction as a result.[30, 31] Reperfusion with blood with slightly increased potassium concentrations appears to antagonize these effects.[25]

Diagnosis of Hyperkalemia

The normal resting potential of the cell membrane is maintained by the transmembrane concentration gradient for potassium.

Cardiac Effects.—An increase in extracellular potassium decreases resting membrane potential (membrane potential becomes more positive and closer to the threshold), shortens action potential duration, and reduces its amplitude in all cardiac tissues (Fig 45–2).[32] Cardiac excitability is increased as the reduction in resting potential toward threshold allows stimuli of lesser magnitude to elicit an action potential. On the ECG these effects appear as shortened PR and QT intervals with peaked T waves in the precordial leads at serum potassium concentrations of 6 to 7 mEq/L (Fig 45–3). The T waveform changes result from inhomogenous reduction of local repolarization duration with more marked reduction in the endocardium than in the epicardium of the left ventricle.[33] The inhomogeneity may favor reentrant dysrhythmias.

Intracardiac conduction is progressively depressed as potassium increases to 8 to 9 mEq/L (Fig 45–3). Unifascicular and bifascicular block are infrequently seen as conduction is globally depressed.[34] Complete heart block can be produced with potassium infusions in experimental animals but is rarely seen in the clinical setting. However, iatrogenic hyperkalemia resulting from excessive infusion of potassium perioperatively and as a consequence of mild renal failure has been reported to produce complete heart block in humans.[34] Usually the atrial myocardium is most sensitive to the depressed conduction, followed by the ventricular myocardium, and last, the sinoatrial node and bundle of His. The P waves disappear and conduction appears to be sinoventricular, although intracardiac electrocardiography demonstrates intra-atrial conduction. The QRS widening and QT-interval prolongation occur at serum potassi-

FIG 45–2.
The effect of hyperkalemia on the membrane and action potentials of a cardiac pacemaker cell. Both action potential duration and resting membrane potential are decreased.

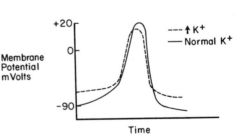

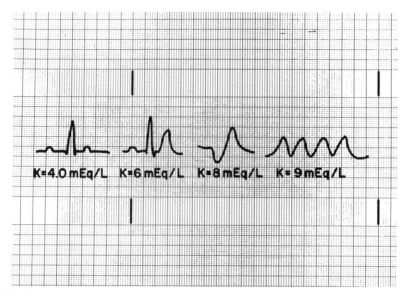

FIG 45–3.
Changes in the electrocardiogram with an increase in serum potassium concentration. An increase in size and peaking of the T wave coupled with decreased intracardiac conduction are the principal changes.

um concentrations of 9 to 10 mEq/L. Escape beats and slow idioventricular rhythms develop as intramyocardial conduction decreases.[35] Further depression of intracardiac conduction merges the QRS and T waves into a sine wave, which usually precedes ventricular asystole or fibrillation at a potassium level greater than 10 mEq/L (Fig 45–3). Cardiac standstill results from inactivation of the sodium channels in the cell membrane, preventing a stimulus from eliciting an action potential. Cardiotoxicity from hyperkalemia is more often seen with an abrupt increase in potassium level than with a more gradual increase. The rate of increase in serum potassium value also determines the ECG findings; more rapid increases produce bradycardia and ventricular fibrillation, while more gradual development enhances the intracardiac conduction problems leading to asystole.[36]

Noncardiac Effects.—Lassitude, fatigue, and weakness occur with serum potassium concentrations above 6.5 mEq/L. Neuromuscular paralysis supervenes at serum potassium levels greater than 8 mEq/L and respiratory failure resulting from hyperkalemia has been reported.[37] Other physical findings are absent or nonspecific, although symptoms of nausea and vomiting secondary to paralytic ileus have been noted. Generally the cardiac effects occur well before the neuromusclar symptoms.

Therapy for Hyperkalemia

Definition of Hyperkalemia.—No additional potassium should be administered if the serum potassium level is greater than 5.5 mEq/L, which is arbitrarily defined as hyperkalemia.[3] A serum potassium value of 5.5 to 6.5 mEq/L has been defined as mild or minimal hyperkalemia.[38] Moderate hyperkalemia exists at levels of 6.5 to 8.0 mEq/L and severe hyperkalemia at concentrations over 8.0 mEq/L.[38] An increased serum potassium concentration unaccompanied by ECG evidence of hyperkalemia requires evaluation as a possible laboratory artifact, the so-called pseudohyperkalemia described earlier.

Initial Treatment.—Since the patient described in the above case report has ECG evidence of hyperkalemia, a laboratory error is unlikely. Discontinuation of the potassium infusion alone, accompanied by the preexisting diuresis, should rapidly restore normal potassium concentrations. Continuous ECG monitoring is essential until normokalemia returns. If the ECG indicates progressively increasing hyperkalemia, the pharmacologic intervention described below should be initiated.

Possibilities other than overinfusion of potassium must also be investigated and corrected. These include: (1) cellular and tissue damage during cardiopulmonary bypass or resulting from incompatible blood transfusion; (2) massive transfusions secondary to blood loss (stored banked blood often has 20 mEq/L or more of potassium); (3) acidosis secondary to low cardiac output; (4) drugs such as propranolol, captopril, or spironolactone that the patient was receiving preoperatively; or (5) early high-output renal failure. If these conditions are absent, maintenance infusion of potassium may be reinstituted when normokalemia ensues.

Therapy for Moderate or Severe Hyperkalemia.—If the serum potassium level is moderately or severely increased or associated with ECG evidence of hyperkalemia, acute therapy is mandatory. The aim of treatment is to reverse membrane abnormalities, restore transcellular gradient by transferring potassium intracellularly, and remove excess body potassium. It includes: (1) calcium chloride, 10 mg/kg; (2) bicarbonate, 0.5 to 1 mEq/kg, or an infusion of 100 to 150 mEq/L over 60 to 120 minutes; (3) 50 ml of 50% dextrose followed by an infusion of 500 to 1,000 ml of 10% glucose with 10 to 15 units of regular insulin given over 60 minutes to adults, particularly if decreased renal function is present; (4) diuretics; and (5) ion exchange resins. By increasing the transmembrane resting potential to restore a more normal differential between threshold and resting potential, calcium inhibits the depressant effects of potassium on the heart. It does not reduce the serum potassium concentration; therefore, other measures must immediately be instituted to reduce the level of serum potassium, as the administered calcium will be excreted or sequestered into bone. Calcium should be avoided in patients with digitalis intoxication. Rapid alkalinization with bicarbonate shifts potassium intracellularly, as do glucose and insulin. Because of the intracellular transfer, the potassium level may slowly increase as pH decreases when the bicarbonate infusion is terminated.[39]

Diuretics will also decrease serum potassium level. Osmotic diuresis with mannitol often removes as much as 2 to 3 mEq within three hours. However, the administration of an osmotically active substance such as mannitol may enhance outward diffusion of potassium from cells, causing hyperkalemia. This probably relates to interference with the exchange pump or membrane permeability.[40] Furosemide, ethacrynic acid, and thiazides also increase sodium and potassium excretion. Ion exchange resins—sodium polystyrene sulfonate (Kayexalate)—are generally too slow acting to be applicable during open heart surgery, although they may be used to treat postoperative hyperkalemia. The usual adult dose is 80 to 200 gm orally or rectally for each milliequivalent of potassium greater than 5 mEq/L. Excess total body potassium can be removed by ion exchange, but hypernatremia may occur as sodium is released in exchange for the potassium bound to the resin. Fluid retention secondary to increased sodium is a consequence of resin use. In patients with resistant hyperkalemia, either peritoneal or hemodialysis may be employed. In fact, hemodialysis can be performed during cardiopulmonary bypass.

REFERENCES

1. Hill AB, Nahrwold ML, Noonan D, et al: A comparison of methods of blood withdrawal and sample preparation for potassium measurements. *Anesthesiology* 1980; 53:60–63.
2. Weissman N, Pileggi VJ, Inorganic ions, in Henry RJ, Cannon DC, Winkelman JW (eds): *Clinical Chemistry: Principles and Technics.* Harper and Row, Hagerstown, Md, 1974, pp 645–646.
3. Reineck HJ: Disorders of potassium homeostasis. *Compr Ther* 1981; 7:12–21.
4. DeFronzo RA, Bia M, Smith D: Clinical disorders of hyperkalemia. *Ann Rev Med* 1982; 33:521–554.
5. Hassan H, Gjessing J, Tomlin PJ: Hypercapnia and hyperkalemia. *Anaesthesia* 1979; 34:897–899.

6. Gennari FJ, Cohen JJ: The role of the kidney in potassium homeostasis: Lessons from acid-base disturbances. *Kidney Int* 1975; 8:1–5.
7. Giebisch G, Stanton B: Potassium transport in the nephron. *Ann Rev Physiol* 1979; 41:241–256.
8. Vick RL, Todd EP, Leudke DW: Epinephrine-induced hypokalemia: Relation to liver and skeletal muscle. *J Pharmacol Exp Ther* 1972; 181:139–146.
9. Hierholzer K, Wiederholt M: Some aspects of distal tubular solute and water transport. *Kidney Int* 1976; 9:198–213.
10. Barratt LJ: Potassium handling by the kidney: Hyperkalemia. *Aust NZ J Med* 1981; 11(suppl 1):16–22.
11. Good DW, Wright FS: Luminal influences on potassium secretion, sodium concentration and fluid flow rate. *Am J Physiol* 1979; 236:F192–F205.
12. Finkelstein FO, Hayslett JP: Role of medullary Na-K-ATPase in renal potassium adaptation. *Am J Physiol* 1975; 229:524–528.
13. Alexander EA, Levinsky NG: An extrarenal mechanism of potassium adaptation. *J Clin Invest* 1968; 47:740–748.
14. Van Ypersele De Strihou C: Potassium homeostasis in renal failure. *Kidney Int* 1977; 11:491–504.
15. Cox M, Sterns RH, Singer I: The defense against hypokalemia: The roles of insulin and aldosterone. *N Engl J Med* 1978; 299:525–532.
16. Morgan DB, Mearns AJ, Burkinshaw L: The potassium status of patients prior to open-heart surgery. *J Thorac Cardiovasc Surg* 1978; 76:673–677.
17. Babka R, Pifarré R: Potassium replacement during cardiopulmonary bypass. *J Thorac Cardiovasc Surg* 1977; 73:212–215.
18. Ebert PA, Jude JR, Gaertner RA: Persistent hypokalemia following open heart surgery. *Circulation* 1965; 31 (suppl 1):137–143.
19. Lim M, Linton RAF, Band DM: Rise in plasma potassium during rewarming in open-heart surgery. *Lancet* 1983; 1:241–242.
20. Williams JR, Morrow AG, Braunwald E: The incidence and management of "medical" complications following cardiac operations. *Circulation* 1965; 32:608–619.
21. Weber DO, Yarnoz MD: Hyperkalemia complicating cardiopulmonary bypass: Analysis of risk factors. *Ann Thorac Surg* 1982; 34:439–445.
22. Azar I, Satyanarayana T, Turndorf H: Urine and serum potassium levels after cardioplegia. *J Thorac Cardiovasc Surg* 1981; 81:516–518.
23. Surawicz B, Chlebus H, Reeves JT, et al: Increase of ventricular excitability threshold by hyperpotassemia. *JAMA* 1965; 191:1049–1054.
24. Lake CL: *Cardiovascular Anesthesia.* New York, Springer-Verlag Publishers, 1985, pp 210, 359.
25. Lake CL, Sellers TD, Nolan SP, et al: Determinants of reperfusion cardiac electrical activity after cold cardioplegic arrest during coronary bypass surgery. *Am J Cardiol* 1984; 54:519–525.
26. Babbs CF, Whistler SJ, Yim GKW, et al: Dependence of defibrillation threshold upon extracellular/intracellular K+ concentrations. *J Electrocardiol* 1980; 13:73–78.
27. Lauler DP: A symposium: Potassium, catecholamines and beta blockade: Introduction. *Am J Cardiol* 1985; 56:1D–2D.

28. Regan TJ, Moschos CB, Lehan PH, et al: Lipid and carbohydrate metabolism of myocardium during the biphasic inotropic response to epinephrine. *Circ Res* 1966; 19:307–316.
29. Kleber AG: Extracellular potassium accumulation in acute myocardial ischemia. *J Mol Cell Cardiol* 1984; 16:389–394.
30. Nordrehaug JE: Malignant arrhythmia in relation to serum potassium in acute myocardial infarction. *Am J Cardiol* 1985; 56:20D–23D.
31. Donaldson RM, Nashat FS, Noble D, et al: Differential effects of ischaemia and hyperkalaemia on myocardial repolarization and conduction times in the dog. *J Physiol* 1984; 353:393–403.
32. Fisch C: Relation of electrolyte disturbance to cardiac arrhythmias. *Circulation* 1973; 47:408–419.
33. Tsutsumi T, Wyatt RF, Abildskov JA: Effects of hyperkalemia on local changes of repolarization duration in canine left ventricle. *J Electrocardiol* 1983; 16:1–6.
34. Przybojewski JZ, Knott-Craig CJ: Hyperkalemic complete heart block. *S Afr Med J* 1983; 63:413–420.
35. Pick A: Arrhythmias and potassium in man. *Am Heart J* 1966; 72:295–306.
36. Surawicz B, Chlebus H, Mazzoleni A: Hemodynamic and electrocardiographic effects of hyperpotassemia: Differences in response to slow and rapid increases in concentration of plasma K. *Am Heart J* 1967; 73:647–664.
37. Barker GL: Hyperkalemia presenting as ventilatory failure. *Anaesthesia* 1980; 35:885–886.
38. Levinsky NG: Management of emergencies: VI. Hyperkalemia. *N Engl J Med* 1966; 274:1076–1077.
39. Newmark SR, Dluhy RG: Hyperkalemia and hypokalemia. *JAMA* 1975; 231:631–633.
40. Makoff DL, DaSilva JA, Rosenblum BJ: On the mechanism of hyperkalemia due to hyperosmotic expansion with saline or mannitol. *Clin Sci* 1971; 41:383–393.

46

Preoperative Hypokalemia

A 60-year-old man with two-vessel coronary artery disease and unstable angina was scheduled to have coronary bypass surgery. He had mild hypertension and had been treated with furosemide (Lasix) for more than three months without potassium supplementation. His preoperative potassium level was 2.9 mEq/L, and because of the unstable angina urgent surgery was considered necessary.

Recommendations by K. C. Wong, M.D., Ph.D.

ANALYSIS OF THE PROBLEM

There are many controversies in clinical medicine. The management of the hypokalemic patient is one that especially impacts on the surgical team. There are sound explanations for the detrimental effects of hypokalemia on the electrophysiology of excitable cells[1] and of the heart,[2] and there are ample clinical reports to suggest that cardiac arrhythmias are made worse by alkalosis,[3, 4] digitalis[5] and myocardial infarction[6] in the presence of hypokalemia. Therefore, it has been traditionally taught that hypokalemia increases risk in the anesthetized patient and a minimal serum potassium level of 3.0 mEq/L without digitalis therapy and 3.5 mEq/L with digitalis therapy is required in the anesthetized patient. In spite of this time-honored recommendation, there is no good evidence to show that anesthetic dysrhythmias are increased in the hypokalemic patient.

APPROACH TO THE PROBLEM

The serum potassium level in this patient is borderline and the result of chronic potassium loss. With no ECG evidence of arrhythmia and urgent surgery requested, the case should be managed without acute potassium replacement (see discussion below).

DISCUSSION

This chapter reviews the electrophysiology of potassium in maintaining homeostasis, the clinical evidence for the concern of anesthetizing the hypokalemic patient, and the perioperative management of the hypokalemic patient who is to receive coronary artery bypass graft surgery.

Electrophysiology of Cardiac Cells and Endogenous Cations

There is increasing evidence to suggest that there is a close interaction of the cations of the body for maintaining homeostasis. Proper distribution of cations between the intracellular and extracellular space is essential for maintaining electrophysiologic function. Potassium is important for maintaining resting membrane potential and repolarization of excitable cells. Proper sodium concentration in the extracellular fluid is essential for depolarization and the production of action potentials of excitable cells. Calcium sets the threshold of excitation and is necessary for muscle contraction. Magnesium is vital for a variety of cellular functions and important for modulating the amount of active intracellular calcium concentration.

The distribution of ions across the cellular membrane is summarized in Table 46–1.[1] The primary extracellular ions are sodium and chloride, while the primary intracellular ions are potassium and anions that represent negatively-charged sites on intracellular proteins and metabolites. It is simplistic but useful to suggest that such an ionic distribution between the intracellular and extracellular sites may have evolved by the following process, ''Protein synthesis occurs intracellularly.'' Anionic sites contributed by protein and phosphate are attracted to cations to maintain electrical neutrality. Potassium, being approximately 200 times more mobile than sodium across the cellular membrane, is attracted into the intracellular compartment. Sodium remains largely in the extracellular compartment with chloride and bicarbonate contributing to the electrical neutrality in the extracellular space. The mobility of potassium ions and their transmembrane concentration gradient are primarily responsible for the resting membrane potential (RMP) of the ventricular cells and is mathematically described by the Nernst equation:

$$E = 60 \times \log (K_o/K_i)$$

where o = extracellular and i = intracellular. This RMP is approximately -90 mV in cardiac ventricular fibers and about -60 mV in cardiac sinoatrial

TABLE 46–1.

Ionic Concentrations and Potentials in Mammalian Muscle Cells and Interstitial Fluid*

	INTERSTITIAL FLUID	INTRACELLULAR FLUID	$E = \dfrac{[ion]_o}{[ion]_i}$	=	$60\left(\log\dfrac{[ion]_o}{[ion]_i}\right)(mV)$
Cations					
Na$^+$	145 μmole/mL	12 μmole/mL	12.1		65
K$^+$	4 μmole/mL	155 μmole/mL	1/39		$^-$95
H$^+$	3.8×10^5 μmole/mL	13×10^5 μmole/mL	1/3.4		$^-$32
[pH]	[7.43]	[6.9]			
Others	5 μmole/mL				
Anions					
Cl$^-$	120 μmole/mL	3.8 μmole/mL	31.8		$^-$90
HCO$_3^-$	27 μmole/mL	8 μmole/mL	3.4		$^-$32
Others	7 μmole/mL	155 μmole/mL			
Potential	0	$^-$90 mV	31.6		$^-$90

*Adapted from Woodbury JM: The cell membrane: Ionic and potential gradients and active transport, in Ruch TC, et al (eds): *Neurophysiology.* Philadelphia, WB Saunders Co, 1962, pp 2–30.
$^\dagger_o$ = extracellular; $_i$ = intracellular.

(SA) and atrioventricular (AV) nodal cells (Fig 46–1). In the SA and AV nodal cells, the RMP is a result of both calcium and potassium gradients.

Excitable cells can change their membrane potential by altering their permeability to certain ions. The SA and AV nodal cells slowly open more calcium channels and gradually close potassium channels. The resultant accumulation of intracellular calcium and potassium causes the RMP to drift toward 0 mV. In ventricular cells, changes in the potassium channels alone account for spontaneous depolarizations. The rate at which spontaneous depolarization occurs determines the "automaticity" of a cell (Fig 46–1).

When the RMP of a pacemaker cell reaches a critical value—threshold potential (TP)—calcium and sodium channels open. The influx of these ions causes a reversal of the resting membrane potential. Now the cytoplasm becomes more positively charged than the extracellular fluid. In ventricular cells this action potential (AP) or depolarization results from activating sodium channels alone; a ventricular AP rises instantaneously to +30 mV as compared with a sinus node with a slower rise to about +10 mV (Fig 46–1). The speed with which the AP rises determines "conduction." Local anesthetics and procainamide reduce the speed of this depolarization phase. The RMP can significantly influence the speed and magnitude of the AP. The closer the RMP is to TP, the fewer sodium channels will open and conduction will be slowed.

The AP stimulates the ventricular fibers to open their calcium channels for the first time. A slow sustained calcium influx causes the membrane potential to be held at a low positive voltage. This produces the "plateau phase" at

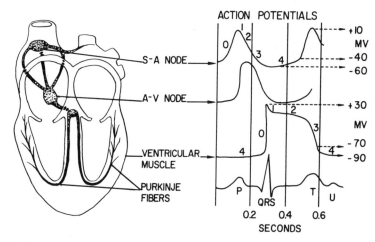

FIG 46-1.
Action potentials of the sinoatrial (SA) node, atrioventricular (AV) node, and ventricular muscle are displayed with respect to time, showing the descending order of importance as pacemakers of the heart. The ECG represents the combined effect of the action potentials.

The SA node shows spontaneous depolarization (phase 4) from calcium influx until the threshold potential (TP) is reached when calcium and sodium channels open to produce rapid depolarization (phase 0). The beginning of repolarization (phases 1 and 2) represent calcium and sodium influx through the "slow channel" with a concurrent influx of chloride. The repolarization phase 3 is completed by a rapid efflux of potassium. Calcium-channel blockers inhibit the influx of calcium into the cells; verapamil is effective to treat supraventricular tachyarrhythmias, while nifedipine is useful to treat myocardial ischemia.

Ventricular muscle maintains a more negative resting membrane potential (RMP) than the SA node and shows no spontaneous depolarization (phase 4). The rapid phase 0 depolarization is from activating sodium channels alone. Phases 1 and 2 are more prolonged in the ventricular muscle in which the calcium influx is also important for contractility. Phase 3 of the ventricular muscle is also generated by rapid potassium efflux.

which contraction begins and the heart beats. Repolarization is accomplished by opening potassium channels and losing positive charges to the extracellular fluid. Calcium is also actively extruded from the cell. In order to maintain electrochemical gradient of the principal cations, sodium is actively pumped out of and potassium into the cell. A diagrammatic representation of these events is depicted in Figure 46-2.

Both calcium and magnesium are important for determining cardiac excitability. Calcium binds negative sites in the channels for sodium and thus sets the level of threshold for excitation (i.e., the opening of the sodium gate). Hy-

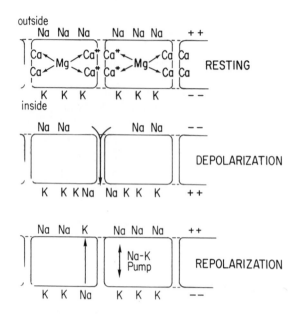

FIG 46–2.
A diagrammatic representation of the interaction of cations during membrane excitation. (1) Sodium (Na) is the primary extracellular cation and potassium (K) is the primary intracellular cation. (2) Calcium (Ca) plays an important role in setting the threshold of excitation by regulating the Na channels, while magnesium modulates the intracellular Ca concentration. (3) Depolarization is accomplished by a rapid influx of Na ions. (4) Repolarization is accomplished by a rapid efflux of K. The electrochemical gradient is maintained by the Na-K pump that pumps K into and Na out of the cell.

percalcemia elevates the threshold for maximal sodium permeability, while hypokalemia lowers the threshold. Magnesium can control calcium ion movements and distribution in several types of muscles, thus it also regulates calcium excitability. High extracellular concentrations of magnesium depress AV and intraventricular conduction, while hypomagnesemia can produce cardiac arrhythmias including ventricular fibrillation and sudden asystole. The physiologic antagonistic effect between calcium and magnesium is exemplified by the rational use of intravenous calcium to antagonize the neurodepressant effect of magnesium during unintentional overdose of magnesium sulfate.

In summary, the interrelationships of potassium, sodium, magnesium, and calcium have been briefly discussed. They are important in maintaining the normal electrophysiologic function of the excitable cell. Abnormalities in concentration gradient of potassium across cell membrane are frequently accompanied by abnormalities of magnesium and sodium concentration gradients.

Therefore, it is germane to focus on concurrent electrolyte abnormalities in addition to the concern of hypokalemia in the surgical patient.

Hypokalemia and Cardiac Arrhythmias

The cellular electrophysiologic data would suggest that hypokalemia should play a significant part in the genesis of cardiac arrhythmias. Hypokalemia has been shown to increase pacemaker discharge rates due to an increase in the slope of phase IV, diastolic depolarization, with a concurrent decrease in the threshold potential (Fig 46–1), thus favoring the emergence of potential pacemakers for the development of arrhythmias. Hypokalemia has also been shown to cause slowing of conduction and unidirectional block, thereby providing an electrophysiologic environment favoring reentrant cardiac arrhythmias. In the isolated rabbit heart preparation, severe hypokalemia of the perfusate has resulted in spontaneous ventricular fibrillation of the heart that can be reversed by the addition of potassium in the perfusate. Furthermore, laboratory studies have demonstrated a decrease in myocardial contractility in the chronically hypokalemic cat and dog.

There are ample clinical reports to suggest that cardiac arrhythmias are made worse by alkalosis, digitalis, and myocardial infarction in the presence of hypokalemia. Other clinical reports suggest that intravenous KCl is antiarrhythmic in hypokalemic patients whose ventricular arrhythmias are unresponsive to lidocaine treatment.[7] Many cardiovascular problems are intensified by hypokalemia, and potassium repletion in such patients tends to improve their ventricular arrhythmias[8] or cardiovascular functions.[9]

Based upon the physiologic and clinical evidence that suggest the correlation between hypokalemia and cardiac arrhythmias, I presented the first refresher course on this topic for the American Society of Anesthesiologists (ASA).[10] I also based the course on the influence of anecdotal experiences of clinicians around the country (e.g., those clinicians who have encountered malignant arrhythmias and difficult resuscitations in patients who from retrospective review of their clinical charts had untreated, chronic hypokalemia. Unfortunately, a critical review of published reports has not revealed any positive correlation between *anesthetic risk* or *increased incidence* of experimental or intraoperative arrhythmias with hypokalemia.

The only prospective study in anesthetized patients has failed to demonstrate an increase in intraoperative arrhythmias associated with chronic hypokalemia.[11] It is important to point out that the results were obtained from chronically asymptomatic, hypokalemic patients, and the results may not pertain to patients with acute potassium loss, patients receiving digitalis, or patients who have preoperative arrhythmias characteristic of hypokalemia. Nevertheless, the results seriously question the common practice of surgical postponement based upon serum potassium values alone and the wisdom of acute intravenous potassium administration. In the author's laboratory, threshold to epinephrine-induced arrhythmias has shown no difference between normokalemic and hypokalemic dogs anesthetized with halothane, enflurane, or methoxyflurane.[12] However, the hypokalemic animals were prone to ventricular tachycardia or ventricular fibrillation when the levels of epinephrine were elevated above the threshold. These results suggest that the hypokalemic animal may tolerate some encroachment upon its cardiovascular system but not severe physiologic trespass. Indeed, subsequent study from this laboratory has shown that chronically hypokalemic dogs are more difficult to resuscitate than normokalemic dogs after an asphyxial challenge.[13]

The controversy about how to manage the hypokalemic patient during diuretic therapy for hypertension also exists among our internal medicine colleagues. In two separate editorials, Harrington et al. "recommends that potassium salts or potassium-sparing diuretics should not be prescribed routinely for diuretic-treated hypertensive patients unless they are also receiving digitalis,"[14] while Kaplan believes that "there should be a universal concern about hypokalemia and hypokalemia should be appropriately corrected in most patients."[9] Underlying their differences is the belief that there is no good correlation per se between hypokalemia and cardiac arrhythmias.

Problems of Interpretation

Hypokalemia is a far more complex problem both physiologically and clinically than most people appreciate. Some of these factors are summarized below:

1. Hypokalemia is only measured clinically from a reduction in serum [K]. This value alone is not an adequate measure of total body [K] or distribution of [K] between the intracellular and extracellular compartments. Intracellular [K] is around 40 times greater than extracellular [K] (i.e., 155 mEq/L to 4 mEq/L).

2. Furthermore, the electrophysiology of excitable cells is dependent upon a complex relationship among the cations potassium, sodium, calcium, and magnesium. It is highly unlikely that changes in electrolyte concentrations involve only one ion. Disturbance of each cation is known to produce cardiovascular and ECG changes. The role of hypomagnesemia in digitalis toxicity and cardiac arrhythmias is becoming better appreciated.[15–17]

3. Potassium homeostasis is also regulated by a multitude of factors.[18] The generalization that alkalemia induces transmembrane shift of potassium ion into the cell and acidemia induces the opposite is valid during *acute* hypocapnia and hypercapnia, respectively.[19] However, chronic respiratory acid-base disturbance is accompanied by renal compensatory mechanisms resulting in

minimal disturbance of potassium ion balance between the intracellular and extracellular compartments. The effects of metabolic acid-base disturbance on serum potassium level are more variable. Lactic acidosis produces minimal change in serum [K] while hydrochloric acid infusion into dogs produces large increases in values of serum [K]. Metabolic alkalosis is associated with a marked kaliuresis without apparent effect on cellular [K]. Potassium homeostasis is also influenced by other factors such as hyperglycemia, insulin, mineralocorticoids, catecholamines, and osmolality of the plasma.

4. The most common cause of hypokalemia is induced by diuretic therapy for treating hypertension. Asymptomatic hypokalemic patients may represent a physiologically or chemically compensated population in contrast to the symptomatic hypokalemic patients. Obviously, it is inappropriate to compare these two populations based upon hypokalemia alone. Likewise, assessment of hypokalemic patients to be anesthetized for surgery should also include all the factors considered for the ASA status classification as well as the contemplated surgery.

5. Published data would imply that chronic potassium loss up to a point is reasonably well tolerated because of physiologic compensatory mechanisms and reestablishment of potassium concentration gradients between body compartments. A chronic hypokalemic level of just below 3 mEq/L may be tolerated, but below 2.5 mEq/L it is associated with cardiovascular collapse.[20-22] Acute loss of potassium from the body (presumably without adequate time for reestablishing proper equilibrium between compartments) may produce cardiovascular problems. Therefore, the *magnitude* and the *rate* of potassium loss are important considerations.

In summary, serum potassium level alone is not a reliable reflection of the extent of the hypokalemic problem in a patient. Inability to control the factors that can influence hypokalemia or other concurrent cardiovascular problems that can coexist in hypokalemic patients makes comparison of results among studies difficult and increases the possibility of arriving at conflicting conclusions.

Preoperative Evaluation

From the above discussion it can be seen that hypokalemia is an enormously complex problem that can contribute to cardiovascular instability. However, experience and published data have shown that hypokalemia alone should not be the cause of alarm in the anesthetized patient. In the patient with coronary ischemic disease and unstable angina, hypokalemia may indeed be an important contributing factor to cardiac arrhythmias. Assuming all of the usual preoperative evaluations such as cardiac catheterization, chest x-ray films, blood chemistry analysis, stress tolerance tests, ECG, echocardiogram, etc. are done before surgery, hypokalemia will add to the anesthetic problems of managing the patient with low ejection fraction, ventricular arrhythmias with multifocal ectopic pacemakers, ventricular akinesis, and cardiac failure.

Anesthetic management of this patient for coronary bypass graft should be aimed at the primary problems of cardiac ischemia and a discussion of these problems is found in other chapters of this book. The remarks here then will be aimed at the contribution of hypokalemia to the patient's cardiac problems. This is a chronic potassium loss from furosemide-induced kaliuresis. Therefore, the clinician would expect there is a proportional loss of potassium from the intracellular as well as the extracellular site. The generally accepted serum potassium value of 3.0 mEq/L required for a nondigitalized patient is reasonable because assuming a total body potassium content of around 4,000 mEq/L for a 70-kg patient, a 25% loss of potassium represents about 1,000 mEq/L. In general, such a chronic loss of potassium does not produce overt cardiac arrhythmias on the ECG except for a reduction in the amplitude of the T wave and sometimes the appearance of a U wave. Without the appearance of cardiac arrhythmias on the ECG, it would not be advisable to administer intravenous potassium as a means of normalizing the serum potassium level. Acute intravenous administration of potassium is not an effective means of replenishing potassium loss from the body because of rapid elimination by the kidneys. Cellular uptake of potassium can be promoted by the administration of glucose and insulin; however, I feel that that mode of treatment should be reserved only for more profound levels of hypokalemia or for patients who are showing cardiovascular instability and arrhythmias as symptoms of hypokalemia. The usual acceptable method of promoting potassium uptake by cells is to use up to 40 mEq/L of potassium in 10% dextrose with 25 units of regular insulin (0.5 units regular insulin per 2 gm dextrose).

Intravenous potassium administration is not innocuous. As many as 1 in 200 patients receiving potassium may suffer a morbid or fatal episode of hyperkalemia.[23] Therefore, the administration of intravenous potassium should always be accompanied by careful monitoring of the patient, by frequent checking of serum potassium level, and continuous monitoring of the ECG in the operating room. When insulin is used to facilitate cellular uptake of potassium, blood glucose values should also be monitored. Intravenous administration of potassium in other settings in the hospital must have adequate surveillance by the nursing staff.

Intraoperative Management

There are no absolute rules as to the type of general anesthetic that must be administered for the patient during coronary revascularization. Both inhalational anesthetics and a primary narcotic anesthetic have been used with equal effectiveness. More importantly, the amount of anesthetic and other intraoperative drugs administered are based upon principles of good management related to hemodynamic stability in the operating room. The major difference of a patient receiving coronary artery bypass grafting is that the principal problem of myocardial ischemia will be improved following the surgery. Under most circumstances hypertension rather than hypotension is the rule following cardiopulmonary bypass or during the immediate postoperative phase.

Hypothermia can induce a mild degree of hypokalemia. The mechanism of this reduction in level of serum potassium is not entirely clear but may be related to cold-induced renal excretion of potassium and cellular uptake of potassium from acute respiratory alkalosis.[24] In any event, it is not unusual to observe hypokalemia as the patient is removed from cardiopulmonary bypass and is gradually rewarmed. It is conceivable that this transient hypokalemia can add to a preexisting hypokalemia, thus producing cardiac instability. Many cardiac anesthesiologists routinely will add potassium chloride in the intravenous fluid during the postbypass period. However, we do not routinely administer potassium at this time unless the serum potassium level is less than 2.9 mEq/L and there is evidence of cardiovascular instability. The clinician should be reminded that a cardioplegic agent containing high concentrations of potassium is commonly used during cardiopulmonary bypass. The routine administration of potassium following cardiopulmonary bypass without actual measurement of the serum potassium level can lead to potassium overdose or cardiovascular collapse.

In summary, hypokalemia will contribute to preexisting cardiovascular problems with regard to cardiac arrhythmias and poor contractility. A slow infusion of potassium may exert an antiarrhythmic effect in a patient who is exhibiting cardiac arrhythmias associated with hypokalemia, but it is not expected to be an effective method of replenishing cellular loss of potassium. Repletion of cellular loss of potassium should be aided by the concurrent intravenous administration of glucose and insulin. The most safe and effective way to replenish potassium loss from the body is by oral administration for at least seven days in the elective surgical patient. Intravenous administration of potassium is not innocuous. An overdose can lead to conduction block, bradycardia, and even cardiovascular collapse.

Postoperative Management

Changes in serum potassium level during the postoperative phase in the intensive care unit are common. Metabolic alkalosis is not uncommon during the immediate postoperative period from the intraoperative administration of large volumes of Ringer's lactate solution, which undergoes metabolic biotransformation to bicarbonate. Since fluid overload is fairly common, furosemide is generally administered to promote diuresis and this could also bring about the loss of potassium from renal kaliuresis. Respiratory alkalosis from continued mechanical ventilatory support is also another source of reducing serum potassium. Nasogastric suction not only enhances metabolic alkalosis from the loss of hydrochloric acid but also from the loss of potassium. For the above reasons, it is important to check the concentration of serum electrolytes frequently and to administer potassium chloride in the intravenous fluid when there is a reduction in serum potassium level.

Summary

There are a large number of factors that can produce a reduction in level of serum potassium. Acute respiratory or metabolic alkalosis can cause a shift of potassium from the serum into the cell, thus producing hypokalemia without the loss of body potassium. A chronic loss of body potassium, most commonly from the use of diuretics, would generally produce a proportional loss of potassium from the intracellular and extracellular compartments. This chronic loss of potassium may allow time for a compensatory mechanisms of the body and, therefore, does not produce overt cardiac arrhythmias or cardiovascular problems. Nevertheless, laboratory evidence suggests that the chronic hypokalemic animal is less able to tolerate severe physiologic trespass. Present data would suggest that the acute loss of body potassium may be more harmful than the transmembrane shift of potassium or the chronic loss of potassium from the body. Hypokalemia is thus a complex problem that cannot be assessed by simply measuring the serum potassium value. The magnitude and the rate of potassium loss are important considerations. The usual limits of acceptable potassium levels for elective surgery (3.0 mEq/L for chronic hypokalemia and 3.5 mEq/L for hypokalemia with digitalis therapy) are useful but arbitrary generalizations. Other information must be utilized to modify these guidelines. Cardiac arrhythmias are common in patients with ischemic heart disease, especially with myocardial infarction associated with hypokalemia. Therefore, special attention must be paid to the serum potassium concentration, but the clinician should not lose sight of concurrent abnormalities in changes of other cation concentrations such as sodium and magnesium. Finally, the intravenous administration of potassium should always be monitored carefully to avoid an acute overdose.

REFERENCES

1. Woodbury JW: The cell membrane: Ionic and potential gradients and active transport, in Ruch TC, Patton HD, Woodbury JW, et al (eds): *Neurophysiology*. Philadelphia, WB Saunders, 1962, pp 2–30.

2. Prys-Roberts C: Electrophysiology: The origin of the heart beat, in Prys-Roberts C. (ed): *The Circulation in Anesthesia*. Boston, Blackwell Scientific Publications, 1980, pp 29–56.

3. Lawson NW, Butler GH, Rat CT: Alkalosis and cardiac arrhythmia. *Anesth Analg* 1973; 52:951–962.

4. Wright BD, DiGiovanni AJ: Respiratory alkalosis, hypokalemia and repeated ventricular fibrillation associated with mechanical ventilation. *Anesth Analg* 1969; 48:467–473.

5. Lown B, Black H, Moore FD: Digitalis, electrolytes and the surgical patient. *Am J Cardiol* 1960; 6:309–337.

6. Solomon RJ, Cole AG: Importance of potassium in patients with acute myocardial infarction. *Acta Med Scand* 1981; 647(suppl):87–93.

7. Katz RL: Bigger JT Jr: Cardiac arrhythmias during anesthesia and operation. *Anesthesiology* 1970; 33:193–208.

8. Holland OB, Nixon JV, Kuhnert L: Diuretic-induced ventricular ectopic activity. *Am J Med* 1981; 70:762–768.

9. Kaplan NM: Our appropriate concern about hypokalemia. *Am J Med* 1984; 77:1–4.

10. Wong KC: *Electrolyte disturbance and anesthetic considerations. ASA Refresher Course in Anesthesiology*. Philadelphia, JB Lippincott Co, 1978, vol 6, pp 187–198.

11. Vitez TS, Soper LE, Wong KC, et al: Chronic hypokalemia and intraoperative dysrhythmias. *Anesthesiology* 1985; 63:130–133.

12. Wong KC, Tseng CK, Puerto BA, et al: Chronic hypokalemia on epinephrine-induced dysrhythmias during halothane, enflurane or methoxyflurane with nitrous oxide anesthesia in dogs. *Anaesth Sinica* 1982; 21:139–146.

13. Wong KC, Port JD, Steffins J: Cardiovascular responses to asphyxial challenge in chronically hypokalemic dogs. *Anaesth Analg* 1983; 62:991–994.

14. Harrington JT, Isner JM, Kassirer JP: Our national obsession with potassium. *Am J Med* 1982; 73:155–159.

15. Seller RH, Cangiano J, Kim KE, et al: Digitalis toxicity and hypomagnesemia. *Am Heart J* 1970; 79:57–68.

16. Iseri LT, Chung P, Tobis J: Magnesium therapy for intractable ventricular tachyarrhythmias in normomagnesemic patients. *West J Med* 1983; 138:823–828.

17. Dycker T, Wester PO: Ventricular extrasystoles and intracellular electrolytes before and after potassium and magnesium infusions in patients on diuretic treatment. *Am Heart J* 1979; 97:12–18.

18. Cox M: Potassium homeostasis. *Med Clin North Am* 1981; 65:363–384.

19. Adrogue HJ, Madias NE: Changes in plasma potassium concentration during acute acid-base disturbances. *Am J Med* 1981; 71:456–466.

20. Simodynes E: Preoperative shock secondary to severe hypokalemia and hypocalcemia from recreational enemas. *Anesth Analg* 1981; 60:762–763.

21. Nardone D, McDonald, Cirard D: Mechanisms in hypokalemia. *Medicine* 1978; 57:435–446.

22. Albrecht PH: Cardiovascular effects of chronic potassium deficiency in the dog. *Am J Physiol* 1972; 222:555–560.

23. Kassirer JP, Harrington JT: Diuretics and potassium metabolism: A reassessment of the need, effectiveness and safety of potassium therapy. *Kidney Int* 1977; 11:505–515.

24. Wong KC: Physiology and pharmacology of hypothermia. *West J Med* 1983; 138:227–232.

47

Perioperative Clonidine Withdrawal Syndrome

A 55-year-old man with a 15-year history of hypertension and three-vessel coronary artery disease was scheduled for coronary bypass surgery. For the last six months the patient had been receiving clonidine 0.2 mg twice a day. His clonidine therapy was discontinued the morning of surgery. He had an uneventful induction and bypass period. Discontinuation of cardiopulmonary bypass was uneventful, but during chest closure, the blood pressure began to rise. At the termination of surgery, the blood pressure was 180/90 mm Hg, despite nitroprusside (10 μg/kg/minute) and nitroglycerine (10 μg/kg/minute).

Recommendations by Byron C. Bloor, Ph.D., Joan W. Flacke, M.D., and Werner E. Flacke, M.D.

ANALYSIS OF THE PROBLEM

In the United States, clonidine is not available in an intravenous form, which makes continuation of this medication often difficult in patients during the perioperative period. The clonidine withdrawal syndrome, a hyperadrenergic state, has been described as being similar to a pheochromocytoma crisis. Therefore, when it is necessary to discontinue clonidine, careful consideration must be given to the possibility of a life-threatening systemic hypertension.

APPROACH TO THE PROBLEM

Once the withdrawal syndrome has been diagnosed, as in the case above, and a further increase in the dose of nitroprusside could prove toxic, certain steps are essential. Monitoring of intra-arterial blood pressure, filling pressures, cardiac output, and systemic vascular resistance is recommended. The first consideration is the acute control of the blood pressure; secondarily, reestablishing the clonidine blood levels is vital, if it is at all possible.

Rapid control of blood pressure will not be accomplished by one predetermined regimen, and the course of action depends on the preoperative medications and the patient's status. Both α- and β-adrenergic components need to be treated; particular attention should be paid to balancing these effects. Hydralazine, which causes direct dilation of arteriolar vascular smooth muscle, can be added to the sodium nitroprusside to assist in counteracting the α-adrenergic vasoconstriction, thus unloading the heart. A β-adrenergic blocking agent should be given to block both cardiac and metabolic effects. If this combination is not successful then, lastly, an α-blocker should be added.

DISCUSSION

Background

Clonidine (Catapres) is a centrally acting antihypertensive agent. It has been suggested that clonidine modulates rather than blocks final efferent sympathetic vasomotor neurones, thereby allowing sympathetically mediated reflex control of blood pressure.[1] Although some peripheral effects are known, the predominant action is through stimulation of the central α_2-adrenergic receptors. Clonidine's effect can be thought of as being similar to activation of the baroreceptor reflex in such a way as to reflexively decrease blood pressure by a decrease of sympathetic and an increase in parasympathetic tone. The hemodynamic consequences of this central action are somewhat dependent on the level of preexisting sympathetic tone, but generally the consequences are manifested by a decreased heart rate, cardiac output, and systemic vascular resistance, leading to a "balanced" reduction in blood pressure. Blood flow to vital organs is maintained.[2] Clonidine is also an agonist at the peripheral presynaptic α_2-adrenergic receptors; this results in a decreased release from the nerve terminal of the sympathetic neurotransmitter, norepinephrine.

The Clonidine Withdrawal Syndrome

Mechanism

The actual physiologic basis of the clonidine withdrawal syndrome is not well understood. Considerable debate exists even as to whether blood pressure "rebounds" rapidly to untreated levels or "overshoots" on withdrawal to levels above those obtained before clonidine treatment. Increased variability (lability) of blood pressure has been a feature of clonidine withdrawal in humans and animals.[3] However, hypertensive patients are known to be hyperdynamic anyway, and perioperative stress provides additional opportunities for substantial blood pressure lability during and after surgery. The relative contribution of this stress, superimposed upon a hyperdynamic baseline, to the clonidine withdrawal syndrome is certainly difficult to determine.

The syndrome is marked by a massive rise in sympathetic tone. Large increases in both circulating and urinary catecholamine levels have been found.[4-6] Physiologic down-regulation of the central α_2-adrenergic receptors has been postulated[7] as the mechanism for this increased central sympathetic outflow. Plasma renin activity, on the other hand, is not increased.[6, 8]

Signs and Symptoms

Anxiety, nervousness, restlessness, tremors, agitation, palpitations, insomnia, severe headache, and nausea and vomiting have been reported, in addition to hypertension.[9] More serious sequelae, such as malignant hypertension with papilledema, accelerating angina, myocardial infarction, ventricular arrhythmias, left ventricular failure, and death, have on occasion been associated with this syndrome.[10]

Occurrence

The incidence and severity of the withdrawal syndrome increases with the dose and duration of clonidine treatment. Normally, the antihypertensive dose for clonidine ranges from 0.3 to 2.4 mg/day. When the last dose of clonidine had been given on the day before surgery,[11] rebound hypertension during surgery has been reported to occur after doses as low as 0.1 mg/day and should be *expected* to occur whenever the daily dose is greater than 1.2 mg. However, duration of therapy is also important. Withdrawal symptoms have not been seen in animal models after treatment for three days.[12] Hokfelt et al. have suggested that 6 to 30 days of clonidine treatment are required before a rebound phenomenon is seen in patients.[13] Several subsequent studies have confirmed that these withdrawal reactions are relatively common in unselected groups of patients who have been treated with higher doses (>0.9 mg/day) for longer periods (>three months). Rebound has been found also to occur more readily in those individuals with severe hypertension before the onset of clonidine treatment.[7] Concurrent therapy with other antihypertensive drugs, particularly nonselective β-adrenergic receptor antagonists, may exacerbate withdrawal symptoms. These may occur within 12 to 18 hours after the last dose of clonidine; withdrawal hypertension may last for up to 7 to 10 days.[14]

Antihypertensive treatment commonly requires a combination of two or more antihypertensive drugs. In these cases it is often impossible to ascribe withdrawal symptoms to a single agent. Other antihypertensives known to be associated with rebound phenomena include propranolol (and other β-adrenergic blockers), methyldopa, and guanfacine. When clonidine treatment is discontinued, as in the case above, the clinician must consider any other concomitantly administered drugs that may or may not have been discontinued. For example, stopping clonidine and continuing therapy with a β-blocker can be detrimental. With increased sympathetic tone and β-blockade of a less than healthy myocardium, the unopposed peripheral vascular α-effects (increased afterload) may push the heart into failure (see discussion below). A frequent offender in this regard is propranolol.

Perioperative Management of Rebound Hypertension

Limitations of Nitroprusside and Nitroglycerin

In the case report above, the patient is being given nitroprusside and nitroglycerin in an effort to bring down the blood pressure. Sodium nitroprusside is a directly acting vasodilator with its primary site of action being the resistance vessels. Thus, it lowers pressure and decreases afterload. Because of cyanide toxicity, the "safe" maximal dosage of nitroprusside in the human has been reported to be between 3.0 and 3.5 mg/kg,[15, 16] with a maximal infusion rate of 10 μg/kg/minute.[17] The patient is already receiving this amount and increasing the dose further cannot be recommended. Nitroglycerin is not immediately toxic; however, as this agent is primarily a venodilator with relatively little effect upon arterioles, increasing the dose would not be expected to produce any further beneficial lowering of blood pressure. The *addition* of a β-adrenergic blocker, such as propranolol, will potentiate the effects of the nitroprusside by blocking reflex β-adrenergic effects.[18] However, treatment with propranolol *alone* is not recommended for the reason mentioned above, and care must be taken not to discontinue the vasodilators (or decrease the amounts greatly) in the presence of this β-adrenergic antagonist.

Treatment Options

Proper treatment should begin by *not* discontinuing the clonidine therapy and, in fact, by making sure that it is given on the morning of surgery. Clonidine therapy should be continued if at all possible, with adherence to the patient's already instituted schedule and doses. Although including clonidine in the list of preanesthetic medications does prevent intraoperative hypertension associated with withdrawal, this alone does not preclude the same events occurring in the postoperative period. Unfortunately, as clonidine is not available in the United States in an intravenous form, certain surgical procedures will require interruption of therapy.

Attempts to wean the patient from clonidine by tapering of the dose in the days prior to operation is not recommended, as even a gradual reduction has been reported to result in withdrawal symptoms.[7] Substituting other antihypertensive medications while tapering clonidine can result in unwanted swings in arterial blood pressure. Drug combinations recommended elsewhere that include prazosin should not be used, as prazosin, like clonidine, is only available in oral form in this country.

Once clonidine therapy has been interrupted and withdrawal symptoms have begun, the most efficacious treatment is clonidine itself. In countries where parenteral forms (IV and IM) of this drug are available, hypertensive episodes have been shown to be controlled within five minutes after injection of additional clonidine.[11] Oral dosing in a nonsurgical setting was found to be effective within two hours. Even in an anesthetized patient, or in one who cannot take medications by mouth for other reasons, clonidine can be administered by nasogastric tube after crushing and mixing it with saline. We have been doing this routinely in patients undergoing coronary artery bypass surgery who have been on prior clonidine therapy, as well as in those in whom we anticipate substantial problems in intraoperative and postoperative blood pressure control. Absorption of clonidine, when given by this route, may vary, of course, according to the patient's condition, being affected by gastrointestinal function, visceral blood flow, hypothermia, and numerous other factors.

Clonidine has recently been approved for administration in a time release transdermal patch (Clonidine TTS). A minimum of two to three days after application is required to obtain adequate clonidine blood levels. Although little literature is available on this subject, it seems likely that a patient could be switched to the transdermal preparation several days prior to surgery and therapy maintained in this fashion throughout the operative period.

Concerning the special situation delineated in the case report above—that is, the patient who has just undergone coronary artery bypass graft surgery—it should be pointed out that a high percentage of these patients receive large doses of narcotics as part of their anesthetic regimen. In light of the known interaction between these agents and clonidine[19] and the known potential of increased adrenergic tone upon narcotic reversal,[20] it would certainly seem prudent to be certain that the patient is not being "withdrawn" from his opioids at the same time that he is experiencing clonidine rebound. Indeed, extra doses of narcotics would seem to be in order until his blood pressure is well under control.

Pharmacologic Options

Optimal treatment would be, as stated, rapid reestablishment of clonidine. Since this option is not open to us, treatment would include the use of both a specific α_1- and a β_1-adrenergic antagonist. However, prazosin is the only pure α_1-blocker available in this country, and it is not available in parenteral form.

The significant disadvantage of a nonselective α-blocking agent (such as phentolamine or tolazoline) in comparison to one that blocks only α_1-receptors, is that the former will block also the same α_2-receptors that are activated by the clonidine. Therefore, these agents may exacerbate the hypertensive episode by displacing any remaining clonidine from its receptors. In fact, adrenergic antagonists with α_2-activity have been shown experimentally to precipitate an acute clonidine withdrawal syndrome and therefore should be avoided.[3] Clonidine has been shown to reduce halothane[21] and narcotic[22] anesthetic requirement. This too is reversed by α_2-antagonist activity. Certainly when parenteral forms of selective α_1-blockers become available, they may well be the drugs of choice, in combination with a β-adrenergic blocking agent. The latter must be added to attenuate the increased myocardial oxygen consumption brought about by reflexively induced tachycardia, increased contractility, and cardiac output.

Just as the use of α-blockers alone must be avoided, so must that of β-blockers. Increased peripheral vascular tone mediated by unopposed α-adrenergic effects may precipitate failure in a marginally competent heart. In addition, nonselective β-adrenergic blockers, such as propranolol, may even increase peripheral vascular resistance. Therefore, a hypertensive crisis after rapid withdrawal of clonidine could be worsened in a patient treated solely with a nonselective β-adrenergic blocking drug. In fact, sotalol, a nonselective β-blocker, has been reported to antagonize clonidine[23]; thus, it should not be used in rebound. The use of a cardioselective β-blocker (β_1) (such as metoprolol) is a safer choice. Atenolol has also been used for this purpose.[7]

Labetalol has been suggested as an appropriate agent for treatment of hypertension associated with clonidine withdrawal. It is unique in that it exhibits both selective α_1- and nonselective β-blocking activity. These actions on adrenergic receptors are about one tenth as potent as phentolamine and one third as potent as propranolol (respectively). Oral doses of 800 to 1,200 mg of labetalol per patient have been used to prevent rebound from clonidine and seem to be effective in alleviating the hypertension.[24] Labetalol treatment did not prevent the subjective symptoms associated with withdrawal.

Hydralazine has been used as a substitute for clonidine.[25] However, as is the case with forced lowering of blood pressure by other direct vasodilators such as nitroprusside, hydralazine will activate baroreceptors. This leads to stimulation of both the α- and β-adrenergic sympathetic system, resulting in tachycardia and increased myocardial contractility, which causes increased oxygen demand as outlined above. Indeed, hydralazine is known to precipitate angina pectoris in patients with coronary artery disease.[26]

Methyldopa, another centrally acting antihypertensive drug that is in part similar to clonidine in its mechanism of action, is available in parenteral form, and, therefore, might seem to be a logical substitute for clonidine. However, in one report, a dose of 500 mg four times a day was given in substitution for clonidine and met with little success in prevention of the clonidine withdrawal syndrome.[6]

Summary

The "best treatment" for clonidine withdrawal is not to let it happen. Under many circumstances the clinician can avoid this crisis (Fig 47–1) with adequate patient preparation. Availability of the transdermal clonidine preparation should benefit situations in elective surgery in which adequate time is available to switch from oral medication to the dermal patch.

Clonidine withdrawal resembles a pheochromocytoma-like hypertensive crisis. Both α- and β-adrenergic components need to be considered. Although treatment may be influenced by the preoperative medications used, pressure reduction in the case presented can be achieved using hydralazine (a direct acting vasodilator) to counteract α-adrenergic vasoconstriction and a β-adrenergic antagonist to block cardiac and metabolic effects. Last, if required, α-adrenergic antagonists can be added. Beta-adrenergic blockade should not be used singly as it results in an unopposed α-adrenergic effect, which increases afterload and thus could push the heart into failure. Similarly, nonselective α-adrenergic antagonists should be used carefully, as they can aggravate the situation by antagonizing clonidine at the α_2 receptor site (see Fig 47–1).

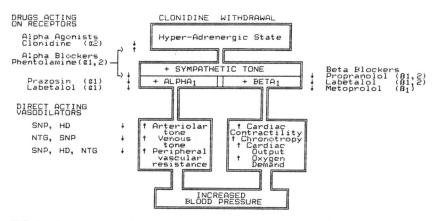

FIG 47–1.
Summary schematic of the important events occurring during clonidine withdrawal. Direct-acting vasodilators indicated are sodium nitroprusside (SNP), hydralazine (HD) and nitroglycerine (NTG). Arrows pointing down and up indicate a reduction and an increase in that event, respectively.

REFERENCES

1. Kobinger W: Central α-adrenergic systems as targets for hypotensive drugs. *Rev Physiol Biochem Pharmacol* 1978; 81:39–100.
2. Abrams WB: In summary: Satellite symposium on central α-adrenergic blood pressure regulating mechanisms. *Hypertension* 1984; 66(suppl II):1187–1193.
3. Thoolen MJ, Timmermans PB, van Zwieten PA: Withdrawal of antihypertensive treatment in rats. *Br J Clin Pharmacol* 1983; 15:491S.
4. Bruce DL, Croley TF, Lee JS: Preoperative clonidine withdrawal syndrome. *Anesthesiology* 1979; 51:90–92.
5. Geyskes GG, Dorhout-Mees EJ, Boer P: Clonidine withdrawal mechanism and frequency of rebound hypertension: A reply to the letters of Dr McMahon (1979) and Drs Whitsett & Chrysant (1979). *Br J Clin Pharmacol* 1979; 8:379–380.
6. Mate TP, Swerdlin AHR, Stone RA, Steinberg SM: Clonidine hydrochloride withdrawal complicating bilateral nephrectomy. *West J Med* 1979; 131:59–62.
7. Reid JL, Campbell BC, Hamilton CA: Withdrawal reactions following cessation of central α-adrenergic receptor agonists. *Hypertension* 1984; 6:1171–1175.
8. Geyskes CCV, Boer P, Darhout Mees EJ: Clonidine withdrawal: Mechanisms and frequency of rebound hypertension. *Br J Clin Pharmacol* 1979; 7:55–62.
9. Hökfelt B, Hedeland H, Dymling JF: Studies on catecholamines, renin and aldosterone following Catapressan (2-2,6-dichlor-phenyl-amine)-2-imidazoline hydrochloride) in hypertensive patients. *Eur J Pharmacol* 1970; 10:389–397.
10. Cummings DM, Vlasses PH: Antihypertensive drug withdrawal syndrome. *Drug Intell Clin Pharm* 1982; 16:817–822.
11. Stevens JE: Rebound hypertension during anaesthesia. *Anaesthesia* 1980; 35:490–491.
12. Barber ND, Reid JL: Studies on clonidine and guanfacine withdrawal after short-term treatment in the rat. *Arch Int Pharmacodyn Ther* 1982; 259:112–118.
13. Hökfelt B, Hedeland H, Dymling JF: Studies on catecholamines, renin and aldosterone following Catapressan (2-(2,6-dichlor-phenylamine)-2-imidazoline hydrochloride) in hypertensive patients. *Eur J Pharmacol* 1970; 10:389–397.
14. Reid JL: The Fourth Lilly Prize Lecture, University of Aberdeen, September 1980; The clinical pharmacology of clonidine and related central antihypertensive agents. *Br J Pharmacol* 1980; 12:295–302.
15. Merrifield AJ, Blundell MD: Toxicity of sodium nitroprusside. *Br J Anaesth* 1974; 46:324.
16. Davies DW, Kadar D, Steward DJ, et al: A sudden death associated with the use of sodium nitroprusside for induction of hypotension during anaesthesia. *Canad Anaesth Soc J* 1975; 22:547–552.
17. Greiss L, Tremblay NAG, Davies DW: The toxicity of sodium nitroprusside. *Canad Anaesth Soc J* 1976; 23:480–485.
18. Niarchos AP, Kritikou PE: Cardiovascular effects of sodium nitroprusside in hypertensive patients before and during acute β-adrenergic blockade. *J Clin Pharmacol* 1979; 19:31–38.

19. Gold MS, Redmond DE, Kleber HD: Clonidine in opiate withdrawal. *Lancet* 1978; 1:929–930.
20. Flacke JW, Flacke WE, Bloor BC, et al: Effects of fentanyl, naloxone, and clonidine on hemodynamics and plasma catecholamine levels in dogs. *Anesth Analg* 1983; 62:305–313.
21. Bloor BC, Flacke WE: Reduction in halothane anesthetic requirement by clonidine, an α-adrenergic agonist. *Anesth Analg* 1982; 61:741–745.
22. Ghignone M, Quintin L, Duke PC, et al: Effects of clonidine on narcotic requirement and hemodynamic response during laryngoscopy and intubation. *Anesthesiology* 1984; 61:A38.
23. Saarimaa H: Combination of clonidine and sotalol in hypertension. *Br Med J* 1976; 1:810.
24. Rosenthal T, Rabinowitz B, Boichis H, et al: Use of labetalol in hypertensive patients during discontinuation of clonidine therapy. *Eur J Clin Pharmacol* 1981; 20:237–240.
25. Kushins L: Clonidine withdrawal, propranolol, and rebound hypertension. *Anesthesiology* 1980; 53:178–179.
26. Moyer JH: Hydralazine (Apresoline) hydrochloride: Pharmacological observations and clinical results in the therapy of hypertension. *Arch Intern Med* 1953; 91:419–439.

48

Protein Binding Changes

A 56-year-old man with severe three-vessel coronary artery disease was scheduled to have coronary artery surgery. He was treated medically with nitroglycerin and propranolol and was anesthetized with diazepam and fentanyl. During surgery after administration of heparin 4 mg/kg, the heart rate (HR) decreased from 55 to 45 beats per minute and the blood pressure (BP) from 100/60 to 90/50 mm Hg.

Recommendations by Robert A. Kates, M.D.

ANALYSIS OF THE PROBLEM

Analyzing intraoperative hemodynamic instability requires a knowledge of the pathophysiology of the patient, the pharmacology of the drugs administered prior to and during surgery, and the effects of surgical stimulation. For this case discussion we will assume that the reduction in heart rate and blood pressure was not due to underlying pathophysiology or to a decrease in the level of surgical stimulation, but resulted from heparin administration.

Several animal investigations have demonstrated that heparin can cause peripheral arterial vasodilation.[1, 2] The mechanism of action remains controversial, probably because of heparin's complex pharmacologic effects as well as the heterogenicity of substances, including histamine precursors present in commercial heparin solutions.[3] Two clinical reports have indicated that heparinization for cardiopulmonary bypass is associated with a mild decrease in peripheral vascular tone; however, in these reports heart rate remained constant while blood pressure decreased.[4, 5] Since heparin has not been shown to produce a negative chronotropic effect, this case, which demonstrates a decrease in heart rate as well as blood pressure, suggests a possible drug interaction between heparin and propranolol. Heparin decreases plasma protein binding of many drugs, including propranolol, resulting in greater plasma levels of the unbound, or biologically active form of these drugs.[6-8] Increased plasma levels of unbound propranolol provide more available drug for diffusion from plasma into tissues, where it can interact with β-adrenergic receptor sites. The resultant increase in β-adrenergic blockade could have decreased heart rate and blood pressure in this case.

APPROACH TO THE PROBLEM

Assuming that the progressive bradycardia experienced by this patient is due to increased plasma levels of unbound propranolol, the pharmacodynamic effect would be identical to that achieved by intravenous administration of additional propranolol. Treatment is required only if increased β-adrenergic blockade produces hemodynamic instability by decreasing heart rate or myocardial pump function. Sinus bradycardia can be therapeutic in patients with ischemic heart disease and presents a problem only if it results in inadequate blood pressure or dangerous ectopic arrhythmia foci. In this patient with severe coronary artery disease, treatment is especially warranted if the reduction in blood pressure produces myocardial ischemia. If cardiopulmonary bypass is to be instituted at this time, the perfusion could be regulated by extracorporeal circulation. If atrial pacing were readily available, this could be used to control heart rate. Atropine sulfate will increase heart rate by decreasing parasympathetic input into the sinoatrial node, but small incremental doses should be administered to avoid tachycardia. Alternatively, coronary perfusion pressure can be restored with phenylephrine; the bradycardia would remain but should not be a problem in patients with normal left ventricular function. If heart failure develops due to the myocardial depressant effects of increased β-adrenergic blockade, cardiopulmonary bypass could be instituted or a direct inotropic drug (calcium chloride 250 mg IV) or β-adrenergic agonist drug (ephedrine 5 to 10 mg IV, epinephrine 5 to 10 μg IV) can be administered. The increase in unbound propranolol levels should be considered to be a temporary problem, however, since unbound drug will redistribute out of the plasma into a large peripheral compartment and plasma concentrations of the unbound drug will be reestablished relatively quickly to preheparin levels. The distribution half-life of propranolol is five to ten minutes, indicating a rapid equilibrium between plasma and tissues, and the apparent volume of distribution is 4 L/kg, indicating a large compartment into which unbound propranolol is diluted.[9]

DISCUSSION

The hemodynamic effects of propranolol are achieved by an interaction between the unbound (active) drug and the β-adrenergic receptor sites in the peripheral (tissue) compartment (Fig 48–1). Drugs such as propranolol, which are reversibly bound to receptor sites, are in continuous equilibrium between drug concentrations in the tissues and unbound drug in the central (plasma) compartment. Equilibrium is also achieved in the plasma compartment between unbound and protein bound propranolol. In the plasma, propranolol is extensively bound to albumin and glycoproteins; however, only the unbound form can diffuse through capillary membranes to reach the site of action. Since plasma protein binding of propranolol is readily reversible, the bound drug (which accounts for 90% of total drug in the plasma) acts as a large reservoir, continu-

a) BEFORE HEPARIN

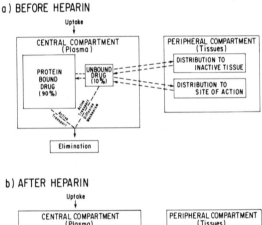

b) AFTER HEPARIN

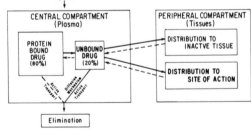

FIG 48–1.
Schematic representation of distribution and elimination of propranolol before *(a)* and after *(b)* heparin administration. Heparin reduces propranolol binding, which results in more available propranolol for diffusion to receptor sites in the peripheral (tissue) compartment.

ously releasing more drug as the unbound (active) drug is metabolized and eliminated. An acute decrease in the binding capacity of plasma proteins for propranolol will result in more drug available for diffusion into the tissue and a greater pharmacodynamic effect. Decreasing the percent protein binding of propranolol from 92% to 84% will effectively double the amount of unbound (active) drug in the plasma, producing a hemodynamic effect similar to an intravenous bolus of propranolol.

The drug-binding capacity of plasma proteins can be affected by physical conditions of the plasma (pH and temperature), competition between different drugs for common binding sites, changes in plasma levels of free fatty acids, hypoalbuminemia, and certain disease states. [10, 11] Heparin decreases plasma protein binding of propranolol because of its effect on plasma concentrations of free fatty acids. Free (nonesterified) fatty acid plasma levels increase due to a heparin-induced augmentation in lipoprotein lipase activity in the blood. [12] Palmitate and oleate, the major free fatty acids in plasma, produce a decrease in the number of available protein binding sites as well as the drug affinity of the protein binding sites. [13]

Heparinization and cardiopulmonary bypass have been shown to produce a threefold increase in free fatty acid levels as well as double the unbound fraction of propranolol (Fig 48–2). [7] Protamine administration, to neutralize the heparin after cardiopulmonary bypass, decreases both the unbound fraction of propranolol and the free fatty acid levels. [7] The decrease in plasma protein binding of propranolol was found to be predominantly due to the heparin-induced increase in free fatty acids and was also accentuated by hemodilution from the cardiopulmonary-bypass pump prime. We also investigated the effect of heparinization on the unbound fraction of propranolol as well as verapamil. [8] In vitro plasma protein binding was tested before anesthetic induction, at surgical skin incision, after heparinization (400 Iu/kg) but before cardiopulmonary bypass, and during cardiopulmonary bypass. The unbound fraction of propranolol and verapamil remained stable prior to heparinization, but increased after heparinization, and further increased during cardiopulmonary bypass. This study demonstrated that heparinization increases the unbound fraction of propranolol before cardiopulmonary bypass, exactly what might have happened to the patient in this case report. Controversy has existed concerning a possible in vitro effect of heparin (in the test tubes) on plasma protein binding that would have artifactually altered the results of these heparin-protein binding interaction studies. We recently evaluated this by adding heparin to aliquots of blood sampled from patients who had not received systemic heparin administration. Our preliminary results (unpublished data; Kates, Bai, 1985) indicated that in vitro heparin (0 to 100 IU/ml) does not affect plasma binding of propranolol or phenytoin. [8] These data [6–8] indicate that intravenous

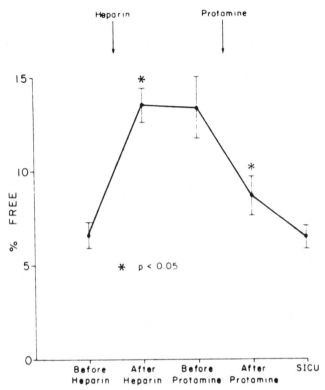

FIG 48–2.
Free (unbound) fractions (per cent) of propranolol (± SEM), before, during, and after cardiopulmonary bypass. Comparisons are with immediately preceding values. (From Wood M, Shand DG, Wood AJJ: Propranolol Binding in Plasma during Cardiopulmonary Bypass. *Anesthesiology* 1979; 51:512–516. Used by permission.)

heparin administration increases the unbound fraction of propranolol and provides a possible pharmacologic mechanism for the decreases in heart rate and blood pressure following heparin administration in this case report.

The heparin-induced decrease in plasma protein binding capacity can also theoretically affect depth of anesthesia. The intravenous anesthetics (diazepam, fentanyl, and sufentanil) are highly protein bound (99%, 85%, and 93%, respectively). Even a 1% decrease in the plasma binding capacity for diazepam after heparinization would effectively double the unbound (active) diazepam concentration, thereby increasing anesthetic depth. This certainly could have decreased heart rate and blood pressure in this patient.

Finally, the effect of heparin on plasma protein binding should be considered when highly protein bound cardiovascular drugs (i.e., propranolol, verapamil, nifedipine, diltiazem, diazoxide) are administered intravenously. A reduced plasma protein binding capacity can substantially increase the intensity of hemodynamic effect when these drugs are administered to heparinized patients. Therefore, cautious incremental dosing to desired effect may be especially important in heparinized patients.

Summary

This case report demonstrates the cardiovascular consequences of heparin-induced changes in plasma protein binding properties and underscores the potential importance of complex pharmacokinetic interactions in patients receiving multiple drugs for cardiac surgery.

REFERENCES

1. Abraham DG, Howarth S: A peripheral action of heparin. *Br Heart J* 1950; 12:429.
2. Gabor M, Antal A, Dirner Z: Effect of anticoagulants on the capillary resistance of internal organs of rats. *J Pharm Pharmacol* 1967, 19:488.
3. Lasker SE: The heterogeneity of heparins. *Fed Proc* 1977; 36:92–97.
4. Seltzer JL, Gerson JI: Decrease in arterial pressure following heparin injection prior to cardiopulmonary bypass. *Acta Anaesthesiol Scand* 1979; 23:575–578.
5. Konchigeri HN: Hemodynamic effects of heparin in patients undergoing cardiac surgery. *Anesth Analg* 1984; 63:175–284.
6. Wood M, Shand DG, Wood AJJ: Altered drug binding due to the use of indwelling heparinized cannulas (heparin lock) for sampling. *Clin Pharmacol Ther* 1979; 25:103–107.
7. Wood M, Shand DG, Wood AJJ: Propranolol binding in plasma during cardiopulmonary bypass. *Anesthesiology* 1979; 51:512–516.
8. Kates RA, Bai SA, Reves JG, et al: Anesthetic and operative effect on plasma protein binding of propranolol and verapamil during cardiac surgery. *Anesthesiology* 1985; 63:A21.
9. Regardh CG: Pharmacokinetics of β-adrenoceptor antagonists, in Poppers, van Dijk, van Elzakker (eds): β-*Blockade and Anaesthesia*. Conference in The Hague, 1979, pp 29–45.
10. Koch-Weser J, Sellers EM: Drug therapy: I. Binding of drugs to serum albumin. *N Engl J Med* 1976; 294:311–315.
11. Koch-Weser J, Sellers EM: Drug therapy: II. Binding of drugs to serum albumin. *N Engl J Med* 1976; 294(10):526–531.
12. Fraser JRE, Lovell RRH, Nestel PJ: The production of lipolytic activity in the human forearm in response to heparin. *Clin Sci* 1961; 20:351–356.
13. Vallner JJ: Binding of drugs by albumin and plasma protein. *J Pharm Sci* 1977; 66:447–464.

49

Calcium Entry Blocker and Hypotension

A 58-year-old man with stable angina pectoris was treated medically with propranolol 80 mg/day and nifedipine 60 mg/day. Both drugs were given the morning of surgery. Induction of anesthesia was accomplished with sufentanil 15 μg/kg and was followed by a decrease in blood pressure from 120/80 to 80/50 mm Hg, while cardiac index remained at 2.2 L/min/m^2. There was subsequent hypotension to 80/50 mm Hg during discontinuation of cardiopulmonary bypass, despite a cardiac index of 2.3 L/min/m^2.

Recommendations by Edward A. Norfleet, M.D.

ANALYSIS OF THE PROBLEM

Preservation of myocardial function and prevention of myocardial ischemia are primary goals in the anesthetic management of patients with coronary artery disease. This particular patient, treated with both a β-antagonist and a calcium-channel blocker, developed hypotension at different times during the course of anesthesia. The etiology of this hypotension is complex and is related to drug-induced interactions that affect the heart, the peripheral vasculature, and neurogenic control mechanisms. Our primary concern in this patient is the potential for the reduction in coronary perfusion pressure to precipitate progressive regional myocardial ischemia and the spiraling cascade of events that may ultimately lead to cardiovascular collapse.

APPROACH TO THE PROBLEM

Hypotension During Induction

Therapy is designed to immediately restore perfusion pressure. The intravascular volume should be increased by administration of an electrolyte solution. Decreased systemic resistance should be treated by the bolus or constant infusion of phenylephrine (see discussion below). Nitroglycerin infusion should be used if ischemia develops or if filling pressures become too high after volume replacement and phenylephrine therapy.

Hypotension at End of Cardiopulmonary Bypass

Therapy here is designed to maintain cardiac output and perfusion (systemic) pressure. Optimal volume should be attained (filling pressures) either by decreasing filling (phlebotomy via the atrial cannula) or increasing filling (transfusing from the pump). Rhythm should be optimized by pacing, if required, and pharmacologic agents should be given to increase both systemic vascular resistance (SVR) and the inotropic state of the heart (see discussion). Calcium chloride and/or epinephrine or dopamine infusions are useful in this situation.

DISCUSSION

The appropriate treatment in this case requires a clear understanding of the underlying cardiovascular pathophysiology integrated with an efficient application of appropriate therapeutic interventions. An analysis of the specific and combined cardiovascular effects of propranolol, nifedipine, and sufentanil will provide insight to allow expedient management of the hypotensive episodes that this patient develops.

Pharmacodynamics

Homeostatic regulation and control of blood pressure is critically dependent on those factors that control cardiac output and systemic vascular resistance. Under normal circumstances, hypotension induced by a decrease in systemic vascular resistance will be compensated for by an increase in cardiac output, whereas hypotension resulting from a decrease in cardiac output will be compensated for by increases in vascular resistance. These cardiovascular responses are mediated by reflex autonomic mechanisms that activate the sympathetic nervous system and α- and β-receptors located on selected target organs. Excitation of the β_1-adrenergic receptors of the heart produces dynamic increases in heart rate and myocardial contractility. Such β-adrenergic responses are mediated by activation of the intracellular enzyme adenylate cyclase. Interestingly, β-stimulation and subsequent adenylate cyclase activation interact to modulate the gating mechanisms of the Ca^{++} channel in myocardial cells. The influx of extracellular Ca^{++} into sensitive cells stimulates the rate and intensity of cellular processes such as depolarization and contractile activity. Thus, β-blockade and calcium-channel blockade together produce synergistic depressant actions on cellular membrane activities that regulate metabolism and function.

Combination therapy with nitrates, β-antagonists, and most recently the calcium-channel blockers have greatly improved the management of ischemic heart disease.[1] Combinations of propranolol and nifedipine have been shown to be more therapeutically effective than either drug by itself.[2, 3] Drug-induced improvement in myocardial oxygen balance occurs as oxygen demand is reduced and oxygen supply is increased. However, combination therapy has been reported to be associated with occasional serious cardiovascular side effects such as hypotension and cardiac failure.[4] Therefore, such drug combinations should be used with caution, particularly in patients with poor ventricular function.

Propranolol, in a dose-related manner, blocks both the β_1- and β_2-receptors. This action effectively diminishes the increases in heart rate and contractility that follow β-stimulation and the vasodilation that is associated with stimulation of β_2-receptors. Propranolol has an elimination half-life of two to three hours.[5] The important interactions of β-blockade with specific anesthetic drugs have been previously reviewed.[5, 6] After two decades of experience with patients undergoing anesthesia who have received β-blockers, there is agreement that adverse anesthetic interactions can be avoided if the clinician understands the potential for side effects. Continuing therapy with β-blockers preoperatively can provide beneficial effects during the stresses imposed by both anesthesia and surgery,[6] while abruptly discontinuing propranolol may induce an acute hypersensitivity to catecholamines, resulting in serious cardiovascular complications associated with a "propranolol-withdrawal syndrome."[7]

The implications of the interactions of calcium-channel blockade with anesthetic management have also been recently reviewed.[8-11] Nifedipine is a very potent coronary and systemic vasodilator that produces its effect by selective dilation of the arterioles (resistance vessels) with minimal effect on the veins (capacitance vessels).[12] Clinically, there is usually little myocardial depression and cardiac output may even improve following the drug-induced decrease in vascular resistance. In patients receiving nifedipine who have also received β-blockers, heart rate and cardiac output usually do not change. Nifedipine has an elimination half-life of five hours.[9] The mechanisms by which calcium-channel blockers such as nifedipine dilate vascular beds is not entirely clear. However, this is an exciting area of investigation that is providing new information that may clarify the therapeutic effects of the calcium-channel blockers.[13] Recent evidence in both animals and man suggests that distinct functionally active subgroups of cellularly located α-adrenergic receptors (α_1 and α_2) may induce vasoconstriction of vascular smooth muscle by different cellular mechanisms (Fig 49–1).[14–16] The α_1-receptors are most readily activated by synaptic release of norepinephrine from sympathetic nerve terminals. Depolarization of the smooth muscle cell membrane via α_1-receptors permits extracellular Ca^{++} to externally "trigger" the release of internal Ca^{++} stores that ultimately produces vasoconstriction. The α_1-receptors are not blocked by the calcium-channel blockers. The α_2-receptors, however, are located on smooth muscle cells on extrajunctional membrane sites and may be preferentially activated by endogenous catecholamines. These receptors differ from α_1 in that activation of the α_2-receptor induces vasoconstriction that is dependent entirely on the influx of extracellular Ca^{++} (see Fig 49–1). Importantly the

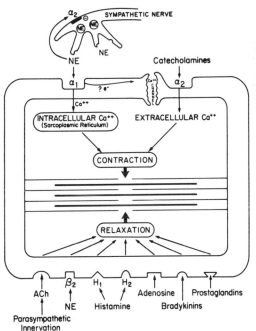

FIG 49–1.
Neurohormonal mechanisms for regulation of vasomotor vascular tone. The α_1-receptors may influence the voltage gate (e-) of the calcium channels associated with the α_2-receptor. *NE*-norepinephrine, *ACH*-acetylcholine (see text for further explanation).

α_2-receptors of vascular smooth muscle can be selectively blocked by calcium-channel blockers such as nifedipine. The α-agonists such as phenylephrine and epinephrine can activate both α_1- and α_2-receptors. These concepts are summarized and illustrated in Figure 49–1. Also, illustrated are those neurohumoral substances that influence smooth muscle cell relaxation and thus oppose α-adrenergic vascular tone. To avoid confusion, it is important to recall that "α_2-receptors" are also located presynaptically, where they decrease the amount of norepinephrine released per nerve impulse. The specific mechanisms by which extracellular calcium entry and depolarization-induced calcium entry affect different α-receptors is still not entirely clear.

Differences in the physiology of α_1- and α_2-adrenergic receptors on vascular smooth muscle may have important clinical implications in our particular patient. It is interesting that although our patient had been treated with nifedipine, the systemic resistance was increased prior to the induction of anesthesia. This suggests increased compensatory α-adrenergic input to the vascular beds, which has not been completely blocked by nifedipine. Such a response may be centrally mediated in an effort to maintain blood pressure in spite of depressed cardiac function (β-blockade) and calcium-channel blockade of the α_2-receptor. This will be important to remember as we review the mechanisms by which narcotic anesthesia induces hypotension.

Sufentanil is a very potent opioid analgesic, which does not depress myocardial contractility. A dose-related decrease in endogenous norepinephrine release is produced with increasing dosages (8 μg to 30 μg/Kg). In general, following induction of anesthesia with sufentanil, cardiovascular stability is usually maintained with only slight decreases in systemic vascular resistance.[17] However, in initial clinical trials, hypotension occurred in 7% of patients.[18] From our experience and from other clinical reports, hypotension with narcotic anesthesia appears to be more common in those patients who are being treated with β-antagonists and Ca^{++}-channel blocking drugs, particularly nifedipine.[19, 20] Such episodes may occur at any time during anesthesia, usually during the induction period prior to surgical stimulation. Hypotension is characteristically associated with a decrease in systemic vascular resistance and little change in heart rate and cardiac index, while ventricular filling pressures may remain stable or significantly decrease.[21] Recently, myocardial blood flow and metabolism have been studied in patients with coronary artery disease who were anesthetized with 10, 20, and 30 μg/Kg of sufentanil.[22] These patients had β- and calcium-channel blocking drugs continued up until the morning of surgery. During the induction of anesthesia, significant reductions in mean arterial pressure occurred at all dosages. In the majority of patients, such reductions in blood pressure were balanced by decreases in myocardial oxygen demand and no evidence of ischemia was found. However, in 10% of these patients (2 of 20), the decrease in perfusion pressure was associated with an increased release of myocardial lactate. Although ischemic biochemical changes did occur, no changes were seen in the electrocardiogram. Such information substantiates our concerns as clinicians whenever significant decreases in blood pressure occur in patients with severely stenotic coronary arteries. Prediction of which patients will develop ischemia is impossible with current monitoring methodology. Therefore, the importance of carefully treating such hypotensive episodes cannot be overemphasized.

Preinduction: Preventative Measures

The proper selection of anesthetic techniques begins with a detailed assessment of the patient's history, physical examination, catheterization data and current drug therapy. The status of cardiovascular changes induced by medical drug therapy and disease must be carefully evaluated and considered when selecting and administering either depressant or nondepressant anesthetics. Preoperatively, medical therapy with β- and calcium-channel blockers should be adjusted to the symptomatology of a particular patient and continued as part of anesthetic preoperative medication.

Successful management of adverse cardiovascular events will depend on certain important preparations prior to the induction of anesthesia. This should include establishment of intravenous access, the application of monitoring devices, and the ready availability of a wide assortment of emergency drugs. A complete hemodynamic profile including cardiac index and calculation of vascular resistance is performed and recorded prior to the induction of anesthesia. This is the most important and relevant cardiovascular information we can obtain. We can then make necessary adjustments of heart rate, preload, afterload, and contractility just prior to and during the anesthetic induction. Interpretation of such information must be integrated to determine what is "normal" for a particular patient.

To recapitulate, our patient has an arterial blood pressure of 120/80 mm Hg, a cardiac index of 2.2 L/min/m^2 and an elevated systemic vascular resistance (1,500 dyne/second/cm^{-5}). These values are typical of patients who are being treated with both a β-antagonist and a calcium-channel blocker. The cardiac index is low, but, by itself, it does not reflect inadequate ventricular function. In such patients, the ventricular filling pressures are usually low or normal. There is no indication that such a cardiac index is not providing adequate oxygen supply to meet the total body metabolic oxygen demands. We have measured the mixed venous oxygen saturation in many such patients and found it to be normal. In fact, following the induction of anesthesia with narcotics, cardiac index does not change or may even decrease as metabolic oxygen demand is even further reduced. This low cardiac index is an indication that our combined medical therapy with propranolol, nifedipine and our other preoperative sedating medications has been successful in depressing both myocardial and total body oxygen demands. Thus, any attempts to increase this index with inotropic drugs prior to the induction of anesthesia are not indicated. The heart is at rest and the patient is fine!

However, the low cardiac index may be associated with a compensatory increase in systemic vascular resistance. Theoretically, although certain vascular receptors (α_2) are preferentially blocked by nifedipine, compensatory sympathetic input to other receptors (α_1) are actively maintaining vascular tone and blood pressure. Therefore, we can anticipate beforehand that any intervention that suddenly depresses efferent sympathetic nervous system influence on vascular tone will likely result in a decrease of blood pressure since all other cardiac and vascular adrenergic compensatory mechanisms will then be effectively blocked. Thus, an increase in systemic vascular resistance will be an important clue to warn the clinician of the potential for narcotic or inhalational anesthesia to induce hypotension.

Hypotension associated with β- and calcium blockade is more likely to occur during the induction of anesthesia, particularly if the patient is volume depleted. Therefore, several preventive measures are essential. In anticipation of the vasodilation associated with narcotic induction, it is useful to carefully preload such patients with 500 to 1,500 cc of lactated Ringer's solution if filling pressures are low. One recent clinical report compared the cardiovascular effect of fentanyl and sufentanil (10 μg/kg) during the induction of anesthesia and found that "without volume loading during the preanesthetic period, sufentanil plus pancuronium produced hypotension associated with a decrease in both pulmonary capillary wedge pressure and systemic vascular resistance."[21] The degree of volume loading required will certainly vary tremendously with each individual patient's ventricular function curve; however, filling pressures of at least 10 to 15 mm Hg should suffice. This preventive measure is most important when the central venous and wedge pressures are initially low, indicating that the patient may be relatively hypovolemic. Although the patient is β- and calcium-channel blocked, such loading may improve the cardiac index via the Frank-Starling mechanism. At the same time volume overloading can be extremely hazardous, as increases in ventricular wall tension from overdistention may induce myocardial ischemia since both myocardial oxygen demand is increased and subendocardial myocardial blood flow is reduced.

The patient is then preoxygenated, and sufentanil is titrated to produce unconsciousness. Very rapid and large quantities of sufentanil initially are more likely to induce hypotension. Therefore, induction should be a controlled and smooth titration of drug effect with the patient's neurologic and cardiovascular response. As we begin to control ventilation, it is also important to remember that the many adverse physiologic effects of positive pressure ventilation and hyperventilation can further decrease preload, particularly in older patients with emphysematous lungs. As cautious as we are during the induction of anesthesia, hypotension may still occur.

Treatment of Drug-Induced Hypotensive Episodes

A complex drug-induced, cardiovascular interaction between propranolol, nifedipine, and sufentanil has resulted in acute hypotension. A simplified mechanism for the development of hypotension during induction of anesthesia is illustrated in Fig 49–2. To summarize, sufentanil anesthesia induces centrally mediated sympathetic depression and a decrease in endogenous catecholamine release. Those α-adrenergic receptors that remain activated and that were maintaining vascular tone are suddenly inactivated as catecholamine release is diminished. The inhibition of such autonomic input results in vasodilation and a decrease in systemic vascular resistance. Since compensatory cardiac reflexes are blocked with propranolol, cardiac index does not change and blood pressure falls. Treatment is important, since systemic perfusion pressure is reduced, and both cerebral perfusion and myocardial blood flow to areas affected by disease are likely to be severely impaired. If not promptly corrected, progressive myocardial ischemia may develop and blood pressure will deteriorate further.

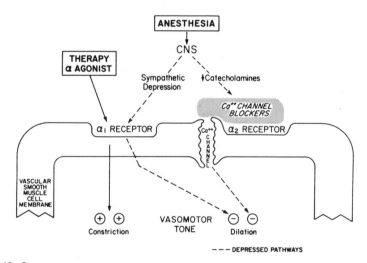

FIG 49–2.
Postulated mechanisms by which narcotic anesthesia and calcium-channel blockers interact to induce reductions in vasomotor tone. Anesthetic-induced sympathetic depression of vasomotor tone can be reversed by therapy with α-agonists.

Therapeutic intervention may be directed at either volume administration, readjusting vasomotor tone, improving cardiac index, or a combination approach. Numerous therapeutic options for restoration of blood pressure are available to the clinician and many factors will influence our philosophy of management. The first episode of hypotension is acute and occurs during the critical period of anesthetic induction. At this time and given the cardiovascular changes, my preference is to first selectively correct the precipitating problem of depressed vascular tone with a careful intravenous titration of an α-adrenergic agonist that activates both α_1- and α_2-receptors. A phenylephrine drip (80 μg/cc) is infused via a central line (0.1 to 1.5 μg/kg/minute) until systemic blood pressure begins to respond. The infusion is carefully titrated to return diastolic pressure to a "normal" preoperative value. Simultaneously, if the central venous pressure and "wedge" pressures have decreased, which frequently occurs, continued preloading with intravenous fluid is appropriate to normalize filling pressures to maintain cardiac index by the Starling mechanism. Combinations of phenylephrine and fluid administration are usually promptly effective in restoring blood pressure. Almost always, very minimal amounts of phenylephrine are needed, and the infusion can usually be discontinued as surgical stimulation begins. A cautious approach is recommended since very harmful effects will occur from such therapy if correction is overzealous. Extreme increases in systemic resistance (afterload) or preload will produce increased myocardial work, oxygen demand, and endocardial ischemia, in a heart already compromised by both ischemic disease and drug-induced depression.

While the systemic resistance is carefully adjusted with phenylephrine if central venous pressure and "wedge" pressure suddenly become elevated, this may indicate that ischemic failure or fluid overload is occurring. Therapy should then be changed to include the addition of an intravenous nitroglycerin infusion (0.5 to 1 μg/kg/minute). With a decrease in vascular resistance and an increase in preload, the simultaneous infusion of phenylephrine and nitroglycerin has a sound physiologic basis in the management of patients with ischemic heart disease. Phenylephrine maintains the diastolic perfusion pressure by constricting the arterioles, whereas nitroglycerin dilates the venous capacitance vessels to reduce preload and improve the coronary microcirculation. Thus, coronary blood supply is maintained as myocardial wall tension and oxygen demand are simultaneously reduced. As vascular resistance and blood pressure is restored, it is important to be most attentive to both drug and fluid management since "roller coaster" effects on blood pressure may be significantly detrimental. The rationale for such an approach is based on past clinical observations and accumulating evidence from the laboratory that may explain cellular mechanisms by which anesthetics, calcium-channel blockers, and β-blockers interact to induce hypotension.

Another usually more unpredictable approach is to select a sympatho-mimetic drug or calcium chloride that would affect both α- and β-adrenergic receptors. This course would be directed at improving vasomotor tone and increasing cardiac function by attempting to override β-blockade and calcium-channel blockade. The competitive reversal of β-blockade with such drugs may be either ineffective at low concentrations or unpredictable at higher concentrations where α-adrenergic activity would predominate. I would caution against such an approach since the requirement for high concentrations of such a drug would risk increasing all of the determinants of myocardial oxygen demand. The simultaneous stimulation of an α- and β-adrenergic activity at this particular time and prior to bypass grafting is unsound and most likely to produce circumstances conducive to initiating myocardial ischemia.

As bypass is discontinued, the patient again experiences hypotension! Our overall clinical situation is now vastly different from the initial episode of hypotension that occurred during the induction period, although propranolol and nifedipine because of their long half-lives, are likely still exerting therapeutic effects as we discontinue bypass. Our primary objectives now are to maintain an acceptable cardiac index, to maintain global oxygen delivery, and to utilize the most efficient means available to balance myocardial work with the least expenditure of myocardial energy. During this very critical recovery period, therapeutic interventions should avoid extreme increases in myocardial oxygen demand at a time when intracellular restoration of depleted energy and other restorative cellular processes are occurring. However, coronary artery blood flow has been surgically improved and increases in myocardial oxygen demand may be better accommodated by increases in myocardial oxygen supply.

We must again examine and reevaluate heart rate, preload, afterload, and contractility to make logical and rational decisions regarding therapy. The blood pressure is 80/60 mm Hg, the cardiac index is 2.3 $L/min/m^2$, and systemic vascular resistance is low. If the central venous and wedge pressures are low, volume loading and infusion of phenylephrine may again be useful. However, if the central venous and wedge pressures are elevated and since the cardiac index is low, other interventions will now become important.

The increased preload may be as a result of volume overload, dysrhythmias, myocardial ischemia, or post-pump myocardial depression from the residual effects of cardioplegia and a long aortic cross-clamp time. It is important to mention initially, as we discontinue bypass, excessive intravascular volume overload will manifest itself with high central venous and wedge pressures and low cardiac index. Simple venous phlebotomy through the atrial venous cannula may sometimes dramatically reverse the vicious cycle of cardiac failure associated with iatrogenic fluid overload.

As we closely examine the heart rate and rhythm, we find a rate of 50 beats per minute associated with intermittent second-degree heart block. An initial approach is to apply atrioventricular pacing to increase heart rate and coordinate atrial emptying with ventricular filling. This is a simple yet most effective and controlled way to greatly improve cardiac function, which may allow us to avoid potent inotropes and pressor drugs. Atrioventricular sequential pacing may be all that is needed to improve blood pressure, reduce filling pressures, and increase cardiac index. If pacing is not immediately effective, we must now select pharmacologic agents that will improve other derangements in cardiovascular function.

Calcium chloride has been an empirically useful and a very popular drug to dramatically improve ventricular function and blood pressure following the discontinuation of cardiopulmonary bypass. Blood pressure increases following administration of calcium chloride, but systemic resistance may increase or decrease depending on the extent of α- and β-blockade.[23] Calcium-channel blockade can be effectively reversed with appropriate dosages of calcium chloride.[24, 25] A bolus dose of 0.5 to 1 gm administered slowly may be quite effective in treating our particular patient. The disadvantages, however, are that the effect is only transient and occasionally extreme increases in myocardial oxygen demand may occur. Other drugs may be more appropriate for long-term management of depressed cardiovascular function.

A sympathomimetic drug that will act on both β- and α-adrenergic activity is indicated at this time. An infusion of epinephrine (4 μg/cc) will produce dose-related and combined β- and α-adrenergic effects. A low dosage, 1 to 2 μg/minute would ordinarily activate only β-receptors, whereas 2 to 10 μg/minute may produce mixed β- and α-effects and 10 to 20 μg/minute would produce primarily α-effects.[26] Since our patient may still have some residual effects of β-blockade, higher dosages of epinephrine may be required to elicit an effective β-response. However, if β-blockade is intense the β-response will be diminished, and the α-adrenergic effects of epinephrine will prevail. This will be true for other drugs such as dopamine, which will also have dose-related β- and α-adrenergic effects. An extreme therapy would be to select a pure β-adrenergic agonist such as isoproterenol. Isoproterenol should effectively and competitively reverse β-blockade, but such a choice may be quite hazardous since further decreases in systemic vascular resistance may occur as β2-receptors are activated. The overall result is detrimental to myocardial oxygen balance since myocardial oxygen demand is greatly increased in disproportion to myocardial oxygen supply. This has been substantiated historically in patients with ischemic heart disease who were treated for lengthy periods with isoproterenol infusion. Such therapy during cardiogenic shock frequently induced lethal subendocardial infarctions as a result of the drug-enhanced disturbances in myocardial oxygen balance.

To return to our clinical situation, my preference would be to gradually titrate either epinephrine (2 to 10 μg/minute) or dopamine (5 to 10 μg/kg/minute) to increase inotropy, improve cardiac index, and restore systemic vascular resistance and blood pressure to normal levels. Our patient responds favorably and soon inotropic support is no longer required as cardiovascular adjustments and normal homeostatic mechanisms recover. During anesthesia, it is important to remember that the negative cardiovascular effects of both the β- and calcium-channel blockers can be reversed by β- and α-agonists, calcium chloride, and AV sequential pacing. Failure to correct cardiovascular disturbances using various combinations of therapy is certainly unusual. Other less commonly used drugs such as glucagon and amrinone may have a role in improving myocardial function in patients who are both β- and calcium-channel blocked and who have myocardial depression following cardiopulmonary bypass. These drugs stimulate cardiac function via metabolic pathways that bypass β-receptors and calcium channels. Glucagon induces a positive inotropic effect on the heart that is related to stimulation of intracellular cyclic adenosine monophosphate (AMP).[27] Amrinone, a newly available drug for the treatment of congestive heart failure, exerts its positive inotropic and vasodilating effects by selectively inhibiting cellular phosphodiesterase and thus increasing intracellular cyclic AMP.[27] When conventional pharmacologic intervention fails, very serious and perhaps permanent pathologic disturbances in ventricular function are likely present. Under such circumstances aggressive therapy with temporary intra-aortic balloon assist therapy may be lifesaving.

In summary, the occurrence of hypotension associated with the interactions of the β-antagonists, calcium-channel blocking drugs, and narcotic anesthesia is well recognized. The physiologic causes for such an event are certainly related to specific cardiovascular disturbances induced by the cardiovascular interactions of such potent drug combinations with adrenergic receptors. The extreme variation in patient response to drug therapy, ventricular function, and the temporally related and everchanging dynamics imposed by the pathophysiology of coronary artery disease must all be balanced when managing a particular hypotensive episode. Therapeutic intervention will require a sophisticated knowledge of the pharmacologic actions of each agonist and antagonist during normal and abnormal cardiovascular events. Success will depend on anticipation, recognition, preparation, and close monitoring of the response to each therapeutic intervention. Therapy must allow flexibility since each intervention has the potential to produce negative responses, which should signal reevaluation and new direction in therapeutic approach. The β-antagonists and the calcium-channel blockers have added new and positive dimensions in the therapy of coronary artery disease. The specific and fascinating mechanisms by which they exert their selective effects on the heart and vascular beds continue to be discovered. Clinically, these drugs continue to exert their positive influence on myocardial oxygen balance during anesthesia and should be considered as important adjuvant drugs to preserve perioperative myocardial function and oxygen balance in patients with coronary artery disease.

REFERENCES

1. Braunwald E: *Heart Disease: A Textbook of Cardiovascular Medicine*. Philadelphia, WB Saunders Co, 1984.
2. Bassan M, Weiler-Ravell D, Shavev O: The additive antianginal action of oral nifedipine in patients receiving propranolol: Magnitude and duration of effect. *Circulation* 1982; 66:710.
3. Dargie HJ, Lynch PG, Krikler DM, et al: Nifedipine and propranolol: A beneficial drug interaction. *Am J Med* 1981; 71:676.
4. Opie LH, White DA: Adverse interaction between nifedipine and β-blockage. *Br Med J* 1980; 281:1462.
5. Kapur PA: Cardiovascular pharmacology: β-Receptor blockers and slow calcium-channel inhibitors, in Katz RL (ed): *Seminars in Anesthesia*. New York, Grune & Stratton, 1982, vol 1, pp 196–206.
6. Lowenstein E: β-adrenergic blockers, in Smith NT (ed): *Drug Interactions in Anesthesia*. Philadelphia, Lea & Febiger, 1981, pp 83–101.
7. Lefkowitz RJ, Caron MG, Stiles GL: Mechanisms of membrane-receptor regulation biochemical, physiological, and clinical insights derived from studies of the adrenergic receptors. *N Engl J Med* 1984; 310:1570–1578.
8. Kapur PA: Calcium channel blockers, in Stoelting RK (ed): *Advances in Anesthesia*. Chicago, Year Book Medical Publishers Inc, 1985, pp 167–205.
9. Reves JG, Kissin I, Lell WA, et al: Calcium entry blockers: Uses and implications for anesthesiologists. *Anesthesiology* 1982; 57:504–518.
10. Kates RA, Kaplan JA: Calcium channel blocking drugs, in Kaplan JA (ed): *Cardiac Anesthesia: Cardiovascular Pharmacology*. New York, Grune & Stratton, 1983, vol 2, pp 209–242.
11. Jenkins LC, Scoates PJ: Anesthetic implications of calcium channel blockers. *Can Anaesth Soc J* 1985; 32:436–447.
12. Braunwald E: Mechanism of action of calcium-channel blocking agents. *N Engl J Med* 1982; 307:1618–1627.
13. Snyder SH, Reynolds IJ: Calcium-antagonist drugs: Receptor interactions that clarify therapeutic effects. *N Engl J Med* 1985; 313:995.
14. Matthews WD, Jim KF, Hieble JP, et al: Postsynaptic adrenoceptors on vascular smooth muscle. *Fed Proc* 1984; 43:2923–2928.
15. Van Brummelen P, Verney P, Timmermans PBMW, et al: Postjunctional α_2 adrenoceptors in the vasculature of the human forearm. *Blood Vessels* 1983; 20:208.
16. Van Meel JCA, Towart R, Kazda S, et al: Correlation between the inhibitory activities of calcium entry blockers on vascular smooth muscle constriction in vitro

after K^+ depolarization and in vivo after α_2-adrenoceptor stimulation. *Arch Pharmacol* 1983; 322:34–37.

17. deLange S, Boscoe MJ, Stanley TH, et al: Comparison of sufentanil-O_2 and fentanyl-O_2 for coronary artery surgery. *Anesthesiology* 1982; 56:112–118.

18. Howie MB, Lingham RP, Lee JJ, et al: Sufentanil-oxygen compared with fentanyl-oxygen anesthesia for coronary artery surgery. *Anesthesiology* 1982; 57:A292.

19. Reves JG: Calcium antagonists and anesthesia, in Stanley TH (ed): *Anesthesia and Cardiovascular System*. Boston, Martinus Nijhoff Publishers, 1984, pp 50–58.

20. Freis ES, Lappas DG: Chronic administration of calcium entry blockers and the cardiovascular responses to high dose of fentanyl in man. *Anesthesiology* 1982; 57:A295.

21. Komatsu T, Shibutani K, Okamoto K, et al: Is sufentanil superior to fentanyl as an induction agent? *Anesthesiology* 1985; 63:A378.

22. Lappas DG, Palacios I, Athanasiadia C, et al: Sufentanil dosage and myocardial blood flow and metabolism in patients with coronary artery disease. *Anesthesiology* 1985; 63.

23. Drop LJ: Ionized calcium, the heart, and hemodynamic function. *Anesth Analg* 1985; 64:432–451.

24. Kates RA, Zaggy AP, Norfleet EA, et al: Comparative cardiovascular effects of verapamil, nifedipine and diltiazem during halothane anesthesia in swine. *Anesthesiology* 1984; 61:10–18.

25. Morris LD, Goldschlager N: Calcium infusion for reversal of adverse effects of intravenous verapamil. *JAMA* 1983; 249:3212–3213.

26. Waller JL: Inotropes and vasopressors, in Kaplan JA (ed): *Cardiac Anesthesia: Cardiovascular Pharmacology*. New York, Grune & Stratton, 1983, vol 2, pp 273–295.

27. Opie LH: *The Heart. Physiology, Metabolism, Pharmacology and Therapy*. London, Grune & Stratton, 1984.

50

Ventricular Arrhythmias Following Coronary Artery Bypass Graft

A 65-year-old man, who had a subendocardial anterior wall myocardial infarction six months previously and who had severe chronic obstructive pulmonary disease, underwent coronary artery bypass surgery for three-vessel disease. A short run of uniform ventricular tachycardia occurred during Foley catheter insertion. This was not treated. The surgical and anesthetic course was uneventful until immediately following termination of cardiopulmonary bypass when the patient had recurring short runs of uniform ventricular tachycardia and multiple, uniform ventricular extrasystoles (Fig 50–1). Blood gas, acid-base, and electrolyte values were normal. The arrhythmias failed to respond to lidocaine, but did to IV verapamil (12.5 mg in divided doses over ten minutes). Two recurrences of the arrhythmia within the first several hours following cardiopulmonary bypass also responded to verapamil (2.5 to 5 mg). There were no further ventricular arrhythmias requiring treatment during the postoperative course.

Recommendations by John L. Atlee III, M.D.

ANALYSIS OF THE PROBLEM

Cardiac arrhythmias may occur in as many as 84% of patients undergoing general anesthesia and surgery, irrespective of the type of surgery.[1] The incidence will be highest when ECG data are continuously recorded for later playback (complete studies).[2] Unfortunately, there are no "complete studies" for patients undergoing cardiac surgical procedures, although it is widely appreciated that such patients are quite likely to have arrhythmias at some time in the perioperative period.

Arrhythmias are serious and warrant drug or electrical management (in addition to other corrective and supportive measures) when they (1) jeopardize a favorable myocardial oxygen balance (tachycardia), (2) impair hemodynamics—arrhythmias associated with atrioventricular (AV) dyssynchrony, or (3) are likely to precipitate/deteriorate into lethal ventricular arrhythmias. The arrhythmias in the case under consideration warranted treatment because they did/could have caused any of the above. Moreover, they did not respond to conventional management (lidocaine). The following discussion focuses on (1) mechanisms for ventricular arrhythmias; (2) drug therapy; (3) electrical management; and (4) management of the case under consideration.

Except for a short run of uniform ventricular tachycardia (different morphology from that occurring postbypass) during insertion of the Foley catheter, the patient had no significant arrhythmias until coming off cardiopulmonary bypass. The arrhythmias produced only modest hemodynamic compromise (Fig 50–1). However, due to the setting of their occurrence (coronary reperfusion following a prolonged period of nonperfusion, possible air in coronaries), their recurring nature, and because the rate (about 140 beats per minute) could have led to myocardial ischemia, it was deemed necessary to treat the arrhythmias.

APPROACH TO THE PROBLEM

As with any arrhythmia, it is first necessary to identify the possible cause(s) and any aggravating factor(s) and correct these. A plausible cause was occlusion/reperfusion injury leading to reentry/abnormal automaticity associated with the depressed fast response secondary to a reduction in resting membrane potential (RMP). Contributing factors could have been myocardial ischemia, acid-base or electrolyte imbalance, although the latter two were ruled out. Also ventilation and oxygenation were normal, and the patient was adequately anesthetized. Next, it is necessary to provide a correct diagnosis for the rhythm disturbance. The arrhythmia under consideration could have been an atrial or AV junctional tachycardia with aberrant ventricular conduction, although this seemed unlikely given the setting and appearance (note that there are no discernible P waves associated with the ventricular complexes in the esophageal electrogram–Fig 50–1). Consequently, the diagnosis of ventricular tachycardia was made, and treatment with *lidocaine* (two 100 mg IV boluses) was provided. Lidocaine is the first-line approach to ventricular tachycardia.

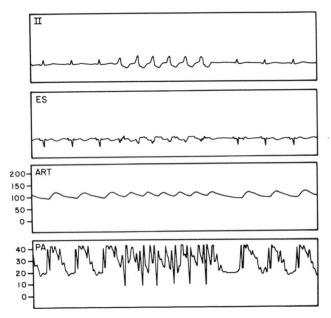

FIG 50–1.
ECG showing recurring short runs of uniform ventricular tachycardia and multiple, uniform ventricular extrasystoles. *II* = surface ECG, lead II; *ES* = esophageal ECG; *ART* = brachial arterial pressure; *PA* = pulmonary arterial pressure.

This had no effect on the arrhythmia. Treatment with *propranolol* was considered (the patient had not been on β-blockers preoperatively, but was receiving diltiazem 90 mg four times a day), but the arrhythmia was not associated with congenital QT prolongation and did not appear catecholamine-mediated. *Phenytoin* was not considered because the patient had received only 1.0 mg of digoxin preoperatively (as a prophylactic measure) and was not hypokalemic. *Bretylium* was not considered for several reasons: (1) the arrhythmias were not life-threatening; (2) initial catecholamine release with bretylium could have aggravated the arrhythmias; and (3) there were several remaining, more conventional options (propranolol, phenytoin, verapamil, and, possibly, procainamide). Given the setting and possible cause (as described above), it was decided to treat with IV verapamil (initial dose 5 mg followed by three repeat doses of 2.5 mg). This treatment was effective and suggests that the etiology of the arrhythmia may indeed have been slow-channel activation with loss of RMP in fast-response (ventricular, Purkinje) fibers. A loss of RMP could then have led to slow conduction, uneven changes in refractoriness and resultant reentrant excitation. Alternatively, it could have caused an abnormal mechanism for automaticity or led to triggering. Regardless of cellular mechanism, block of the slow-inward current (Ca^{++}) by verapamil was effective in terminating the arrhythmia and preventing its recurrence. However, it should be noted that therapy of ventricular tachycardia with verapamil is *not conventional treatment*. Based on known electrophysiologic actions, verapamil would probably only be effective against ventricular arrhythmias associated with loss of RMP in normally fast-response type fibers. Also, the efficacy of verapamil in the case under consideration does not rule out the possibility that the arrhythmia was supraventricular in origin and associated with aberrant ventricular conduction.

DISCUSSION

Causes

Cardiac arrhythmias are considered disorders of *automaticity* (either normal or abnormal), *triggered activity* (either from stimulated or automatic action potentials, or as the result of after-depolarizations), *conduction* (heart block, reentrant excitation), or both *automaticity and conduction* (parasystole). [2-5] Any of these electrophysiologic mechanisms could have been responsible for the ventricular arrhythmias described in the case report.

Normal automaticity is spontaneous phase 4 (diastolic) depolarization. It is a normal property of cells found in the SA node, along the sulcus terminalis (subsidiary atrial pacemakers), in the AV junctional tissues, and in the His-Purkinje network. These pacemaker sites are listed in order of decreasing inherent automaticity. *Abnormal automaticity,* also spontaneous phase 4 depolarization, is exhibited by fast-response fibers (atrial/ventricular muscle, Purkinje fibers) with reduced levels of resting membrane potential (RMP)—that is, their RMP is reduced from normal values of from -80 to -90 mV to between -40 and -60 mV. Abnormally low levels of RMP may be due to drugs or pathophysiologic processes (see discussion below). *Triggered activity* is sustained rhythmic activity that is critically dependent on prior impulses for its initiation, and without which there is electrical quiescence. In addition to automatic or stimulated impulses, the inciting event for triggering could be early or late after-depolarizations. Triggering has been observed in most cardiac fiber types and varied and assorted conditions, including digitalis excess and disease states. [2] However, because both triggered and reentrant arrhythmias (below) may be initiated by critically timed prior impulses, it is difficult to clinically distinguish between these two mechanisms. *Reentrant excitation,* which requires uneven changes in refractoriness and unidirectional block of conduction, is a possible mechanism for many clinical arrhythmias, including those occurring in the setting of myocardial ischemia and infarction. Concerning any of the above possible mechanisms for tachyarrhythmias, it is unlikely that tachycardia with rates in excess of 200 beats per minute can be due to enhanced normal automaticity. However, it could be due to any of the other cited arrhythmia mechanisms.

Loss of RMP, in addition to causing abnormal automaticity, may also contribute to reentrant excitation. This is because fast-channel fibers with reduced RMP have largely inactivated Na channels, so that conduction velocity (dependent on the rate of rise of the upstroke of the action potential during phase 0) is slowed even to the point of conduction block. Such fibers exhibiting slow conduction as the result of reduced RMP are termed *depressed fast-response* fibers.[6] Thus, the depressed fast response could provide the conditions for reentry of excitation in atrial or ventricular muscle. Indeed, abnormal automaticity and slowed conduction as the result of the depressed fast response may explain many ventricular tachyarrhythmias that occur in the setting of myocardial ischemia and infarction. Cellular hypoxia, increased extracellular K^+, and excess catecholamines associated with myocardial ischemia and infarction—all may contribute to loss of RMP, the depressed fast response, and consequent arrhythmias.

A basic understanding of mechanisms for cardiac arrhythmias is important to arrhythmia management for at least two reasons. *First,* antiarrhythmic drugs have been designed to affect one or more of the proposed arrhythmia mechanisms. Hence, their efficacy in the clinical setting will in large part be determined by discovery of the mechanism responsible for the arrhythmia. Thus, it is unlikely that lidocaine, which inhibits the fast-channel (Na^+) and may also affect repolarization currents (K^+) in fast-channel fibers (atrial/ventricular muscle, Purkinje fibers), would be effective in terminating tachycardia due to sinoatrial (SA) or AV nodal reentry. *Second,* misdiagnosis of the mechanism for a particular arrhythmia could lead to adverse results with treatment. An example would be use of direct current (DC) cardioversion to terminate paroxysmal atrial tachycardia in an overly digitalized patient. The DC cardioversion either would have no effect or could precipitate new and potentially more dangerous arrhythmias (e.g., ventricular fibrillation). However, DC cardioversion is indicated management for arrhythmias due to reentrant excitation (see discussion below).

Pharmacologic Therapy

Any of the four classes of antiarrhythmic drugs[7] (Table 50–1) can be effective against ventricular arrhythmias, depending on the setting in which they occur. Class I drugs have as their principal action the ability to block the fast inward (Na^+) current. Class II drugs include all of the β-receptor antagonists, although most are not approved antiarrhythmics. Class III drugs prolong action potential duration. Class IV drugs block the slow inward current carried mainly by Ca^{++} (calcium-channel blockers). However, not all drugs listed in Table

TABLE 50–1.

Antiarrhythmic Drugs

CLASS I	CLASS II	CLASS III	CLASS IV
Disopyramide	Esmolol	Amiodarone	Verapamil
Lidocaine	Propranolol	Bretylium	(Other calcium-channel
Phenytoin	Labetalol*		blockers†)
Procainamide	(Other β-blockers†)		
Quinidine			
Tocainide			

*Combined α-, β-antagonist.
†May or may not be approved for antiarrhythmic use.

50–1 possess single class actions.[8] Lidocaine (I) and propranolol (II) affect K^+-repolarization currents, and phenytoin (I) affects both the fast (Na^+) and slow inward (Ca^{++}) currents. Also, antiarrhythmic properties of some drugs may be in part related to extracardiac actions. Quinidine (I) and related (disopyramide, procainamide) antiarrhythmics possess varying anticholinergic actions, while vasodilation with procainamide is the result of mild ganglionic blockade. Amiodarone and bretylium (following initial catecholamine release), both Class III drugs, have sympatholytic properties, and verapamil (IV) has some local anesthetic potency and may exert an α-adrenergic blocking action.[9]

Of the drugs listed in Table 50–1, bretylium, lidocaine, phenytoin, propranolol, and verapamil are useful for the acute management of ventricular arrhythmias in cardiac surgical patients. Lidocaine has a rather narrow antiarrhythmic spectrum and is used almost exclusively for the management of ventricular arrhythmias in the setting of acute myocardial infarction, cardiac surgery, anesthesia, and digitalis toxicity. It suppresses abnormal automaticity in ventricular muscle fibers that have survived experimental infarction,[10] and reduces the temporal dispersion of refractoriness in those portions of the specialized ventricular conducting system where the duration of the action potential is longest.[9] These actions could explain lidocaine's antiarrhythmic efficacy against ventricular arrhythmias due to abnormal automaticity or reentrant excitation. Lidocaine should be considered the initial drug of choice for the management of most ventricular arrhythmias. The others (listed above) have rather special applications, and should be considered as second-line or last-resort (bretylium) therapy. Bretylium, which has a direct effect on the cell membrane and antiadrenergic action (following initial catecholamine release which could aggravate arrhythmias), increases action potential duration and refractoriness in atrial and ventricular muscle and Purkinje fibers. There is some evidence that bretylium can reduce the disparity in action potential and refractoriness between normal and infarcted myocardium,[11] which may account for some of the antifibrillatory effects of bretylium in the setting of myocardial ischemia. Bretylium should be used only for the treatment of life-threatening, recurrent ventricular tachyarrhythmias not responsive to conventional drugs. Phenytoin has been shown to be effective in abolishing abnormal automaticity due to digitalis-induced delayed after-depolarizations in Purkinje fibers,[12] and in suppressing atrial and ventricular arrhythmias caused by digitalis in man. It should be considered (after lidocaine) for the management of ventricular arrhythmias when digitalis (with or without associated hypokalemia) could be the cause. The antiarrhythmic effects of propranolol have been attributed to competitive β-adrenergic blockade and to membrane stabilizing ("quinidine-like") properties, although the latter are not important at clinically useful levels. Propranolol is most commonly used in the management of supraventricular tachyarrhythmias. It should be considered (after lidocaine) for the management of ventricular arrhythmias due to catecholamine excess, sympathetic imbalance (congenital long QT syndrome), and hyperthyroid states. Verapamil blocks the slow-inward (Ca^{++}) current in slow-response (SA, AV nodes) or depressed fast-response (atrial/ventricular muscle or Purkinje fibers with reduced RMP) fibers. It has become the drug of choice for terminating reentrant supraventricular tachyarrhythmias (RSVT). However, it is not usually effective treatment for ventricular arrhythmias. It may be of value in selected cases,[13] perhaps because the arrhythmia is due to reentrant excitation (slow conduction secondary to depressed fast response) or abnormal forms of automaticity/triggering associated with loss of RMP. It is interesting to note that verapamil and the potent, modern volatile anesthetics are about equally efficacious against ventricular fibrillation in the canine, acute, coronary occlusion/reperfusion arrhythmia model.[14]

Electrical Management

Electrical management for ventricular arrhythmias can include cardiac pacing, DC cardioversion, and defibrillation.[2] Ventricular overdrive pacing ("overdrive suppression") is indicated management for torsade de pointes, tachycardia associated with the prolonged QT syndrome,[15] particularly when it is drug-induced (acquired) as opposed to the congenital form.[2, 9] Increasing the ventricular rate by pacing ameliorates disparate ventricular refractoriness, which possibly serves as the substrate for this arrhythmia.[16] However, it should be cautioned that ventricular overdrive pacing, in the presence of myocardial ischemia, could increase the degree of conduction block in the ischemic zone and, as a direct result, increase the temporal dispersion of refractoriness. If this were the case, overdrive ventricular pacing could worsen the tachycardia or initiate ventricular fibrillation ("overdrive excitation").

DC cardioversion differs from *defibrillation* in that with the former, a time-delay circuit permits synchronization of the shock with the R wave of the surface ECG. Synchronized shocks are used for the management of all tachyarrhythmias amenable to electrical conversion, except ventricular fibrillation and ventricular tachycardia when the QRS is wide and cannot be distinguished from T waves. DC cardioversion is effective only in terminating reentrant tachyarrhythmias. It does this by depolarizing all excitable myocardium, including automatic foci, and interrupting the circuit(s) involved in reentry. By establishing electrical homogeneity, conditions for reentry are removed, at least temporarily. However, the reentrant tachycardia may be reinitiated by factors that provoked it in the first place. Correction of these by the institution of drug and other therapeutic measures may help to prevent such recurrences. DC cardioversion is not usually effective in terminating automatic tachycardia (e.g., that caused by digitalis). This is because it only resets the cycle of the automatic focus so that tachycardia can resume after attempted cardioversion. In general, any ventricular tachyarrhythmia due to reentry that produces severe hemodynamic compromise and/or myocardial ischemia and has not responded to drugs or other indicated management should be terminated by DC cardioversion. DC cardioversion is first-line therapy if ventricular tachycardia is such that there is the possibility that the arrhythmia will progress to ventricular fibrillation if not terminated immediately. Only the lowest energy shocks should be used, and often 50 joules (watt-sec) or less will be effective in terminating ventricular tachycardia.

REFERENCES

1. Bertrand CA, Steiner NV, Jameson AG, et al: Disturbances of cardiac rhythm during anesthesia and surgery. *JAMA* 1971; 216:1615–1617.
2. Atlee JL: *Perioperative Cardiac Dysrhythmias: Mechanisms, Recognition, Management.* Chicago, Year Book Medical Publishers, 1985.
3. Cranefield PF: *The Conduction of the Cardiac Impulse.* Mt Kisco, NY, Futura Publishing Co, 1975.
4. Hoffman BF, Rosen MR: Cellular mechanisms for cardiac arrhythmias. *Circ Res* 1981; 49:1–15.
5. Zipes DP: Genesis of cardiac arrhythmias: Electrophysiological considerations, in Braunwald E: *Heart Disease,* ed 2. Philadelphia, WB Saunders Co, 1984, pp 605–647.
6. Wit AL, Rosen MR, Hoffman BF: Electrophysiology and pharmacology of cardiac arrhythmias: II. Relation of normal and abnormal electrical activity of cardiac fibers to the genesis of arrhythmias. *Am Heart J* 1974; 88:798–806.
7. Vaughan Williams EM: Classification of antidysrhythmic drugs, part B. *Pharmacol Ther* 1975; 1:115–138.
8. Hauswirth O, Singh BN: Ionic mechanisms in heart muscle in relation to genesis and the pharmacological control of arrhythmias. *Pharmacol Rev* 1978; 30:5–63.

9. Zipes DP: Management of cardiac arrhythmias, in Braunwald E (ed): *Heart Disease,* ed 2. Philadelphia, WB Saunders Co, 1984, pp 648–682.

10. Kupersmith J: Electrophysiological and antiarrhythmic effects of lidocaine in canine acute myocardial ischemia. *Am Heart J* 1979; 97:360–366.

11. Waxman MB, Wallace AG: Electrophysiological effects of bretylium tosylate on the heart. *J Pharmacol Exp Ther* 1972; 183:264–274.

12. Ferrier GR: Digitalis arrhythmias: Role of oscillatory after-potentials. *Prog Cardiovasc Dis* 1977; 19:459–474.

13. Singh BN, Collett JT, Chew CY: New perspectives in the pharmacologic therapy of cardiac arrhythmias. *Prog Cardiovasc Dis* 1980; 22:243–301.

14. Kroll DA, Knight PR: Antifibrillatory effects of volatile anesthetics in acute occlusion/reperfusion arrhythmias. *Anesthesiology* 1984; 61:657–661.

15. Khan MM, Logan KR, McComb JM, et al: Management of recurrent ventricular tachyarrhythmias associated with Q-T prolongation. *Am J Cardiol* 1981; 48:1301–1308.

16. Han J, Millet D, Chizzonitti B, et al: Temporal dispersion of excitability in atrium and ventricle as a function of heart rate. *Am Heart J* 1966; 71:481–487.

PART SEVEN

Coagulation and
Blood Products

51

Streptokinase Patient for Surgery

A 50-year-old man with an isolated left anterior descending coronary artery stenosis of 95% was scheduled to have angioplasty. The procedure was considered successful, but after the procedure he complained of chest pain and had ST changes. On repeat angiography, the lesion was found occluded by a fresh clot. At that time, 1.5 million units of streptokinase was administered intravenously and a repeat angioplasty performed. These procedures were unsuccessful in reopening the vessel and emergency surgery was scheduled. Of note on physical examination was the fact that bleeding was observed at the site of catheterization and around the intravenous catheter site on the arm.

Recommendations by Judith A. Fabian, M.D.

ANALYSIS OF THE PROBLEM

This case presents the not uncommon dilemma of a patient recently given intravenous streptokinase who needs emergency surgery. Questions regarding management of a patient given streptokinase are raised by this case. Complications of streptokinase therapy are: fever, allergic reactions, and hemorrhage. Of these, the threat of excessive bleeding is the most disturbing in this case.

APPROACH TO THE PROBLEM

Generally, when a patient arrives in the operating room directly from the cardiac catheterization lab in an emergency situation, he will be apprehensive. This and the possibility of hemodynamic instability are strong reasons *not* to waste time. If the anesthesiologist has not dealt with the situation previously, it is well to have a management plan so that things will proceed quietly and calmly.

Electrocardiography (ECG) leads should be attached and oxygen administered by mask. If the Judkins technique was used, the indwelling catheter should be used for monitoring arterial blood pressure. The existing intravenous catheter in the arm should be used for induction of anesthesia with 50 μg/kg fentanyl. Vecuronium (0.1 to 0.125 mg/kg) is administered intravenously to prevent rigidity and facilitate endotracheal intubation. Intravenous fentanyl is then given continuously 10 to 20 μg/kg/hour.

After endotracheal intubation is accomplished, lines more appropriate for cardiac surgery are established *if the patient is hemodynamically stable.* A single intravenous catheter in the arm is inadequate for the administration of inotropes, fluid, and/or blood. An internal jugular vein (IJV) cannulation may be accomplished, even in the patient who has had high-dose streptokinase therapy, provided it is performed by a clinician who is experienced and adept. Multiple attempts at locating IJV should be avoided.

It is our routine to place two 8.5 F sheaths in the IJV approximately 1 cm apart for cardiac surgery, one for the insertion of a pulmonary artery catheter (PAC) and one for a triple lumen venous catheter.[1] The PAC should not be placed in the wedge position in this patient, but rather advanced just into the pulmonary artery. When cardiopulmonary bypass (CPB) is initiated, the PAC should be withdrawn 3 to 5 cm. If the radial artery cannot be easily cannulated with a 20- or 22-gauge Teflon catheter, the sheath through which the Judkins catheter was inserted will suffice for measuring arterial pressures during surgery. At the end of the procedure, the sheath should be removed and the artery surgically repaired if bleeding is a problem.

The usual dose of heparin is administered prior to CPB and its effectiveness confirmed with the activated clotting time. After termination of CPB, if the patient continues to bleed despite adequate heparin reversal and no discrete vessels are determined to be responsible, platelets and fresh frozen plasma should be administered. Epsilon aminocaproic acid (EACA) should be reserved for cases of hemorrhage unresponsive to the above measures.

DISCUSSION

Background

Streptokinase is the metabolic product of β-hemolytic streptococci of Lancefield group C. It was first used intravenously in acute myocardial infarction (AMI) by Fletcher et al.[2] in 1959, but a number of subsequent clinical trials met with mixed results.[3] However, treatment was delayed for 12 to 72 hours postinfarct due to the prevalent belief that myocardial necrosis occurs within 45 to 60 minutes of total coronary occlusion. Following the demonstration that ischemic tolerance time for myocardial necrosis is usually three to six hours or longer,[4, 5] and the successful recanalization of the infarcted vessel in four of five patients treated with selective intracoronary (IC) infusion of streptokinase by Rentrop et al.,[6] there was a resurgence of interest in the use of streptokinase in AMI. Lee and associates were the first to demonstrate angiographically the efficacy of intravenous (IV) streptokinase for coronary thrombolysis in AMI.[7]

Streptokinase Activity

Hemostasis is brought about by the interrelated action of the vasculature, platelets, and the coagulation cascade to form a clot. In pathologic intravascular thrombosis, platelets adhere to the endothelium and aggregate to form a thrombus. Although both reactions may be initiated by platelet aggregation, it is the formation of fibrin strands that lends support to the platelet plug and prevents its rapid disintegration.

The final common pathway is the activation of factor X and its cofactor, factor V, by the intrinsic and/or extrinsic pathways of the coagulation cascade, details of which may be reviewed elsewhere.[8] Activated factor X then converts prothrombin to thrombin, which cleaves fibrinogen to fibrin and two pairs of fibrinopeptides. The fibrin monomers polymerize and stabilize catalyzed by factor XIII, forming a tight clot.

In order to reestablish circulation in an injured blood vessel, the fibrin clot must be removed once the vessel has healed. This is accomplished by the lytic system, which parallels the coagulation cascade in that it has intrinsic and extrinsic pathways (Fig 51–1). Factor XIIa activates the intrinsic system, while tissue activators stimulate the extrinsic system to cleave plasminogen to plasmin. Plasmin, similar to thrombin in chemical composition, is a serine protease capable of breaking down fibrin into fibrin degradation products, or fibrin split products (FSP). These products serve as anticoagulants in that they inhibit cross-linking of fibrin monomers, inhibit thrombin, and, in large concentrations, produce platelet dysfunction. Their presence indicates clot lysis in both normal and pathologic situations.

Thrombolysis may be enhanced by factors that act directly on fibrin (trypsin), drugs that promote the release of naturally occurring plasminogen activators (nicotinic acid), and drugs that activate plasminogen directly or indirectly (urokinase and streptokinase).[3]

Streptokinase, as with other streptococcal proteins, has the ability to act as an antigen in man. Antistreptokinase is present in varying titers in man and reacts with part of an injected dose of streptokinase to form an inert complex.

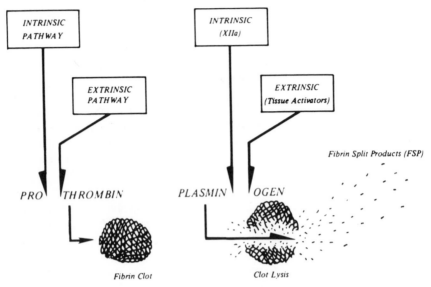

FIG 51–1.
The parallel clotting and lytic system. Streptokinase forms an equimolar complex with plasminogen that generates plasmin by peptide-bond cleavage of other circulating plasminogen. (From Fischbach DP, Fogdall RP: *Coagulation: The Essentials*. Baltimore, Williams & Wilkins, 1981. Used by permission.)

That part of a streptokinase dose that has not been immunologically neutralized interacts with plasminogen to form an equimolar complex within which an active serine center, or plasminogen-activating site, is exposed.[9] This active site may then generate plasmin by peptide-bond cleavage of plasminogen. Urokinase, on the other hand, directly activates plasmin by cleavage of plasminogen at the same peptide site. Theoretically, the two-step mechanism of action of streptokinase means that a small dose of streptokinase can result in high levels of plasmin because more free plasminogen is left to be activated, whereas a high dose of streptokinase may, by forming complexes with the available plasminogen, leave only small amounts free for conversion to plasmin.[3]

Management Concerns

The two main concerns in a patient about to undergo cardiac surgery following high-dose IV streptokinase therapy are insertion of lines and postoperative hemorrhage.

Insertion of Venous Catheters
There are no reports in the literature of hemorrhagic complications from IJV and radial artery cannulation following streptokinase therapy, perhaps be-

cause the number of patients undergoing surgery with 24 hours of therapy is relatively small. Goldberg et al. reported a patient who required platelets, fresh frozen plasma, cryoprecipitate, and EACA to control a coagulopathy after CPB.[10] Prior to CPB, they inserted IJV and radial arterial lines and reported no bleeding from those sites even though the patient's blood did not clot at the time of insertion.

Of 209 nonsurgical patients treated with IC streptokinase at six medical centers, Weinstein reports six had bleeding/hematoma at the puncture site, two had retroperitoneal bleeding, and five had gastrointestinal bleeding.[11] However, five of the bleeding complications occurred after the first day and were attributed to heparinization. Whether or not the others were related to heparin was unclear.

In five of six studies of patients undergoing cardiac surgery within 24 hours of streptokinase therapy, hemorrhage was not reported to be a problem. In a single study excessive bleeding was noted in 17 of 24 patients, 5 of which bled in excess of 2,000 ml (Table 51–1).[12–17] Why these differences exist is not apparent.

Perioperative Hemorrhage

Whether or not patients who have had IV streptokinase (dose range 1 to 1.5 million units) are at greater risk for bleeding complications than those having IC therapy (dose range 100,000 to 300,000 units) is unclear. Cowley et al. found an 88% incidence of systemic thrombolysis in patients receiving IC streptokinase.[18] Although Rogers and associates noted a more profound, acute drop in serum fibrinogen levels in patients receiving IV streptokinase compared to those receiving IC streptokinase, there was no difference in incidence of bleeding complications, which was low.[19] Earlier reports of a high percentage of hemorrhagic complications with IV streptokinase therapy may have been due to a longer duration of administration, rather than the brief, high-dose

TABLE 51–1.

Hemorrhage and EACA Administration in Patients Undergoing Cardiac Surgery After Coronary Thrombolysis With Streptokinase

INVESTIGATOR	NO. OF PATIENTS	HEMORRHAGE (NO. OF PATIENTS)	EACA ADMINISTRATION (NO. OF PATIENTS)
Walker et al.[12]	?	0	NR*
Krebber et al.[13]	14	NR	NR
Skinner et al.[14]	24	17	6
Mathey et al.[15]	8	0	NR
Lolley et al.[16]	5	0	1
Krebber et al.[17]	5	0	NR

*NR = not reported

therapy currently used.[20] Although current data are inconclusive, it appears that patients may safely undergo cardiac surgery within 24 hours of IV or IC streptokinase therapy.

REFERENCES

1. Fabian JA, Jesudian MCS, Rah KH: Double internal jugular vein cannulation in pediatric and adult cardiac surgery patients: An easy and convenient technique. *Anesth Analg* 1986; 65:419–420.
2. Fletcher A, Sherry S, Alkjaersig N, et al: Maintenance of a sustained thrombolytic state in man: II. Clinical observations on patients with myocardial infarction and other thromboembolic disorders. *J Clin Invest* 1959; 38:1111.
3. Brogden RN, Speight TM, Avery GS: Streptokinase: A review of its clinical pharmacology, mechanism of action and therapeutic uses. *Drugs* 1973; 5:357–445.
4. Rentrop P, Blanke H, Karsch KR, et al: Selective intracoronary thrombolysis in acute myocardial infarction and unstable angina pectoris. *Circulation* 1981; 63:307–316.
5. Ginks WR, Sybers HD, Maroko PR, et al: Coronary artery reperfusion. *J Clin Invest* 1972; 51:2717.
6. Reimer KA, Lowe JE, Rasmussen MM, et al: The wave front phenomenon of ischemic cell death. *Circulation* 1977; 56:786.
7. Lee G, Amsterdam EA, Low RL, et al: Coronary thrombolysis in acute myocardial infarction. *Am Heart J* 1981; 102:783–786.
8. Fischbach DP, Fogdall RP: *Coagulation: The Essentials.* Baltimore, Williams & Wilkins Co, 1981.
9. Bell WR, Meek AG: Guidelines for the use of thrombolytic agents. *N Engl J Med* 1979; 301:1266–1270.
10. Goldberg M, Colonna-Romano P, Babins NA: Emergency coronary artery bypass surgery following intracoronary streptokinase. *Anesthesiology* 1984; 61:601–604.
11. Weinstein J: Treatment of myocardial infarction with intracoronary streptokinase: Efficacy and safety data from 209 United States cases in the Hoechst-Roussel registry. *Am Heart J* 1982; 104:894–898.
12. Walker WE, Smalling RW, Fuentes F, et al: Role of coronary artery bypass surgery after intracoronary streptokinase infusion for myocardial infarction. *Am Heart J* 1984; 197:826–829.
13. Krebber HJ, Mathey DG, Schofer J, et al: Indication for early aorto-coronary bypass surgery after successful intracoronary lysis. *J Thorac Cardiovasc Surg* 1983; 31:50–53.
14. Skinner JR, Phillips SJ, Zeff RH, et al: Immediate coronary bypass following failed streptokinase infusion in evolving myocardial infarction. *J Thorac Cardiovasc Surg* 1984; 87:567–570.
15. Mathey DG, Rodeward G, Rentrop P, et al: Intracoronary streptokinase thrombolytic recanalization and subsequent surgical bypass of remaining atherosclerotic stenosis in acute myocardial infarction: Complementary combined approach effecting reduced infarct size, preventing reinfarction, and improving left ventricular function. *Am Heart J* 1981; 102:1194–1201.

16. Lolley DM, Fulton R, Hamman J, et al: Coronary artery surgery and direct coronary artery thrombolysis during acute myocardial infarction. *Am Surg* 1983; 49:296–300.

17. Krebber HJ, Mathey D, Kuck KJ, et al: Management of evolving myocardial infarction by intracoronary thrombolysis and subsequent aorto-coronary bypass. *J Thorac Cardiovasc Surg* 1982; 83:186–193.

18. Cowley MJ, Hastillo A, Vetrovec GW, et al: Fibrinolytic effects of intracoronary streptokinase administration in patients with acute myocardial infarction and coronary insufficiency. *Circulation* 1983; 67:1031–1038.

19. Rogers WJ, Mantle JA, Hood WP Jr, et al: Prospective randomized trial of intravenous and intracoronary streptokinase in acute myocardial infarction. *Circulation* 1983; 68:1051–1061.

20. European Cooperative Study Group: Streptokinase in acute myocardial infarction. *N Engl J Med* 1979; 30:797–802.

52

Heparin-Induced Platelet Agglutination

A 56-year-old woman had a myocardial infarction prior to scheduled operation for unremitting chest pain. Her infarct had been complicated by left ventricular failure and she required three days of heparinization and intra-aortic balloon pump (IABP) circulatory assistance. After the IABP removal, she continued to receive subcutaneous heparin. The night before surgery, she suffered vertebral artery occlusion. Her platelet count was measured at that time and found to be 50,000/cu mm, compared to an admission count of 360,000/cu mm.

Recommendations by Norbert P. de Bruijn, M.D.

ANALYSIS OF THE PROBLEM

Heparin, an antithrombotic agent used to prevent or treat thrombosis, is a negatively charged mucopolysaccharide. Its anticoagulant action is exerted in the presence of a cofactor, antithrombin III. The heparin-antithrombin III complex binds to and inactivates certain anticoagulation factors.

Heparin-induced thrombocytopenia, the most likely diagnosis in this patient, is an entity that ranges from an asymptomatic decrease in the platelet count to a dramatic thrombocytopenia, of as low as 5200/cu mm, accompanied by extensive arterial thrombosis. Heparin-induced thrombocytopenia occurs during the use of both bovine and porcine heparin, although the incidence of this disorder due to porcine heparin has been reported to be lower than that during the use of bovine heparin. [1-4] The mild thrombocytopenia, the incidence of which has been reported to be as high as 31%, [5, 6] occurs frequently on the second to fourth day of heparin therapy with platelet counts around 100,000/cu mm. The patients do not develop thrombotic or hemorrhagic manifestations. [5, 7] The severe type occurs after several days of heparin treatment. The platelet count rises rapidly after discontinuation of heparin therapy and rechallenging with the drug causes a recurrence of the thrombocytopenia, sometimes with thrombosis. This pattern suggests an underlying immunologic mechanism and these cases have a high incidence of heparin-dependent antiplatelet antibodies.

The majority of patients with the severe thrombocytopenia have thrombotic complications including major arterial occlusions, like our patient; myocardial infarction; recurrent venous thrombosis; and recurrent pulmonary embolization. Hemorrhagic complications are less frequent. Heparin-induced thrombocytopenia appears to be independent not only of the origin of the heparin (beef lung or porcine mucosa), but also of the dosage and route of administration.

Heparin-induced, "true" immunologic reactions are unusual. Nevertheless, heparin-dependent antiplatelet antibodies have been detected in most patients with severe thrombocytopenia. Drug-related antiplatelet antibodies can be detected using platelet aggregation studies in which heparin is added to the patient's platelet-rich plasma, as well as by using a variety of other techniques.

The proposed mechanism for the development of thrombocytopenia and the associated thrombosis is that platelet membrane antibody, in the presence of heparin, induces platelet aggregation with the release of platelet granule contents. Also a release of platelet factor 4 occurs that has heparin neutralizing activity. This may explain the commonly observed tachyphylaxis for heparin. Green et al. [8] were unable to show an antibody that could bind to heparin alone but found that platelet lysates absorbed an immunoglobulin-heparin complex. This suggests that the heparin, acting as a hapten, induced an immune response against the heparin-platelet complex. Platelet aggregation may activate the intrinsic pathway of blood coagulation and thus may contribute to the development of thrombosis. Green et al. [8] observed that aspirin inhibited heparin-induced platelet aggregation.

There is an abundance of case reports describing heparin-induced thrombocytopenia with arterial thrombosis. The incidence of this serious complication is not well established, but it is much lower than heparin-induced thrombocytopenia. When arterial thrombosis is present there is significant morbidity and mortality associated with it. King and Kelton [9] reviewed the literature and reported 29% mortality and 21% limb amputation in patients with this complication. Because arterial thrombosis complicating a drug-induced thrombocytopenia is such a unique complication, some authors have speculated that there would be a different pathophysiologic basis for heparin-induced thrombocytopenia than for classic drug-induced thrombocytopenias.

APPROACH TO THE PROBLEM

Patients with heparin-induced thrombocytopenia, who are candidates for cardiac surgery in which high-dose heparin treatment during cardiopulmonary bypass is unavoidable, present the surgical team with a number of issues that require management decisions. The first question that arises is one of timing of the operation. In general, attempts should be made to postpone surgery until the patient's clinical situation due to the arterial thrombosis has resolved or stabilized and until the patient has had a thorough workup in regard to the coagulation status. Most authors have discontinued heparin therapy once heparin-induced thrombocytopenia has been recognized and patients have started to receive oral anticoagulants. If the indication for surgery is not emergent, the patient may be put on antiaggregative therapy until in vitro platelet aggregation studies have normalized. Olinger et al.[10] reported a four- to eight-week period required before the antiplatelet antibody reaction had vanished in the presence of antiaggregating therapy, after which the surgery was performed with full heparinization, and further heparin exposure in the postoperative phase was avoided. In the three cases that they reported, the patients had no perioperative evidence of intravascular thrombosis or bleeding diathesis and in vitro heparin-dependent aggregation did not recur.

Pansard et al.[11] successfully performed cardiac surgery on two patients one and two months following heparin-induced thrombocytopenia. In one patient no heparin was used in the postoperative phase; in the second patient heparin with a low molecular weight was used postoperatively.

Our own experience consists of two patients with heparin-induced thrombocytopenia, one of whom suffered anterior spinal artery occlusion with paralysis of both legs. Both patients required urgent coronary artery bypass grafting for unremitting angina pectoris. Platelet aggregation studies were positive for antiplatelet antibodies. The patients were treated with aspirin for 12 to 24 hours and when the repeat platelet aggregation studies proved to be negative they were scheduled for coronary revascularization under full heparinization. In both patients porcine heparin was used during cardiopulmonary bypass. There were no complications. In vitro platelet aggregation studies performed during the period of heparinization remained negative. Postoperatively, dextran with a low molecular weight was used for the continuous flush systems of the central venous and arterial catheters. In our view, therefore, it is not absolutely necessary to postpone surgery requiring high-dose heparin treatment, provided that the platelet aggregation studies have become negative prior to heparinization.

DISCUSSION

In our view the single most important determinant of whether or not it is safe to proceed with cardiac surgery requiring cardiopulmonary bypass and systemic heparinization in patients with heparin-induced thrombocytopenia is the absence of a positive platelet aggregation test. Even though patients have been rechallenged with heparin after a documented episode of heparin-induced thrombocytopenia without a recurrence of the thrombocytopenia, it seems advisable to institute antiaggregative therapy in all these patients before reheparinization.

It has not been established whether substitution of porcine heparin for the commonly used bovine heparin in patients that are being rechallenged decreases the risk of recurrence of thrombocytopenia. There is no doubt that cross-sensitivity exists between heparins of porcine intestinal mucosal and bovine sources,[12] both in vivo and in vitro. However, the incidence of severe thrombocytopenia reactions to porcine heparin appears to be less.

There are a number of possible alternatives for systemic anticoagulation in patients with heparin-induced thrombocytopenia. Org 10172 is a new sulphated mucopolysaccharide from pig intestinal mucosa, with a bimodal molecular weight with means of 4,200 and 14,000. In animal models the compound has proved to be an effective antithrombotic agent. Harenberg et al.[13] described its use in a patient with heparin-induced thrombocytopenia accompanied by extensive thrombosis of the right leg. A second possible alternative is the use of low-molecular-weight heparin. In two patients with heparin-induced thrombocytopenia complicated by pulmonary embolism, Roussi et al.[14] used subcutaneous low-molecular-weight heparin fraction (CY-216). The platelet count reverted to normal in three to five days, and the pulmonary embolism resolved. Heparin-dependent platelet aggregating factor was not active in the presence of low-molecular-weight heparin. We are not aware of the use of any of these agents during cardiopulmonary bypass but consider them possible alternatives in case of emergency cardiac surgery in a patient with heparin-induced thrombocytopenia in which platelet aggregation would not be readily reversible with anti-aggregative agents, so that regular heparin might be used.

Kappa et al. used Iloprost (ZK 3637 4) in two patients with heparin-induced thrombocytopenia. Iloprost is a new prostacyclin analogue that prevents platelet aggregation. Iloprost induces less vasodilatation and is more potent than prostacyclin. They demonstrated that Iloprost effectively prevented platelet aggregation in their patients.[15]

We conclude that heparin-induced thrombocytopenia is an entity that is being recognized with increasing frequency as the use of heparin increases. It has potentially disastrous complications with a relatively high incidence. Preparation of these patients for cardiac surgery that necessitates systemic anticoagulation consists of treatment with antiaggregating agents until in vitro heparin-induced platelet aggregation becomes negative, at which time heparinization appears to be safe.

REFERENCES

1. Ansell J, Hepchuk N Jr, Kumar R, et al: Heparin-induced thrombocytopenia: A prospective study. *Thromb Haemost* 1980; 43:61–65.
2. Bell WR, Royall RM: Heparin-associated thrombocytopenia: A comparison of three heparin preparations. *N Engl J Med* 1980; 303:902–907.
3. Kwaan HC, Kampmeier PA, Gomez HJ: Incidence of thrombocytopenia during therapy with bovine lung and porcine gut mucosal heparin preparations. *Thromb Haemost* 1981; 46:680A.
4. Powers PJ, Carter C, Kelton J, et al: Heparin-associated thrombocytopenia: A randomized trial comparing beef lung and pork intestinal mucosal heparin. *Blood* 1981; 58:720A.
5. Bell WR, Tomasulo PA, Alving BM, et al: Thrombocytopenia occurring during the administration of heparin: A prospective study in 52 patients. *Ann Intern Med* 1976; 85:155–160.
6. Cines DB, Kaywin P, Bina M, et al: Heparin associated thrombocytopenia. *Arch Intern Med* 1978; 138:548–552.
7. Nelson JC, Lerner RG, Goldstein R, et al: Heparin-induced thrombocytopenia. *Arch Intern Med* 1978; 138:548–552.
8. Green D, Harris K, Reynolds N, et al: Heparin immune thrombocytopenia: Evidence for a heparin-platelet complex as the antigenic determinant. *J Lab Clin Med* 1978; 91:167–175.
9. King DJ, Kelton JG: Heparin-associated thrombocytopenia. *Ann Intern Med* 1984; 100:535–540.
10. Olinger GN, Hussey CV, Olive JA, et al: Cardiopulmonary bypass for patients with previously documented heparin-induced platelet aggregation. *J Thorac Cardiovasc Surg* 1984; 87:673–677.
11. Pansard Y, de Prost D, Hvass U, de Brux JL, et al: Problèmes posés par les thrombopénies induites par l'héparine dans une service de chirurgie cardiovasculaire. *Ann Chir Thorac Cardiovasc* 1984; 38:119–123.
12. Guay DRP, Richard A: Heparin-induced thrombocytopenia: Association with a platelet aggregating factor and cross-sensitivity to bovine and porcine heparin. *Drug Intell Clin Pharm* 1984; 18:398–401.
13. Harenberg J, Zimmerman R, Schwarz F, et al: Treatment of heparin-induced thrombocytopenia with thrombosis by a new heparinoid. *Lancet* 1983; I:986–987.
14. Roussi JH, Houbouyan LL, Goquel AF: Use of low-molecular-weight heparin in heparin-induced thrombocytopenia with thrombotic complications. *Lancet* 1984; I:1183.
15. Kappa JR, Ellison N, Fisher CA, et al: The use of Iloprost (ZK 3637 4) to permit cardiopulmonary bypass in two patients with heparin-induced thrombocytopenia. *Anesthesiology* 1985; 63:A32.

53

Postoperative Prolongation of Activated Clotting Time

A 60-year-old man underwent coronary artery bypass grafting for three-vessel disease. The entire procedure was uneventful except for considerable clinical oozing postbypass. The patient had been taking only nitroglycerin and propranolol for his heart disease; he was on no other medication. Activated clotting time (ACT) was used to calculate protamine administration. The ACT had initially returned to baseline, but one hour after arrival in the CCU the ACT was slightly prolonged. The computed protamine dose (50 mg) was administered; however, moderate chest drainage continued and the ACT remained slightly prolonged.

Recommendations by Norig Ellison, M.D.

ANALYSIS OF THE PROBLEM

If a normal screening hemostatic profile and a negative history for bleeding have been obtained preoperatively, including an activated partial thromboplastin time (APTT), the possibility of a preexisting defect can essentially be ruled out. The best way to detect a hemorrhagic diathesis is by a properly taken history. Particularly important in the history is determining the hemostatic response to any prior surgical experience. Also, keep in mind that defects in platelet quantity or quality will not be detected by an ACT.

For these reasons in this patient the probable cause of bleeding can be attributed to either of two mechanisms: coagulation factor deficiency or heparin effect. Furthermore, the description of ". . . considerable clinical oozing postbypass. . ." also suggests a nonsurgical cause rather than one or more discrete bleeders that require surgical attention. The most likely problem in this patient is heparin rebound.

APPROACH TO THE PROBLEM

In a patient whose ACT returns to normal and is later prolonged and that prolongation is associated with excessive bleeding, heparin rebound is the most likely explanation. Heparin rebound was originally described by Kolff et al. as "a treacherous phenomenon in which heparin is neutralized by protamine and the protamine leaves the bloodstream first, thereby leaving the heparin uncovered."[1] The entity remains controversial in that some authorities deny its existence and others find rebound in the majority of their cases. We believe that heparin rebound is a rare, but real, entity that should be considered in patients whose clinical course is similar to that described in this case.[2] The entity is easily diagnosed with a protamine titration (as discussed below) and responds rapidly to the administration of a small dose of protamine, usually less than 50 mg.[3-4] Table 53–1 lists the several theories that have been proposed to explain why heparin rebound occurs.

DISCUSSION

Causes of Bleeding in the Postbypass Period

The leading cause of excessive bleeding following cardiopulmonary bypass is inadequate surgical hemostasis.[5] Other potential causes are (1) preexisting diseases, (2) platelet deficiencies, (3) acquired coagulation factor deficiencies, and (4) heparin effect.[6]

Two types of acquired defects in coagulation factors, other than inhibition of coagulation factors by heparin anticoagulation, can theoretically produce a similar picture to that seen in this patient. However, as mentioned above, in both types the deficiency produced must be very severe to produce prolongation of the ACT. The first is disseminated intravascular coagulation (DIC), which is a pathologic syndrome in which the deposition of thrombin and fibrin within the vascular tree suggests the onset of a widespread intravascular coagulation.[7] In this patient the procedure is described as otherwise uneventful, and in the absence of shock, hemoglobinuria suggesting an incompatible blood transfusion, or some other obvious mechanism for initiating DIC, it is not a likely cause of this patient's prolonged ACT and continued bleeding. Second, if the patient continues to bleed whole blood, which is replaced with packed

TABLE 53–1.

Proposed Theories to Explain Why Heparin Rebound Occurs*

DATE	SUGGESTED CAUSE OF REBOUND
1957	Heparin may be released by red blood cell breakdown.
1958	Heparin may escape from the circulation into the extravascular space and return via the lymphatics and thoracic duct to the circulation many hours later.
1959	Heparin may be injected into tissues instead of intravenously, forming a depot source for prolonged absorption.
1961	A part of the heparin level may be temporarily neutralized by an endogenous antagonist, not otherwise specified.
1962	Protamine may be removed by metabolism or may be combined with other plasma proteins before heparin is removed.
1966	Protamine chloride does not produce heparin rebound, although protamine sulfate does, possibly due to more rapid metabolism of protamine sulfate.
1970	Heparin rebound is seen more commonly with hypothermia, possibly because heparin levels do not decay as rapidly during hypothermic perfusions.
1974	For a given heparin level, low levels of platelets result in a more pronounced effect of that heparin level on the coagulation mechanism. Since thrombocytopenia is a common occurrence following open heart surgery, it is quite possible that heparin activity may be enhanced.
1981	Mechanical devices used to measure heparin levels may produce false-positive results.

*Adapted from Ellison N, Beatty CP, Blake DR, et al: Heparin rebound: Studies in patients and volunteers. *J Thorac Cardiovasc Surg* 1974; 67:723–729.

red blood cells (RBCs) and crystalloid, a decrease in coagulation factor levels will be produced. However, such a drop is not likely to be of the magnitude required to affect the ACT. Producing RBCs from whole blood increases the hematocrit from 35%–45% to 60%–70%. Therefore, RBC units do contain plasma sufficient to keep coagulation factor levels well in excess of 1.0%. Accordingly, sufficient coagulation factors should be present to produce a normal ACT and make a coagulopathy on this basis alone most unlikely.[8]

Tests of Coagulation

There are a number of tests available of the coagulation system.

Hattersley introduced the activated coagulation time (ACT) of whole blood in 1966 as ". . . a simple, reliable and reasonably sensitive bedside test of the coagulation mechanism" and stated that "immediate activation of freshly drawn blood by an inert diatomite greatly shortens the coagulation time (normal mean, 1 minute 47 seconds; standard deviation 13 seconds) and produces a rather sensitive test for coagulation defects."[9] Clearly, the ACT was a giant step forward from the Lee-White whole blood coagulation time originally described in 1903 by two men, one of whom (Paul Dudley White) went on to receive greater recognition in cardiology than in hematology.[10] Nevertheless, today the ACT is considered but a poor screening test of the intrinsic system and informative only if significantly prolonged—e.g., factor levels greater than 1.0% will usually provide normal values.[11] As reported by Hattersley, factor VII levels and platelet deficiencies are not detected by the ACT. Because of these intrinsic limitations, the ACT has been replaced in large measure by the activated partial thromboplastin time (APTT) as a screening test.

Why then has the test gained such great popularity for monitoring anticoagulation with heparin during cardiopulmonary bypass? There are two reasons: (1) The classic work of Bull and associates, which clearly demonstrated that treatment of all patients with 300 units heparin/kg may produce instances where the blood is inadequately or excessively anticoagulated, was performed with the *manual* ACT as the monitoring test.[12] (2) The introduction of *automated* ACT devices, in which electrical, magnetic, mechanical, or optical means are used to detect the end point, has resulted in a very convenient method of monitoring the effect of administered heparin on the coagulation mechanism.[13] For the anesthesiologist who is also concerned with the administration of anesthesia and other drugs, ensuring adequacy of ventilation and normovolemic status, and monitoring hemodynamic values, the convenience of the automated ACT is probably paramount in explaining its widespread acceptance. The characteristics of the ideal test of hemostasis designed for use in the operating room by an anesthesiologist are listed in Table 53–2.

One final point in monitoring heparin anticoagulation: is it more important to monitor the concentration of heparin or its effect on the coagulation mecha-

TABLE 53–2.

Characteristics of the Ideal Operating Room Test of Hemostasis for Use by an Anesthesiologist*

Necessary maneuvers are simple and yield reproducible results.
Equipment is compact, inexpensive, and operates quietly.
Results are available quickly, even when clotting is markedly prolonged.
Test is performed on whole blood rather than plasma.
Test does not require prolonged attention away from the operator's usual duties.

*Adapted from Jobes DR, Schwartz AJ, Ellison N, et al: Monitoring heparin anticoagulation and its neutralization. *Ann Thorac Surg* 1981; 31:161–166.

nism? In addition to being more convenient to monitor, the latter would seem to be more important—i.e., it matters not how many units of heparin per cubic centimeter are present if sufficient paralysis of the hemostatic mechanism does not ensue.[14] While measurement of heparin level is highly desirable in all cases, such measurement is highly essential in cases in which excessive bleeding ensues, to rule out one of the major potential causes of bleeding.

Protamine Titration

The question of heparin effect can readily be answered by means of a protamine titration, which can be performed in a qualitative or quantitative manner.[13] In the former, 10μg of protamine is added to one of two test tubes to each of which 1.0 cc of blood is subsequently added. If blood in the tube containing protamine clots first, heparin was present and neutralized so that the blood clotted before that in the tube containing no protamine. Conversely, if the blood in the tube containing protamine clots more slowly, no heparin was present and the protamine exerted an in vitro anticoagulant effect so that the blood clotted first in the tube without protamine. By adding protamine to several test tubes in 10μg increments, usually from 0 to 50μg, this test can be made quantitative. Multiplying the concentration in the test tube whose blood clots first and the estimated blood volume will determine an accurate protamine dose to be administered to that patient. This includes multiplying by 0 if blood in the tube containing no protamine clots first, indicating that there is no heparin effect.

REFERENCES

1. Kolff WJ, Effler DB, Groves LK, et al: Disposable membrane oxygenator (heart-lung machine) and its use in experimental surgery. *Cleve Clin Q* 1956; 23:69–79.
2. Ellison N, Beatty CP, Blake DR, et al: Heparin rebound: Studies in patients and volunteers. *J Thorac Cardiovasc Surg* 1974; 67:723–729.
3. Pifarré R, Babka R, Sullivan HJ, et al: Management of postoperative heparin rebound following cardiopulmonary bypass. *J Thorac Cardiovasc Surg* 1981; 81:378–381.
4. Jobes DR, Schwartz AJ, Ellison N: Heparin rebound, letter. *J Thorac Cardiovasc Surg* 1981; 82:940–941.
5. McKenna AR, Bachman F, Whittaker B, et al: The hemostatic response after open heart surgery: II. Frequency of abnormal function during and after extracorporeal circulation. *J Thorac Cardiovasc Surg* 1975; 70:298–308.
6. Ellison N: Practical control of hemostasis. *Cleve Clin Q* 1981; 48:104–111.
7. Ellison N: Diagnosis of bleeding disorders. *Anesthesiology* 1977; 47:171–180.
8. Greenwalt TJ (ed): *General Principles of Blood Transfusion.* Chicago, American Medical Association, 1977.

9. Hattersley PG: Activated coagulation time of whole blood. *JAMA* 1966; 1986:436–440.
10. Lee RI, White PD: A clinical study of the coagulation time of blood. *Am J Med Sci* 1913; 145:495–503.
11. Weintrobe MW, Lee CR, Boggs DR, et al (eds): *Clinical Hematology,* ed 8. Philadelphia, Lea & Febiger, 1981, 1057.
12. Bull BS, Huse WM, Brauer FS, et al: Heparin therapy during extracorporeal circulation: II. The use of a dose-response curve to individualize heparin and protamine dosage. *J Thorac Cardiovasc Surg* 1975; 69:685–689.
13. Jobes DR, Schwartz AJ, Ellison N, et al: Monitoring heparin anticoagulation and its neutralization. *Ann Thorac Surg* 1981, 31:161–166.
14. Ellison N, Jobes DR, Schwartz AJ: Implications of anticoagulant therapy. *Intl Anesthesiol Clin* 1982; 20:121–136.

54

Platelet Infusion and Hypotension

A 55-year-old male with ischemic heart disease underwent an uneventful coronary artery bypass grafting operation. However, there appeared to be more bleeding than normal and the platelet count was 100,000/cu mm. Administration of a unit of platelet concentrate was begun, and shortly thereafter the patient's blood pressure decreased to 60/50 mm Hg, with a pulmonary artery wedge pressure of 2 mm Hg.

Recommendations by James H. Diaz, M.D.

ANALYSIS OF THE PROBLEM

The temporal relationship of platelet concentrate administration and the development of severe, life-threatening hypotension suggests that the platelets caused vasodilation. Vasodilation is the most likely problem since there is hypotension and an abnormally low pulmonary artery wedge pressure.

APPROACH TO THE PROBLEM

To avoid hypotension, platelets should be thawed, if frozen, or allowed to warm to room temperature, if fresh. They should be infused slowly and unfiltered at a rate of 10–20 ml/minute into a warmed patient through a large bore intravenous cannula in a peripheral vein. Rapid infusion of platelets into the central circulation may overwhelm the patient's capacity after CPB to inactivate vasoactive substances liberated by the platelet release reaction. Should

TABLE 54–1.

Complications of Platelet Infusion

ACUTE COMPLICATIONS	
Allergic	Nonallergic
Allergic hypotension	Nonallergic hypotension
IgE-mediated	Protamine-mediated
IgA deficiency	Kinin-mediated
	Heparin-mediated
Pulmonary hypersensitivity	
Transfusion reaction	
Nonhemolytic	
Hemolytic	

CHRONIC COMPLICATIONS
Serum sickness
Rh isoimmunization
Platelet isoimmunization

hypotension occur on platelet infusion, volume loading with blood or crystalloid can be initiated and guided by right atrial pressures. After hemodynamic stabilization, platelet infusion can be resumed slowly and through a more peripheral site if possible. The slower the platelet infusion, the warmer the patient after CPB, and the more time elapsed between protamine reversal and platelet infusion, the lower the likelihood of hypotension on platelet infusion.

Prolonged severe hypotension on platelet infusion suggests an allergic or anaphylactic reaction. These reactions are mediated by anti-IgA or IgE antibodies to plasma proteins that direct the massive release of histamine, serotonin, and prostaglandins from mast cells and basophils. Such reactions will require cessation of platelet infusion, volume resuscitation, correction of metabolic acidosis, and intravenous administration of H_1- and H_2-receptor antagonists, glucocorticoids, and epinephrine. Subsequent determination of the etiology of the allergic response will provide valuable information for patients who are likely to require further blood component therapy (Table 54–1). Patients with IgA deficiency should be identified by serum electrophoresis postoperatively and treated with IgA-deficient blood products in the future.

DISCUSSION

Hemostatic abnormalities are commonly associated with cardiopulmonary bypass (CPB) and may include thrombocytopenia, clotting factor deficiencies, disseminated intravascular coagulation (DIC), and primary fibrinogenolysis.

These abnormalities are often reflected in hemostatic screening tests as prolongation of the prothrombin time (PT), activated clotting time (ACT), and activated partial thromboplastin time (APTT), reduced platelet counts, and platelet dysfunction. Primary fibrinogenolysis and DIC are rarely encountered with modern-day cardiopulmonary bypass.[1] Thrombocytopenia, platelet dysfunction, and clotting factor deficiencies occur often after CPB. Thrombocytopenia and platelet dysfunction are now the most commonly reported hemostatic abnormalities after discontinuance of CPB and heparin reversal with protamine sulfate.[2] Less widely appreciated than the decline in platelet numbers after CPB is platelet dysfunction, a disturbance in platelet effectiveness in promoting clot formation. Besides CPB, preoperative medications, heparin anticoagulation and its reversal with protamine, and even anesthetic agents may reduce platelet numbers and limit platelet effectiveness after CPB.

Platelet quantity is reflected by the platelet volume of distribution and a normal total platelet count of 150,000 to 300,000/cu mm. Platelet functional activity can be directly assessed by tests of platelet aggregation, adhesiveness, or clot retraction. Special assays for such platelet-specific chemicals as platelet factor 4 (PF4), thromboxane B_2 (TXB$_2$), thromboxane A_2 (TXA$_2$), prostacyclin (PGI$_2$), and β-thromboglobulin (BTG) have now been developed but are not in widespread clinical use. Platelet functional activity may also be assessed by bleeding time and, possibly, by the ACT.[3]

At the time of surgery, cardiac patients may have a variety of preexisting deficits in platelet numbers or function caused by their medications or other diseases. Platelet deficiency or dysfunction can often be disclosed by a preoperative history of petechiae; tendency to bruise easily; and prolonged bleeding from minor cuts, abrasions, or dental extractions. Preexisting platelet abnormalities in cardiac patients will be aggravated by subsequent CPB and should be evaluated by preoperative assessment of platelet number and function.

Drugs and their metabolites that can induce autoimmune platelet destruction include quinine, quinidine, sulfonamides, digoxin, rifampin, morphine, heroin, α-methyldopa, and even heparin (see Chapter 52).[4] Quinidine, digoxin, α-methyldopa, and "minidose" heparin therapy may often be prescribed in cardiac patients. Drug withdrawal usually reverses these drug-induced immune thrombocytopenias. Steroid therapy may be indicated for rare persistent cases of drug-induced thrombocytopenia. Drugs that limit platelet function by inhibition of prostaglandin (TXB$_2$, TXA$_2$, PGI$_2$) synthesis include aspirin, indomethacin, phenylbutazone, sulfinpyrazone, and ibuprofen.[4] Large doses of most penicillins can coat platelet membranes and impair platelet interaction with disrupted vascular endothelium.[4] Decreased platelet production may characterize bone marrow depression by radiation, industrial toxins, chronic infections, or neoplastic infiltration. Several studies have now documented augmented platelet adhesiveness and aggregability in diabetes, a common condition in cardiac surgical patients.[5] Other disease states associated with alterations of platelet function include autoimmune diseases, liver disease, renal failure, vitamin deficiencies, and viral infections.

Anesthetic agents, heparin and protamine, and the biomechanical effects of CPB may all act to reduce platelet numbers and effectiveness during cardiac surgery. Ueda has shown that nitrous oxide (N_2O) and halothane are capable of inhibiting platelet aggregation induced by adenosine diphosphate (ADP) at clinical doses.[6] Kalter and colleagues[1] also described impaired ADP aggregation during halothane-N_2O anesthesia for cardiac surgery. In their study, impaired platelet aggregation occurred only during CPB and not during induction or sternotomy, suggesting that CPB—not anesthesia or surgery alone—was also responsible.[1] Large-dose heparin boluses for CPB can promote platelet aggregation and release with transient thrombocytopenia.[7] Thrombocytopenia during CPB may also result from mechanical destruction of platelets, platelet adhesion to pump hardware, hepatic sequestration of platelets, and dilution of the circulating platelet pool by pump primes and blood transfusions. Platelet dysfunction after CPB may result from platelet refractoriness to ADP stimulation,[1] platelet membrane changes or coatings,[3] and hypothermia.[5] Even protamine reversal of heparin anticoagulation for CPB can induce platelet aggregation with pulmonary and hepatic sequestration of aggregates and transient thrombocytopenia.[8–10] The transient accumulation of radioactively labeled platelets has now been clearly demonstrated in dog lungs (^{51}Cr-labeled)[9] and human livers (^{111}In-labeled)[10] following administration of protamine.

With perioperative deficits in platelet numbers and function so common in the cardiac patient, it is no surprise that cardiac surgery is the most frequent surgical indication for platelet transfusions.[1] Other indications for platelet transfusions include massive hemorrhage, massive blood transfusion, patients about to undergo surgery with platelet counts below 50,000/cu mm, and nonsurgical patients with platelet counts less than 20,000/cu mm.

Acute complications on platelet infusion may include hemolytic and nonhemolytic transfusion reactions, pulmonary hypersensitivity response with pulmonary edema, allergic hypotension, and nonallergic hypotension.[11] Chronic complications of platelet transfusion may include serum sickness, Rh isoimmunization, and isoimmunization to platelet antigens. Allergic and nonallergic hypotension and platelet isoimmunization appear to be the most common complications of platelet infusions. Serum sickness and Rh isoimmunization are rare results of contamination of platelet concentrates with incompatible plasma or red blood cells (see Table 54–1).

Allergic hypotension and pulmonary hypersensitivity response are usually the results of allergic reaction to plasma proteins in the 40 to 50 ml of plasma in which 5.5×10^{10} platelets per pack are suspended. Incompatible plasma proteins and antileukocyte antibodies have been suggested as being responsible for these reactions by promoting direct release of vasoactive mediators from basophils and mast cells with systemic vasodilation and hypotension. [11] Other groups susceptible to the development of allergic reaction when given blood or platelets are those with a deficiency of IgA antibodies in their plasma. [11] These patients develop anti-IgA antibodies that provoke an anaphylactic reaction when blood products such as plasma or platelets are administered. [10] Should platelet transfusion be indicated in these patients, the use of fresh or frozen platelet concentrates prepared from IgA-deficient donors is indicated. [11]

Although not a true allergic reaction, hypotension on rapid infusion of platelets, plasma, or heat-treated plasma protein fraction may occur after CPB due to impaired inactivation of bradykinin-like substances in the lungs. [11, 12] Other causes of nonallergic hypotension on platelet infusion after CPB may result from platelet interaction with either heparin or protamine. Apart from "minidose" heparin-induced autoimmune thrombocytopenia, heparin bolus doses for CPB can result in aggregation and release of both circulating and infused platelets. As noted, this platelet-release reaction liberates such vasoactive substances as histamine, serotonin, PGI_2, and TXA_2.

Protamine-platelet interaction was first described in dogs in 1949. [8] Like heparin, protamine also appears to be a powerful stimulator of platelet aggregation and release, especially in the massively heparinized patient recently weaned from CPB. [8] The infusion of fresh platelets shortly after heparin reversal with protamine may provide such a sizable bolus of platelets to be aggregated and released by protamine that large quantities of histamine, serotonin, PGI_2, and thromboxanes are liberated. [8] Systemic vasodilation with severe hypotension may result. Impaired pulmonary inactivation of vasoactive substances may prolong the hypotensive response to platelet-protamine interaction. Platelet-protamine interaction appears to be a very common cause of hypotension on platelet infusion in the period immediately following CPB. [8]

Platelet transfusions are indicated following prolonged CPB and after heparin reversal, if bleeding continues with prolonged bleeding time and ACT in the absence of heparin activity to protamine titration. Platelet transfusions in cardiac surgery should be based on preoperative assessment for platelet-related bleeding tendencies, should not be administered for hypovolemia or moderate hemorrhage, and are best withheld until heparin reversal and stabilization of circulating blood volume after CPB. The platelet counts may be low, but, as in the case presented, a platelet count does not evaluate platelet function. As platelet function tests are time consuming and expensive, plasma and platelet infusions are often begun empirically after CPB because of continued bleeding and such prolonged nonspecific tests as ACT or bleeding time. [3]

SUMMARY

Platelet infusions are often indicated for thrombocytopenia or platelet dysfunction after CPB. Continued bleeding, prolonged bleeding time and ACT, absence of heparin activity on automated protamine titration, and a platelet count over 50,000/cu mm suggest thrombasthenia or platelet dysfunction. Hypotension on platelet infusion may occur with rapid infusion into the central circulation of hypothermic patients shortly after decannulation from CPB and heparin reversal with protamine. Slow, peripheral intravenous infusion of platelets into normothermic patients 30 minutes or more following administration of protamine will reduce the likelihood of hypotension on platelet infusion. Although serious hypotension on platelet infusion may be mediated by drugs, immunoglobulins, or kinins, the pathophysiologic mechanisms are the same—vasodilation and shock—as are the treatments—volume expansion and epinephrine (see Table 54–1).

REFERENCES

1. Kalter RD, Saul CM, Wetstein H, et al: Cardiopulmonary bypass: Associated hemostatic abnormalities. *J Thorac Cardiovasc Surg* 1979; 77:427–435.
2. Salzman WE: Blood platelets and extracorporeal circulation. *Transfusion* 1963; 3:274–277.
3. Moorehead MT, Westengart JC, Bull BS: Platelet involvement in the activated clotting time of heparinized blood. *Anesth Analg* 1984; 63:394–398.
4. Moake JL, Funicella T: *Common Bleeding Problems: CIBA Clinical Symposia.* Summit, NJ, CIBA Pharmaceutical Co, vol 35, 1983.
5. Hammerschmidt DE: Platelets and the environment. *JAMA* 1982; 247:345–350.
6. Ueda I: The effects of volatile general anesthetics on adenosine diphosphate-induced platelet aggregation. *Anesthesiology* 1971; 34:405–408.
7. Bjoraker DG, Ketcham TR: Hemodynamics and platelet release with heparin. *Anesthesiology* 1981; 55:A25.
8. Bjoraker DG, Ketcham TR: In vivo platelet response to clinical protamine sulfate infusion. *Anesthesiology* 1982; 57:A7.
9. Radegran K, Bergentz SE, Lewis DH, et al: Pulmonary effects of protamine-induced platelet aggregation: Intravascular obstruction or vasoconstriction. *Scand J Clin Lab Invest* 1971; 28:423–427.
10. Heyns AD, Lotter MG, Badenhorst PN, et al: Kinetics and in vivo redistribution of [111]Indium-labelled human platelets after intravenous protamine sulphate. *Thromb Haemost* 1980; 44:65–68.
11. Stoelting RK: Allergic reactions during anesthesia. *Anesth Analg* 1983; 62:341–356.
12. Bland JHL, Laver MD, Lowenstein E: Vasodilator effect of commercial 5% plasma protein fraction solutions. *JAMA* 1973; 224:1721–1724.

55

Management of Hematocrit of 25%

A 55-year-old woman underwent coronary artery bypass for three-vessel disease. The procedure was uneventful except that her preoperative hematocrit value was 40%, and postbypass it was 25%. Although the anesthetic and hemodynamic states were without complication, the question of whether to transfuse this patient arose.

Recommendations by Norman J. Starr, M.D.

ANALYSIS OF THE PROBLEM

This case raises the question of whether a patient with a normal hematocrit reading preoperatively requires transfusion during a well-conducted operation.

APPROACH TO THE PROBLEM

Patients undergoing primary operation do not require transfusion if care is given to hemostasis and if blood scavenging techniques are employed.

DISCUSSION

Although patients with coronary artery disease have a reduced blood volume,[1, 2] most adult patients scheduled for primary cardiac revascularization procedures do not require transfusion of blood or blood products.[3, 4] When a composite of conservation techniques is practiced, blood or blood product administration should only result from a demonstrable patient need. The data demonstrating the cardiac surgical patients' tolerances of a nonblood prime[5, 6] for use during cardiopulmonary bypass and for normovolemic anemia following bypass[7, 8] have been available for several years. However, the recent alarm among clinicians over potential spread of communicable diseases through transfusion and the potential detrimental cardiovascular responses to blood or blood products[9, 10] have renewed interest in eliminating patient exposure to blood products on a routine basis. Blood conservation is not associated with unusual morbidity or mortality.[11]

Rather than requesting a complete crossmatch, there is a very good possibility this patient would require only an order for blood typing and screening during this hospitalization. It is now quite predictable that primary myocardial revascularization patients will require blood intraoperatively.[11] Those patients with a red blood cell volume greater than 1,600 ml and under age 70 have a greater than 90% chance of not requiring blood throughout their hospitalization, provided a few clear principles are followed rigorously.

These principles include:

1. Appropriate discontinuation of those drugs that interfere with coagulation.

2. Meticulous surgical hemostasis.

3. Acceptance of normovolemic anemia with substitution of appropriate volume expanders for blood or blood products.

4. Reinfusion of all pump oxygenator contents into the patient following cardiopulmonary bypass.

5. Reinfusion of the patient's washed and concentrated red blood cells that were collected in a heparinized suction apparatus.

6. Retransfusion of shed mediastinal blood.

7. Philosophy by the surgical and anesthesia team that most patients will not receive blood or blood products.

Surgical hemostasis must be meticulous from the initial skin incision. The dictum that "if the patient is dry going in, the patient will be dry coming out" carries great weight. Surgical hemostasis cannot wait until the interval following cardiopulmonary bypass. By then the coagulation cascade may be activated by the coagulation debris prior to systemic heparinization. Until proved otherwise, the philosophy should exist that any primary cardiac surgical patient who remains in the operating room (OR) for extensive bleeding, or is returned to the OR because of extensive bleeding, has a lesion correctable by surgical technical expertise. To further maximize effects, all attempts to stop "surgical bleeding" should be made prior to the administration of blood.

Acute normovolemic anemia in cardiac surgical patients has been proven to be well tolerated during the bypass and postoperative period.[8] The absolute degree of anemia tolerated below a hematocrit reading of 20% is not well documented and requires patient individualization. With a reduced hematocrit reading, cardiac output is increased as a consequence of the vasodilation noted with decreased viscosity and increased venous return, not as compensation for inadequate oxygen delivery to tissues.[12,13] Therefore, the hemodynamic response to normovolemic anemia is primarily passive and accountable on the basis of decreased viscosity. As a result, when removing the patient from cardiopulmonary bypass, support of blood pressure may require some intermittent and temporary pharmacologic vasopressor support. However, the diuresis that patients routinely undergo following bypass is associated with the hematocrit reading rising to a level near 30% prior to their transfer from the operating room.

Because the patients are vasodilated, they can accept large volumes of fluid in the postbypass period. This can be accomplished by returning the oxygenator plus tubing contents[14] to the patient either directly from the pump or through sterile transfer into bags that the anesthesia team may transfuse intravenously. If the previous steps have been followed, little or no advantage is gained by removing blood from the patient prior to bypass for subsequent reinfusion following bypass.

If there are further volume requirements, the use of the less expensive hydroxyethyl starch should be considered. It has been documented to be equal in all parameters to albumin during administration to patients undergoing myocardial revascularization.[15] These parameters include fluid administration, urine output, weight change, colloid osmotic pressure, intrapulmonary shunt, coagulation profiles, hemoglobin levels, and chest drainage.

When a heparinized collecting system is used intraoperatively to salvage blood from the surgical field during the intervals the patient is not heparinized, the red blood cells may be separated and washed. Depending upon the urgency, those red blood cells can be reinfused during or immediately following surgery to increase the hematocrit reading and reduce homologous blood utilization.[16, 17]

Through the use of a closed-circuit collection and reinfusion system, shed mediastinal blood can be reinfused for up to 24 hours postoperatively, although it is rarely needed that long. Shed mediastinal blood does not clot and does not affect the patient's coagulation system. The clinical safety of this technique is confirmed by the lack of septic, hematologic, pulmonary, renal, or hepatic complications.[18] Though not well documented for its ability to reduce blood utilization in cases in which blood conservation is aggressively practiced,[19] it is of significant value in those patients that do bleed suddenly and in larger amounts.

Consistent with the philosophy of requiring the patient to demonstrate a need for the administration of blood, rather than administering the blood routinely, is a similar philosophy concerning use of blood products, such as fresh frozen plasma and platelets.[20] The known alterations in coagulation status can be used to advantage in making decisions concerning administration of blood coagulation products when no homologous blood has been used.[21] The platelet count may be expected to drop by 37% during cardiopulmonary bypass, but following operation the count will quickly recover to 75% of the preoperative level. Absolute platelet counts in the range of 60,000/ml do not necessarily predispose hemorrhage requiring transfusion. The largest reduction in a coagulation factor is V, which is reduced approximately 31% following surgery; however, it rapidly increases to 15% greater than preoperative levels within 48 hours. Factor VIII does increase reflecting the stress of operation. Fibrin split products rise immediately following median sternotomy, secondary to bone marrow embolization, activating thromboplastin. However, this does not contribute to bleeding following cardiopulmonary bypass bleeding if there is meticulous surgical care.

Summary

When a patient scheduled for primary myocardial revascularization has an adequate red blood cell volume prior to the operation, with the acceptance of normovolemic anemia, the need for blood or blood products is not established.

REFERENCES

1. Hanson EL, Kane PB, Askanazi J, et al: Comparison of patients with coronary artery or valve disease: Intraoperative differences in blood volume and observations of vasomotor response. *Ann Thorac Surg* 1976; 22:343.
2. Cohn LH, Kloverkorn P, Moore FD, et al: Intrinsic plasma volume deficits in patients with coronary artery disease. *Arch Surg* 1974; 108:57.
3. Weniger J, Shanahan R: Reduction of bank blood requirements in cardiac surgery. *J Thorac Cardiovasc Surg* 1982; 30:142.
4. Cosgrove DM, Thurer RL, Lytle BW, et al: Blood conservation during myocardial revascularization. *Ann Thorac Surg* 1979; 28:184.
5. Panico FG, Neptune WB: A mechanism to eliminate donor blood prime from the pump oxygenator. *Surg Forum* 1959; 10:605.
6. Verska JJ, Ludington LG, Brewer LA III: A comparative study of cardiopulmonary bypass with non-blood and blood prime. *Ann Thorac Surg* 1974; 18:72.

7. Cooley DA, Bloodwell RD, Beal AC, et al: Cardiac valve replacement without blood transfusion. *Am J Surg* 1966; 112:743.

8. Hallowell P, Bland JHL, Dalton BC, et al: The effects of hemodilution with albumin or Ringer's lactate on water balance and blood use in open-heart surgery. *Ann Thorac Surg* 1978; 25:22.

9. Fresh frozen plasma: Indications and risks. Consensus Conference, NIH. *JAMA* 1985; 253:551.

10. Bove JR: Fresh frozen plasma: Too few indications—too much use, editorial. *Anesth Analg* 1985; 64:849.

11. Cosgrove DM, Loop FD, Lytle BW, et al: Determinants of blood utilization during myocardial revascularization. *Ann Thorac Surg* 1985; 40:380.

12. Crowell JW, Ford RG, Lewis VM: Oxygen transport in hemorrhagic shock as a function of the hematocrit ratio. *Am J Physiol* 1959; 196:1033.

13. Keats AS: Hemodynamic consequences of hemodilution. *Cleve Clin Q* 1978; 45:39.

14. Moran JM, Babka R, Silberman S, et al: Immediate centrifugation of oxygenator contents after cardiopulmonary bypass: Role in maximum blood conservation. *J Thorac Cardiovasc Surg* 1978; 76:570.

15. Kirklin JK, Lell WA, Kouchoukos NT: Hydroxyethyl starch versus albumin for colloid infusion following cardiopulmonary bypass in patients undergoing myocardial revascularization. *Ann Thorac Surg* 1984; 37:40.

16. Johnson RG, Rosenkrantz KR, Preston RA, et al: The efficacy of postoperative autotransfusion in patients undergoing cardiac operations. *Ann Thorac Surg* 1983; 36:173.

17. Winton TL, Charrette EJP, Salerno TA: The cell saver during cardiac surgery: Does it save? *Ann Thorac Surg* 1982; 33:379.

18. Thurer RL, Lytle BW, Cosgrove DM, et al: Autotransfusion following cardiac operations: A randomized prospective study. *Ann Thorac Surg* 1979; 27:500.

19. Bayer WL, Coenen WM, Jenkins DC, et al: The use of blood and blood components in 1,769 patients undergoing open-heart surgery. *Ann Thorac Surg* 1980; 29:117.

20. Milam JD, Austin SF, Martin RF, et al: Alteration of coagulation and selected clinical chemistry parameters in patients undergoing open heart surgery without transfusions. *Am J Clin Pathol* 1981; 76:155.

21. Tector AJ, Gabriel RP, Mateicka WE, et al: Reduction of blood usage in open heart surgery. *Chest* 1976; 70:454.

56

Patient Refractory to Heparinization

A 45-year-old woman underwent coronary artery bypass surgery for two-vessel disease. Just prior to cardiopulmonary bypass, the calculated dose of heparin (4 mg/kg) was administered. An activated clotting time (ACT) performed five minutes later revealed an ACT of 280 seconds; baseline was 80 seconds. The patient had no history of clotting disorders and was on no medications other than nitroglycerin and atenolol.

Recommendations by Ron Ruff, M.D.

ANALYSIS OF THE PROBLEM

This patient did not respond normally to a generous heparin dose. Because an ACT of at least 300 seconds is desired before instituting cardiopulmonary bypass, a strategy for patient anticoagulation must be outlined and followed.

APPROACH TO THE PROBLEM

The initial step in patient management is creation of a dose-response heparin vs. ACT graph and extrapolating the additional necessary dose of heparin this patient would require to prolong the ACT to 300.

Alternatively, or if additional heparin does not acceptably prolong the ACT, the clinician could consider administering fresh frozen plasma as an exogenous source of antithrombin III to "normalize" this patient's heparin and ACT dose-response curve. Sabbath et al. state that patients treated in this manner will require less protamine sulfate to reverse the heparin effect.[1] However, there are multiple risks associated with blood and blood product transfusion and I would be very hesitant to employ this treatment in this patient.

DISCUSSION

Control of blood coagulation and its prolongation due to heparin has allowed extracorporeal circulation to be used for cardiac operations. Heparin is a complex acid mucopolysaccharide, isolated from mast cells particularly in pork intestinal mucosa or beef lung tissue.

The mechanism of anticoagulation due to heparin involves heparin's ability to dramatically accelerate the action of antithrombin on thrombin.[2–8] Antithrombin is the principal plasma antagonist of thrombin by binding to thrombin at its active serine center in a 1:1 stoichiometric complex.[9,10] It is also known that heparin interacts with other components of the coagulation cascade such as clotting factors IX-A and X-A, which may also prolong coagulation.[11]

Hattersley described the procedure for the activated clotting time (ACT)[12] and it appears to be an ideal coagulation technique for monitoring heparin therapy as there is a linear correlation between whole blood coagulation time and the ACT.[13,14] Optimal level of the ACT during cardiopulmonary bypass has been arbitrarily selected to be 480 seconds, although clinically it has been observed that blood clots do not occur if the ACT is greater than 300 seconds.[14,15]

It is known that there is a wide range of sensitivity to heparin given to patients as measured by the ACT, and this may be due to the fact that there is not a linear relationship between plasma heparin concentration and the ACT.[16] Bull and associates have shown that a given dose of heparin may prolong the clotting time over a threefold range.[14] Esposito et al. noted in their study of patients receiving an initial heparin dose of 4 mg/kg for anticoagulation that only 47% of the patients would have been adequately anticoagulated as measured by an ACT over 400 seconds.[16] It is also known that there is a margin of product variability in heparin lots that may partially account for apparent patient response variability.[17]

The clinician should be aware that there are populations of patients who may appear resistant to the effects of heparin. Predictably, the patient with low antithrombin III levels (as in congenital anti-thrombin deficiency),[18] or decreased antithrombin III activity associated with the intake of oral contraceptives[19] will appear resistant. Patients with sepsis or disseminated intravascular coagulation (DIC) may appear resistant by generating serine proteases such as thrombin or plasmin that may act to bind antithrombin and lower its plasma concentration, often to 10% of that considered normal.[10, 20–22] It is also known that patients receiving intra-aortic balloon pump therapy may be resistant to heparin.[21]

Patients who have received heparin treatment preoperatively have been shown retrospectively to exhibit a lower ACT response to heparin that is not attributable to antithrombin III activity, fibrinogen concentration, or platelet count. The only predictive parameter of this resistance was a lower baseline ACT.[23]

Children and infants have also been shown to require more heparin than adults to prolong the ACT.[15, 24] To address the problem of the patient described above who was refractory to the 4 mg/kg dose of heparin, it should be noticed that she has none of the predisposing factors that we have discussed to explain her resistance except for her low baseline ACT of 80 seconds.

REFERENCES

1. Sabbath AH, Chung GKT, et al: Fresh frozen plasma: A solution to heparin resistance during cardiopulmonary bypass. *Ann Thorac Surg* 1984; 37:466–468.
2. Contejean CH: Recherches sur les injections intraveineuses de peptone et leur influence sur la coagulabilite du sang chez le chien. *Arch Physiol Norm Patho* 1985; 17:45–53.
3. Howell WH: The coagulation of blood. *Harvey Lect* 1917; 2:272–323.
4. Morawitz P: *Chemistry of Blood Coagulation.* Springfield, Ill, Charles C Thomas Publisher, 1968.
5. Brinkhous KM, Smith HP, Warner ED, et al: The inhibition of blood clotting: An unidentified substance which acts in conjunction with heparin to prevent the conversion of prothrombin into thrombin. *Am J Physiol* 1939; 125:683–687.
6. Waugh DF, Fitzgerald MA: Quantitative aspects of antithrombin and heparin in plasma. *Am J Physiol* 1956; 184:627–639.
7. Monkhouse FC, Frances ES, Seegers WH: Studies on the antithrombin and heparin cofactor activities of a fraction adsorbed from plasma by aluminum hydroxide. *Circ Res* 1955; 3:397–402.
8. Abildgaard U: Highly purified antithrombin III with heparin cofactor activity prepared by disc electrophoresis. *Scand J Clin Lab Invest* 1968; 21:89–91.
9. Rosenberg RD, Damus PS: The purification and mechanism of action of human antithrombin-heparin cofactor. *J Biol Chem* 1973; 248:6490–6505.
10. Rosenberg R: Actions and interactions of antithrombin and heparin. *N Engl J Med* 1975; 292:146–151.
11. Thaler E, Lechner K: Antithrombin III deficiency and thromboembolism. *Clin Haematol* 1981; 10:369.
12. Hattersley PG: Activated coagulation time of whole blood. *JAMA* 1966; 196:436.
13. Schriever HG, Epstein SE, Mintz MD: Statistical correlation and heparin sensitivity of activated partial thromboplastin time, whole blood coagulation time, and an automated coagulation. *Am J Clin Pathol* 1973; 60:323–329.

14. Bull BS, Korpman RA, Huse WM, et al: Heparin therapy during extracorporeal circulation: I. Problems inherent in existing heparin protocols. *J Thorac Cardiovasc Surg* 1975; 69:674.
15. Doty DB, Knott HW, Hoyt JL, et al: Heparin dose for accurate anticoagulation in cardiac surgery. *J Cardiovasc Surg* 1979; 20:597–604.
16. Esposito RA, Culliford AT, Colvin SB, et al: The role of the activated clotting time in heparin administration and neutralization for cardiopulmonary bypass. *J Thorac Cardiovasc Surg* 1983; 85:174–185.
17. Brozovic M, Baugham DR: Standards for heparin, in Bradshaw RA, Wessler S (eds): *Heparin-Structure, Function and Clinical Implications*. New York, Plenum Press, 1975, p 163.
18. Barrowcliffe TW, Johnson EA, Thomas D: Antithrombin III and heparin. *Br Med Bull* 1978; 34:143–150.
19. Zuck TF, Bergin JJ, Raymond JM, et al: Implications of depressed antithrombin-III activity associated with oral contraceptives. *Surg Gynecol Obstet* 1971; 133:609–612.
20. Blauhut B, Necek S, Kramar H, et al: Activity of antithrombin III and effect of heparin on coagulation in shock. *Thromb Res* 1980; 19:775–782.
21. Kamath BS, Fozard JR: Control of heparinisation during cardiopulmonary bypass. *Anaesthesia* 1980; 35:250–256.
22. Chung F, David T, Watt J: Excessive requirement for heparin during cardiac surgery. *Canad Anaesth Soc J* 1981; 28:280–282.
23. Esposito RA, Culliford AT, Colvin SB, et al: Heparin resistance during cardiopulmonary bypass. *J Thorac Cardiovasc Surg* 1983; 85:346–353.
24. Akl BF, Vargas GM, et al: Clinical experience with the activated clotting time for the control of heparin and protamine during cardiopulmonary bypass. *J Thorac Cardiovasc Surg* 1980; 79:97–102.

57

Hemolytic Transfusion Reaction

A 63-year-old man was undergoing triple coronary artery bypass surgery. Following cardiopulmonary bypass the patient was doing well, except for persistent hemodilution (hematocrit value of 20%). To raise the hematocrit, a blood transfusion of packed red blood cells was started. One unit of appropriately checked packed red blood cells was administered without event and then a second unit of whole blood was started. The arterial blood pressure, which had been normal, decreased to 70/60 mm Hg; heart rate increased to 90 beats per minute; cardiac index was 2.1 L/min/m^2; lungs became difficult to ventilate, and the patient's face became red. The urine, which had been clear until this point, became red in color. The blood administration was stopped immediately and a careful check revealed a clerical error and that type A blood had been infused into this type O patient.

Recommendations by Paul Finer, M.D., and Jerrold H. Levy, M.D.

ANALYSIS OF THE PROBLEM

This case presentation represents a major ABO mismatch. The patient, type O, received type A blood and subsequently developed hypotension, tachycardia, hemoglobinuria, bronchospasm, and flushing. This is a typical presentation of a hemolytic transfusion reaction (HTR) in a patient under general anesthesia. Most major ABO mismatches are clerical errors, and thus should be preventable. Although the incidence is low, it is a major hazard with high morbidity and mortality. In a recent Mayo Clinic study, it occurred in 1 out of 6,232 transfusions, with a 17% mortality overall, or 1 death following 33,500 transfusions. Fortunately we are able to recognize the problem early and treat it before more serious complications occur.

APPROACH TO THE PROBLEM

If an HTR is suspected, immediately stop the transfusion. Management at this point is directed toward resuscitation of the patient with prompt intravascular volume expansion and administration of epinephrine to correct hemodynamic instability as follows:

1. Stop the transfusion. This will prevent additional hemolysis and liberation of vasoactive mediators.

2. Administer 100% oxygen.

3. Expand the intravascular volume. Hypovolemia results following anaphylactic reactions due to the acute increases in capillary permeability. Therefore, intravascular volume expansion is important to treat hypotension.

4. Administer epinephrine. With acute hypotension, epinephrine serves several functions. The α-adrenergic effects support blood pressure during volume administration. The β_2-adrenergic effects act as bronchodilators and inhibit mast cell and basophil activation, while the β_1-adrenergic effects increase myocardial contractility. The dose varies and should be administered according to clinical judgment; however, an infusion of 0.02 to 0.05 μg/kg/minute (2 to 4 μg/minute in an adult) are reasonable starting administration rates in a hypotensive patient. The epinephrine infusion should be titrated to correct hypotension.

5. Check blood gas determinations. Hypoxemia may rapidly ensue from ventilation/perfusion abnormalities and bronchospasm. In addition, persistent acidemia may require bicarbonate administration.

6. Administer bronchodilators if necessary. If bronchospasm persists despite epinephrine, additional bronchodilators may be needed. Aminophylline, 5 to 6 mg/kg, administered as a loading dose over a period of 20 minutes followed by an infusion of 0.9 mg/kg/hour may be required with persistent bronchospasm.

7. Recheck blood. A quick clerical check of all blood-containing solutions should be checked and all used blood units should be sent to the blood bank. Blood samples should be drawn for a complete blood cell count, platelet

count, electrolytes, clotting studies, fibrinogen, and fibrin split products. A serum sample should be checked for a pinkish tinge, indicating hemolysis.

8. Maintain urine flow. Mannitol historically has been the diuretic of choice to prevent the oliguria and subsequent renal failure following an HTR. Mannitol is presently thought to be of little benefit, because while it does increase urine flow, simple diuresis may only convert an oliguric renal failure to a nonoliguric renal failure, and furthermore it does not increase renal perfusion. Since ischemia and altered distribution of renal blood flow are significant in the pathogenesis of acute renal failure (ARF), furosemide is thought to be more beneficial because it will increase renal cortical blood flow and urine flow but may not prevent acute tubular necrosis (ATN). Since renal ischemia is present, therapy is best directed at intravascular volume expansion.

DISCUSSION

To understand ABO incompatible transfusion reactions, specific immunologic processes involved and the pathophysiologic abnormalities that occur will be reviewed.

Pathophysiology

The blood group antigens are water-soluble carbohydrates found on the red blood cell (RBC) membrane. Although present on other cells and tissues, their functional role is unknown. Individuals with blood group A have A antigen on the RBC membrane, and anti-B in the serum; while blood group B individuals have B antigen on the RBC membrane and antibodies to the A antigen (Table 57–1). Blood group O individuals lack these antigens and thus have anti-A and anti-B antibodies. If a type O patient receives type A or type AB blood, the naturally occurring antibodies to A antigen present in the recipient will react with the foreign RBC, setting in motion the HTR.

The HTR can be defined as the occurrence of rapid or increased intravascular RBC destruction of either donor or recipient cells following transfusion.

TABLE 57–1.

Blood Group Antigens and Corresponding Antibodies

BLOOD GROUP ANTIGEN	MAJOR SERUM ANTIBODIES
A	Anti-B
B	Anti-A
AB	None
O	Anti-A, anti-B

It may present acutely, occurring within 24 hours of transfusion, or be delayed, presenting 4 to 10 days later. Delayed rates of donor RBC destruction are usually associated with few or no symptoms and may not be recognized unless the life span of the donor cells is reduced.

Differential Diagnosis

True immune-mediated hemolysis must be differentiated from pseudohemolysis or nonimmune mediated hemolysis. Conditions that involve immediate lysis of donor cells include hypotonic solutions (gastric or bladder irrigants), exposure to excess heat greater than 50° C, administration of blood infected with bacteria, concomitant administration of blood and drugs through a common administration set, and transfusion of aged red blood cells. Conditions that involve RBC lysis independent of transfusions include administration of penicillin, quinidine, α-methyldopa, congenital and acquired hemolytic anemias, infections, large hematomas, and finally mechanical trauma from vascular or arterial prostheses.

Pathogenesis

Complement and coagulation pathway activation are responsible for the organ dysfunction that occurs following an HTR. Type O patients seem to be at the greatest risk for severe reactions because the antibodies present seem to be more hemolytic than those of the other blood types. These patients have both anti-A and anti-B, consisting of both IgM and IgG, while patients of other blood types have only one other type of ABO antibody, and it is mainly composed of IgM. In general, the naturally occurring alloantibodies (isohemagglutinins) of the ABO system are mainly IgM. Those antibodies that appear as a result of acquired blood group immunization are mainly IgG. Both IgM and IgG are able to bind complement to produce hemolysis, but anti-A and anti-B of the IgM type bind complement more efficiently than those of the IgG type. Other antibodies besides anti-A and anti-B that can cause hemolysis include some IgM cold agglutinins, and IgG antibodies in the Kidd, Kell, Duffy and Rh groups.

Complement activation results following an ABO incompatible transfusion due to antibodies binding to the foreign blood group antigens. This antigen-antibody interaction liberates a spectrum of physiologically active complement peptides (Fig 57–1). Fragments of C_3 and C_5 (C_{3a} and C_{5a}), called anaphylatoxins, release histamine from mast cells, increase capillary permeability, and contract smooth muscle. In addition, C_{5a} produces aggregation of leukocytes and platelets that embolize to the pulmonary microvasculature to produce endothelial injury, increased capillary permeability, and respiratory dysfunction.

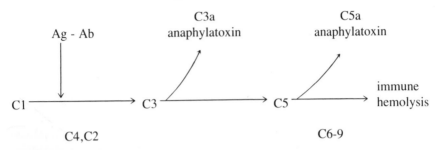

FIG 57–1.
Complement activation pathway.

When the complete complement complex is formed, it penetrates the RBC membrane to produce functional membrane holes. These holes are 8 to 10 nm in diameter by electron microscopy; they result in loss of intracellular electrolytes and small molecules but retention of osmotically active hemoglobin. Cellular destruction and lysis then proceed by an osmotic mechanism with cellular swelling, rupture of the membrane, and release of hemoglobin. Complement activation is also responsible for liberation of other vasoactive mediators as shown in Figure 57–2.

Complications

Renal Failure

The two main complications with major implications for survival are disseminated intravascular coagulation (DIC) and acute renal failure (ARF), and they are intimately related. In general, the larger the amount of incompatible RBCs infused, the more severe the reaction. The most severe manifestations occur following intravascular hemolysis and may result following small volumes of incompatible blood. However, most fatal cases are associated with infusion of more than 50 ml. Prompt recognition and immediate cessation of the incompatible infusion will help limit the amount of damage done.

Acute renal failure, most likely occurring following acute hemolysis, represents the most frequent complication, and in its most severe form still carries a mortality of 50% despite therapeutic advances. Three types of renal failure are recognized as sequelae of HTR. First and most common is an acute transient functional renal shutdown. This can occur following transfusion of a very small amount of incompatible RBCs. Second is acute renal failure due to acute tubular necrosis (ATN). This is more serious and usually requires the transfusion of 200 to 500 ml of incompatible blood. Importantly, this lesion requires vigorous and perhaps prolonged therapy, but it may still be reversible at this stage. The third and most severe form of renal impairment is bilateral renal cortical necrosis. Although rare, it is an irreversible lesion.

The pathogenesis of ARF is believed to represent primary ischemic damage to the tubules, with preferential renal cortical ischemia. Alteration of glomerular afferent/efferent arteriolar tone has been proposed as the most likely mechanism for the decreased glomerular blood flow. The renal insufficiency appears to be the result of decreased glomerular filtration secondary to impaired cortical blood flow. The decreased glomerular filtration rate explains the decrease in urine output, and the decreased glomerular blood flow leads to tubular ischemic necrosis.

The renal tubular ischemia is a result of a combination of factors. Renal deposition of fibrin and renal vascular thrombosis have been demonstrated after incompatible transfusion. This led to the association between DIC and ARF, as will be discussed later. Marked vasomotor alterations also occur that result in glomerular capillary stasis with thrombi formation. The vasomotor changes that are responsible for localization of fibrin appear to be mediated largely by norepinephrine, but the other vasoactive amines released also cause hemodynamic changes within the kidney microcirculation. The release of norepinephrine from the adrenal medulla is either a direct effect of the antigen-antibody reaction or a response to associated hypotension and shock. The com-

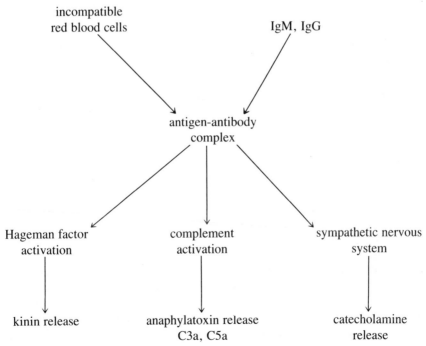

FIG 57–2.
Pathways for liberation of vasoactive mediators during a hemolytic transfusion reaction.

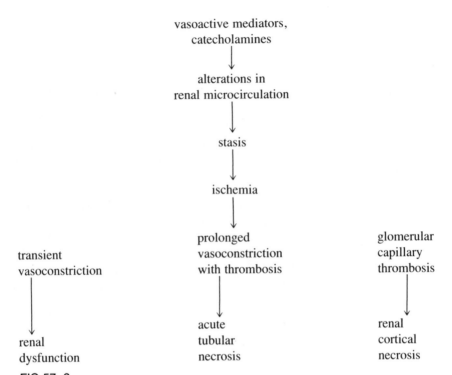

FIG 57–3.
Sequence of events leading to acute renal failure following a hemolytic transfusion reaction. (Modified from Goldfinger D: Acute hemolytic transfusion reactions: A fresh look at pathogenesis and considerations regarding therapy. *Transfusion* 1977; 17:85–97.)

bination of vasoconstriction, stasis, fibrin deposition, thrombosis, and generalized hypotension alters renal microcirculatory flow producing renal tubular ischemia (Fig 57–3). Furthermore, pathologic lesions will correlate with the clinical severity. Transient renal failure, the most common lesion, is the result of vasoconstriction with or without thrombosis, while ATN will demonstrate stasis and thrombosis. Renal cortical necrosis occurs following severe and persistent glomerular capillary thrombosis.

It is important to realize that free hemoglobin alone does not produce ARF. Schmidt and Holland demonstrated renal failure by infusion of hemoglobin-free RBC stroma. This and other studies led to disproval of the theory that hemoglobin by itself had a direct negative effect on renal tubular cells. Obstruction of the tubules by precipitated hemoglobin casts or ''acid hematin'' was also disproved by micropuncture experiments.

Disseminated Intravascular Coagulation

The HTR may also develop into a hemorrhagic diathesis that is often life threatening. In an anesthetized patient, excess bleeding from the surgical site may be the first sign of DIC. Any form of intravascular hemolysis can initiate DIC, by either complement-dependent or complement-independent pathways as shown in Figure 57–4. Erythrocytes contain a phospholipid with procoagulant activity known as "erythrocytin." This is released following RBC lysis and has activity similar to platelet factor 3. The antigen-antibody complex, complement activation, and erythrocytin will activate the clotting cascade to produce DIC.

Diagnosis

Following an incompatible RBC infusion, the host response may be masked in an anesthetized or narcotized patient. It may present as diffuse as oozing or un-

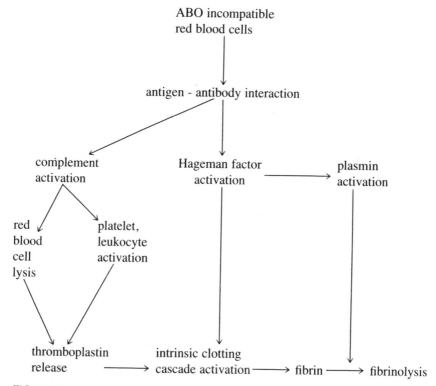

FIG 57–4.
Pathogenesis of disseminated intravascular coagulation during a hemolytic transfusion reaction.

controlled bleeding from the surgical site. Associated findings include hypotension, tachycardia, respiratory dysfunction (bronchospasm and/or hypoxemia), hemoglobinuria, and oliguria. In an otherwise stable patient receiving blood, development of any one of these signs warrants immediate suspicion and treatment. An awake patient may complain of fever, chills, chest pains, burning sensations at the site of infusion, nausea, flushing, and lumbar or sternal pains. Laboratory tests demonstrate evidence of RBC destruction with free hemoglobin in the urine and/or plasma, decreased serum haptoglobin, increased unconjugated bilirubin, decreased platelet count, decreased fibrinogen, decreased fibrin, increased clotting times (prothrombin time and partial thromboplastin time), and increased fibrin split products. The amount of free hemoglobin in plasma directly correlates with the severity of the reaction. Grossly, free hemoglobin in the plasma and urine can easily be checked for at the bedside by examining them for pink discoloration.

Controversial Therapy

In experimentally produced immune reactions, α-blockers have prevented renal glomerular deposition of fibrin by antagonizing norepinephrine. Dopamine and nitroprusside are theoretically beneficial and also under study. Alkalinization of the urine, thought to neutralize the acid hematin from RBC breakdown blocking the tubules, is probably of little benefit.

Heparin has been proposed in the prevention of DIC and its sequelae. In theory, heparin can prevent fibrin formation and its subsequent deposition but to be of any benefit, it must be administered early in the course of the reaction. The development of a hemorrhagic diathesis indicates that a severe DIC and HTR have already occurred. In addition, when given to a patient who is bleeding, anticoagulated, hypotensive, and in need of more blood, heparin represents a significant risk. Therefore, its use should be considered controversial.

BIBLIOGRAPHY

1. Goldfinger D: Acute hemolytic transfusion reactions: A fresh look at pathogenesis and considerations regarding therapy. *Transfusion* 1977; 17:85–97.
2. Greenwalt TJ: Pathogenesis and management of hemolytic transfusion reactions. *Semin Hematol* 1981; 18:84–94.
3. Levy JH, Roizen MF, Morris JM: Anaphylactic and anaphylactoid reactions. *Spine* 1986; 11:282–291.
4. Miller RD: Complications of massive blood transfusions. *Anesthesiology* 1973; 39:82–93.
5. Myre A: Fatalities from blood transfusion. *JAMA* 1980; 244:1333–1335.

6. Pineda AA, Brzica SM, Taswell HF: Hemolytic transfusion reaction: Recent experience in a large blood bank. *Mayo Clin Proc* 1978; 53:378–390.
7. Pineda AA, Taswell HF, Brzica SM: Delayed hemolytic transfusion reaction: An immunologic hazard of blood transfusion. *Transfusion* 1978; 18:1–7.
8. Schmidt PJ, Holland PV: Pathogenesis of the acute renal failure associated with incompatible transfusion. *Lancet* 1967; 2:1169–1172.
9. Toy PT, Vyas GN, Girish N: Blood transfusion reactions, in Englefriet CP, Van Loghem JJ, von dem Borne AE (eds): *Immunohematology*. New York, Elsevier Science Publishing Co Inc, 1984, pp 84–94.
10. Webster BH: Clinical presentation of hemolytic transfusion reactions. *Anaesth Intensive Care* 1980; 8:115–119.
11. Widmann FK: *Technical Manual of the American Association of Blood Banks*. Philadelphia, JB Lippincott Co, 1981.

PART EIGHT

Intensive Care Unit

58

Weaning a Patient From Ventilatory Assistance

A 40-year-old woman with severe mitral stenosis underwent mitral valve replacement. She had a history of recurrent pulmonary infection and at catheterization the pulmonary artery (PA) pressure was 60/25 mm Hg. Cardiac index was 1.8 L/min/m^2 on the first postoperative day, while she was receiving epinephrine, 0.05 mg/kg/minute. Attempts at weaning the patient from ventilatory assistance at this time were complicated by Pao$_2$ of 100, with a fractional inspiratory oxygen level (Fi$_{O2}$) of 0.6, Paco$_2$ of 50, pH of 7.32, and, with an intermittent mandatory ventilation (IMV) of 4, a respiratory rate of 30 breaths per minute.

Recommendations by Robert J. Marino, M.D.

ANALYSIS OF THE PROBLEM

This is a common problem in patients with long-standing mitral valve disease. The weaning process may be long and difficult.

APPROACH TO THE PROBLEM

Figure 58–1 contains the systematic approach to weaning this and other patients from ventilatory dependence. It is crucial that logical steps be followed if weaning is to be expeditious and safe (see discussion below).

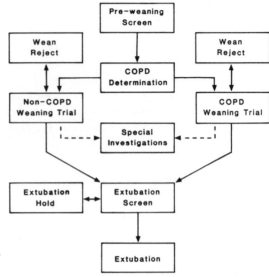

FIG 58–1.
Ventilator weaning flow diagram.

DISCUSSION

Pulmonary Pathology in Mitral Stenosis

Given the direct relationship between pressure and flow, the hemodynamic consequences of a stenosed mitral valve affect not only left ventricular filling and left atrial function but also the pulmonary function and circulation.

Pathology

The stenosed mitral valve leads to an increase in the pressure upstream, which in turn leads to pulmonary congestion, fibrosis, and hypertension. Although infarcts and hemorrhages around the pulmonary arteries are seen later in the disease, the early changes are seen in the pulmonary capillaries and alveoli. Narrowing of the muscular pulmonary arterioles as well as fibrosis are not uncommon findings. In addition, pulmonary interstitial fibrosis secondary to recurrent pulmonary infections is also a frequent pathologic finding.

Pathophysiology

The hydraulic orifice formula of Gorlin and Gorlin is as follows:

$$VA = \frac{BF}{K \times 44.5 \times V_{P1-P2}}$$

where VA = valve area; BF = blood flow (cardiac output); K = constant;

V_{P1-P2} = mean pressure on each side of valve; and 44.5 = calculated from an acceleration factor.

The formula shows us the relationship between blood flow, pressure gradient, and valve area across a stenotic valve. Because of the constant (44.5) in the denominator, a normal valve of 4 to 6 sq cm can tolerate a large increase in blood flow before increased pulmonary venous pressure results. As the stenosis increases, the left atrial pressure increases according to Gorlin's formula. The increased pressure is reflected back into the pulmonary circulation, causing progressive elevation of the pulmonary venous pressure. Eventually perivascular edema results from the elevated pressure, with congestion beginning in the dependent areas of the lung. Elevation of the pulmonary artery pressure is also seen and both results from and adds to the perivascular edema as well as to a redistribution of pulmonary blood flow to previously less perfused areas. The pulmonary artery pressure continues to rise until the mitral obstruction is relieved and then begins to fall gradually over a period of months. When the mitral valve area decreases to 0.5 sq cm or less, the slightest increase in cardiac output or blood flow across the valve will lead to a significant elevation in pulmonary venous pressure. Pulmonary edema and chronic perivascular changes are the results. The pulmonary capillary pressure and subsequently the pulmonary arterial pressure become elevated. Chronic elevation of right ventricular afterload can cause decreased compliance of the right ventricle and ultimately ventricular failure.

Because of the common septum between the right and left ventricles, a decrease in left ventricular compliance results from right ventricular failure and the pulmonary vascular changes seen with mitral stenosis. The left ventricular changes, in turn, affect the left atrium and the pulmonary vascular network, creating a vicious circle leading to biventricular failure.

Pulmonary Function

A decrease in pulmonary compliance and a decrease in lung distensibility are characteristic features of the pulmonary component of mitral stenosis secondary to redistribution of pulmonary blood flow as well as to the perivascular congestion and the frequently present pulmonary edema. Because of the decreased compliance, the work of breathing is significantly increased, even to the point of dyspnea. Pulmonary function studies reveal a decreased vital capacity and total lung capacity early in mitral stenosis secondary to venocapillary congestion and pulmonary arterial hypertension. The constant vascular overload of the pulmonary circulation eventually leads to irreversible fibrotic changes and poor pulmonary function, ventilation-perfusion (V/Q) abnormalities, and impairment of alveolar capillary diffusion.

Related Pulmonary Physiology

The pulmonary pathophysiologic changes are manifested in several ways in mitral stenosis. Ventilation perfusion mismatch and compliance changes are probably the most pronounced. In the later stages increases in physiologic dead space and acid-base changes are seen.

As described by Nunn, *compliance* is the volume change per unit change of transmural pressure gradient. *Static compliance* is the volume change divided by transmural pressure gradient change, at the point of zero air flow after thorough distribution of air. *Dynamic compliance* is the volume change divided by transmural pressure gradient change, at the point of zero air flow, but which is influenced by dynamic factors such as air flow.

Many factors affect compliance among which is lung volume or functional residual capacity (FRC). In mitral stenosis, following cardiopulmonary bypass (CPB) and with the patient in the supine position, lung volumes are decreased resulting in a decreased compliance. Adequate ventilation is also necessary to maintain compliance. Clearing of secretions and expansion of alveoli according to the hysteresis relationship with adequate ventilation can contribute to an improved compliance. Pulmonary vascular congestion as seen in mitral disease is associated with a reduced compliance and an increased work of breathing.

Dead space is the fraction of the tidal volume that does not penetrate to those regions of the lungs in which gas exchange occurs and is therefore exhaled unchanged. While this fraction of the tidal volume has been known as dead space, the effective part of the minute volume is known as the alveolar ventilation (V_A). Physiologic dead space comprises both anatomical and alveolar dead space and is defined as that part of the tidal volume that does not participate in gaseous exchange. Because physiologic dead space is the sum of alveolar and anatomical dead space, any increase in physiologic dead space will cause a decrease in alveolar ventilation.

$$V_A = \text{Respiratory rate} \times (\text{tidal volume} - \text{physiologic dead space})$$

Since the $PaCO_2$ is directly related to the physiologic dead space and minute ventilation, changes in either will be reflected in the blood gases. In addition, reduction of alveolar ventilation due to an increase in physiologic dead space produces changes in alveolar gas tensions, with an increase in PCO_2 and a fall in PO_2. Because changes in both the physiologic dead space and the minute ventilation can cause similar changes in alveolar and, therefore, blood gas tensions, it is important to measure both variables. Samples from expired gas and blood are measured and inserted in the Bohr equation, resulting in calculation of the physiologic dead space. This is a simple clinical tool and is important in determining the failure to wean.

When weaning a patient from the ventilator, the work of breathing is gradually increased to normal. Because of certain iatrogenic and pathophysiologic factors, the work of breathing may become in excess of normal, resulting in a decrease in minute ventilation and an increase in physiologic dead space. The work of breathing can be described as the amount of energy expended moving the mass of air in the tidal volume from the beginning of the upper airway to the alveoli. The amount of work is equal to the product of force $\times$ distance or pressure $\times$ volume. According to Nunn, normally, the work of breathing is minimal, requiring only 2% of the metabolic rate. The energy system in breathing work is extremely inefficient, reaching its maximum effectiveness soon, because most of the energy is lost as heat. Breathing work is normally comprised of the work to overcome the lung and chest wall compliance and gas flow resistance. But with active respiration with high minute volumes and when breathing against high pressures, work increases. Malfunctions in breathing apparati may also cause an increased work of breathing. Investigation into the breathing apparatus must be included into the protocol for a patient unable to wean.

Blood Gas Analysis

Blood gas analysis is of utmost importance in this patient as well as in all patients in the critical care environment. It must be determined whether there is metabolic or respiratory acidosis. Basically, the clinician can look at the P_{CO_2} level to evaluate the respiratory disturbance and the reported value of bicarbonate (HCO^-_3) to diagnose and quantitate metabolic disturbances. Utilizing the Henderson-Hasselbalch equation, this patient with a pH of 7.32 and a P_{CO_2} of 50 mm Hg should have an actual bicarbonate of 25 mEq/L. Indeed, this patient, therefore, has a mild respiratory acidosis with CO_2 retention.

A Pa_{O_2} of 100, although providing adequate oxygenation for this patient, must be considered abnormal with an FI_{O_2} of 0.6. In order to determine what P_{O_2} should be expected with this or any FI_{O_2}, the clinician must refer to the alveolar air equation and to the alveolar arterial oxygen difference to assess the degree of abnormality. With inspiration of 60% oxygen, the alveolar P_{O_2} should be approximately 378 mm Hg. The A-aD_{O_2} then in this patient would calculate to be about 278 mm Hg. Although this is at the upper limits of acceptable, there is not evidence of severe venous admixture and shunting. This moderate abnormality can usually be attributed to an increased lung water resulting from hemodilution and extracorporeal circulation in the early postoperative period or secondary to mitral stenosis pulmonary vascular pathophysiology later in the postoperative period. While this seems not to be the paramount problem with this patient, continued weaning past IMV 4 would have demonstrated further shunting and a falling Pa_{O_2}.

The blood gas determinations then reveal a patient with respiratory acidosis and moderately increased pulmonary venous admixture. These findings are consistent with a failure to wean.

The patient failing to wean also indicates the present ventilator settings are producing unacceptable physiologic results. Increasing the ventilator rate can quickly correct the respiratory acidosis. The addition of positive end expiratory pressure (PEEP) may also improve patient oxygenation, reduce venous admixture, and, most importantly, increase pulmonary compliance. An increased compliance can decrease the work of breathing by lowering the transpulmonary pressure required for inspiration. In addition, with an improved inspiration, a decreased respiratory rate results with its accompanying decrease in dynamic compliance and lower work of respiration.

The PEEP, on the other hand, is a double-edged sword that can be detrimental to the weaning process. Excessive PEEP can result in a decreased cardiac output, and aberration of arterial oxygenation and delivery. In addition, a decreased compliance with its increased work of breathing can result from excessive PEEP. An optimal PEEP setting, then, should be sought that will optimize the measured respiratory variables and the weaning process. Once optimal compliance and oxygen delivery are accomplished with the balance of PEEP and hemodynamic manipulations, the patient's breathing ability should improve and frequently the ventilator rate can then be reduced. It then seems more proper to wean the ventilator rate before the PEEP because the patient's ability to breathe properly is aided by the PEEP. Once the ventilator rate is completely weaned, it is time to wean from the PEEP.

Weaning

Weaning a patient with long-standing respiratory and cardiovascular failure from a ventilator can be an involved process and therefore is best approached in an organized manner. A haphazard approach may result in failure to wean because of simply forgetting a small but important aspect of the patient's pathophysiology. As a model for an organized weaning approach, a simulation to a computer program is useful. An important step in writing a program and in an organized weaning approach is to first construct a flow diagram. See Figure 58–1 as an example of a weaning flow diagram.

Before beginning the actual weaning process, it is necessary to know if the patient is capable of weaning. Because of the many factors that can influence the patient's ability to wean, a preweaning screen is most helpful. Included in a preweaning screen should be some basic pulmonary criteria and some general physiologic and anatomical criteria (Table 58–1). The pulmonary criteria include an evaluation of the patient's pulmonary function status and mechanical

TABLE 58–1.

Preweaning Screen

Basic pulmonary criteria
  A-aDO$_2$ < 300 mm Hg
  Peep ≤ 10 cm H$_2$O
  Vital capacity > 12 ml/kg
  Negative inspiratory force > −20 cm H$_2$O
General physiologic and anatomical criteria
  Acid-base status, pH > 7.35
  Chest wall integrity intact
  Chest x-ray film to rule out significant abnormality
  Stable and optimized hemodynamic status
  Abdominal pathology absent, e.g., distention
  Intact CNS, maintain minute ventilation
  Neuromuscular junction intact
  Bronchospasm optimized
  Sepsis or anaphylaxis absent

ability. An alveolar arterial oxygen difference (A-aDO$_2$) of 300 mm Hg corresponds approximately to a pulmonary shunt fraction (Q$_s$/Q$_t$) of 15% and is more easily obtained than calculating a true shunt. Gazitua et al. demonstrated that in patients with significant changes in Pvo$_2$ and arteriovenous oxygen difference (a=vO$_2$), the A-aDO$_2$ is more reliable as an indicator of pulmonary function than is the calculated shunt. Although not absolutely necessary, a reasonable reserve in mechanical ability is usually required to successfully wean completely from the ventilator. A vital capacity of >12 ml/kg or a negative inspiratory force of >−20 cm H$_2$O usually indicates adequate pulmonary mechanical ability.

In addition to pulmonary criteria certain general physiologic and anatomical criteria are necessary to successfully wean from the patient from the ventilator (see Table 58–1). Of these criteria, a chest x-ray film to rule out a significant abnormality, hemodynamic status, and intact CNS are of special importance to the postoperative cardiovascular patient. A pneumothorax, pleural effusion, or a hemomediastinum would certainly affect the ability to spontaneously breathe and maintain proper oxygenation. It has already been demonstrated by Gazitua et al. that a low cardiac output can decrease arterial oxygenation and oxygen delivery to the tissues. When the work of breathing is added to total oxygen requirement in a compromised delivery system, the oxygen deficit is felt in the tissues needing the greatest oxygen such as the CNS and the heart. It is, therefore, beneficial to optimize oxygen delivery before beginning the weaning process. In the postanesthetic period, especially when large doses of narcotics are used, an intact CNS and the ability to adequately control respiration and maintain a minute ventilation must be documented before any significant weaning begins.

Once these criteria are met, a patient's chances of weaning are reasonable and the weaning process is ready to begin. In order to evaluate the success of weaning, the appropriate criteria must be set in accord with their preoperative pulmonary status. In general, patients can be divided into two groups: those with a previous history of chronic obstructive pulmonary disease (COPD) with CO_2 retention, and those without a history of COPD and CO_2 retention. The CO_2 retention is the most important factor in determining proper weaning parameters. For these parameters see Table 58–2.

The actual weaning process may take numerous forms but with a patient with a long history of cardiac and related pulmonary illness, a slow deliberate process seems to have the most success. Such a weaning protocol should be similar to that of the training schedule of a marathon runner. Progressive exercise, rest, and proper nutrition are the prime ingredients. Patients with such a history seem to eventually succeed when slowly weaned at an IMV rate of approximately two to four breaths per minute per day and rested overnight at an IMV rate of two breaths per minute above where they ended weaning that day. The next day the weaning rate starts immediately at the point the patient left off the prior day and is again advanced two to four breaths per minute that day and each day until the weaning is complete. A blood gas determination is made and pulmonary criteria are checked with each step and applied to the successful weaning criteria described in Table 58–2. Advances are made only if the criteria are met.

Failure to wean is described as not meeting the criteria for successful weaning. According to the weaning flow diagram, a logical next step is to investigate why the patient has failed to wean. To do this it is necessary to begin some special investigations. In this step we systematically examine in a more in-depth manner those factors that affect a patient's ability to wean. Table

---

TABLE 58–2.

Successful Weaning Criteria

Non COPD, no CO_2 retention
1. $Pao_2 \leq 20$ mm Hg fall
2. $A\text{-}aDO_2 \leq 300$ mm Hg
3. pH > 7.35
4. $Paco_2$ $35 \leq Pco_2 \leq 55$ mm Hg
5. Respiratory rate < 30 breaths per minute
COPD, CO_2 retention
1. Pao_2 $55 \leq Pao_2$ 65 mm Hg
2. $Paco_2 \leq 65$ mm Hg
3. pH ≥ 7.30
4. Respiratory rate $\leq 20\%$ increase

TABLE 58–3.

Special Investigations

Fluid balance
  Patient weight—compare with prior weights
  Intake/output balance—must be even or negative
  Fluid restriction—1 ml/kg/hr of total IV fluids
  Diuresis—use to maintain urine output > 100 ml/hr
  Rationale: decrease total body water and thereby
    lung water, thereby improving compliance
Dead space evaluation
  Direct determination of dead space-tidal volume ratio (V_d/V_t)—Bohr equation
  Requirements
    $V_d \leq 175$—200 ml
    $V_d/V_t \leq 0.4$
  If $V_d/V_t > 0.5$:
    Minimize airway resistance—bronchodilators
    Remove all external dead space possible
    PEEP level may be excessive
    Cardiac output improvement—decreases ventilation-perfusion (V/Q)
Compliance evaluation
  Direct measurement—"static" test
  Approximate dynamic compliance = peak inspiratory pressure
  With low compliance measurement:
    Bronchodilator agents
    Clear secretions
    Remove pleural or pericardial effusions
    Increased lung water—most common
Hemodynamic evaluation
  Document PA pressure, Pao_2, CO_2, Pvo_2
  Optimize hemodynamic status
    Manipulate preload, afterload, etc.—vasopressors
  Determine colloid osmotic pressure and correct

58–3 provides an illustration of the special investigation step in the weaning flow diagram. The patient in the given case history had begun a weaning process and failed to wean at IMV 4. The next step, then, is to begin gathering more investigative data, rectify any abnormalities, and return to a weaning trial. But before investigation is to begin, the patient's ventilator rate must be adjusted to a level more physiologically within normal limits.

Of the major factors influencing the weaning process, the fluid status is the simplest to investigate and correct. Every effort should be made to keep such a patient with a compromised pulmonary capillary fluid balance in even or negative fluid balance to minimize lung water and optimize compliance. Patients with mitral stenosis may have elevated pressures in the right and left sides of the heart and pulmonary hypertension even into the postoperative period making fluid balance critical.

Dead space is an important contributor to the work of breathing, for if the dead space-tidal volume ratio (V_d/V_t) were greater than 0.5, the work of breathing becomes elevated in a exponential manner in order to maintain an adequate minute ventilation and a normal $Paco_2$. Dead space can be easily determined clinically utilizing the Bohr equation listed below.

$$\frac{\text{Physiologic}}{\text{dead space}} = \frac{(Pa_{CO_2} - PE_{CO_2})VE}{Pa_{CO_2}}$$

Unfortunately, little can usually be done about a true increase in physiologic dead space. The clinician must also keep in mind that factors other than dead space can contribute to elevated PCO_2 such as an increased CO_2 production and an elevated respiratory quotient secondary to an excess of carbohydrates in the patient's nutritional support formula. These variables can also be easily determined with a metabolic respiratory screen.

Poor compliance is usually one of the factors involved in the failure to wean. Accurate compliance measurements are difficult to obtain clinically, but close approximation of the dynamic compliance can be estimated from the peak inspiratory pressure of the ventilator circuit. Pulmonary compliance can be altered by resolution of the pulmonary pathology and certain physiologic manipulations such as fluid balance and bronchodilatation. Extrapulmonary compliance can be affected by pericardial and pleural masses such as effusions.

Probably of most significance in this patient and in those with long-standing valvular heart disease is proper evaluation and manipulation of the hemodynamic status. If not already present, insertion of a pulmonary artery catheter is indicated along with determinations of observed and derived hemodynamic values. Improvement of the cardiac output, reduction of the pulmonary artery pressure and cardiac filling pressures can only benefit the pulmonary status. Unfortunately in patients with long-standing mitral stenosis, pulmonary hypertension cannot be immediately decreased and may only gradually decrease over weeks and may not ever fall significantly. Certain vasopressors used in the postoperative period may exacerbate the pulmonary vascular disease and should be used with caution. Epinephrine in high doses can result in elevation of the pulmonary vascular resistance. Isoproterenol and dobutamine are more beneficial with preexisting pulmonary hypertension. Dopamine in even small doses should be avoided to prevent further increase in pulmonary vascular resistance (PVR). With the proper combination of vasodilators and inotropic agents, the cardiac function and hemodynamic function may be improved to a significant degree so that reduction in lung water and improved pulmonary compliance may result as well as a more successful weaning trial. Colloid osmotic pressure, although usually not as critical a value in most forms of respiratory failure, is especially significant in mitral stenosis patients with

TABLE 58–4.

Extubation Criteria

Tidal volume $\geq$ 6 ml/kg; vital capacity $\geq$ 12 ml/kg
Negative inspiratory force $>$ -30 cm H_2O
Respiratory rate $<$ 30 breaths per minute
A-aDO$_2$ $\leq$ 300 mm Hg; Q_s/Q_t $<$ 16%
Capable of airway control
Capable of adequate pulmonary toilet

---

their preexisting pulmonary hypertension. Values should be kept close to normal limits, for even minor negative deviations can result in increased lung water and failure to wean.

After fully utilizing the special investigation loop of the weaning flow diagram, most intervention efforts at accomplishing a successful wean should have been completed. Hopefully the complicating factors preventing a successful wean will have been eliminated or at least minimized. The patient is now ready to be returned to a weaning trial, hopefully with more success. Realistically patients with long-standing mitral stenosis not uncommonly require a prolonged postoperative recovery and weaning period. For this reason every effort should be made to proceed with a slow organized approach to weaning, especially in a patient who has already failed to wean on a conventional trial. Within days to weeks such patients should have a reasonable chance to wean, provided they are given daily ventilatory exercise, adequate nutrition, and nightly rest. Once weaning is complete, extubation criteria must be met that have greater CNS and pulmonary mechanical requirements than those of weaning (Table 58–4).

BIBLIOGRAPHY

Civetta JM: *Intensive Care Therapeutics*. New York, Appleton-Century Crofts, 1980.
Conn HL, Horwitz O: *Cardiac and Vascular Diseases*. Philadelphia, Lea & Febiger, 1971.
Gazitua R, Goodfellow R, Villar L, et al: An analysis of the components of the pulmonary shunt equation: Significance of the alveolar-arterial oxygen gradient, arterio-venous oxygen content difference, and mixed venous oxygen pressure. *J Trauma* 1979; 19:81.
Nunn JF: *Applied Respiratory Physiology*. London, Butterworth & Co, 1975.
Thomas J, Lowenstein E: Anesthetic management of the patient with valvular heart disease. *Int Anesthesiol Clin* 1979; 17:67–96.

59

Prolonged Drowsiness

A 65-year-old man underwent coronary artery bypass surgery during which he received four vein grafts. Anesthesia was induced and maintained with fentanyl 100 μg/kg and diazepam 10 mg. Bypass time was two hours and overall anesthesia time was five hours. The postoperative course was uncomplicated, except that the patient remained somewhat somnolent and totally ventilator-dependent. Sixteen hours after operation, the patient was arousable on vigorous stimulation and was grossly intact neurologically.

Recommendations by Donald S. Prough, M.D., and K. C. Angert, M.D.

ANALYSIS OF THE PROBLEM

Prolonged drowsiness following coronary artery bypass surgery presents three problems. The first two, those of differential diagnosis and therapy, are specific patient-related problems that must be addressed. The third, which is the economic implication of a prolonged stay in an intensive care unit, is one that confronts every physician and hospital involved in the management of patients undergoing open heart surgery.

Differential Diagnosis

The differential diagnosis of prolonged drowsiness following coronary artery bypass surgery includes the entire range of nontraumatic causes of disturbed consciousness. However, from a practical standpoint, the differential diagnosis is brief. The two most probable explanations are neurologic dysfunction related to cardiopulmonary bypass and the prolonged effects of anesthetic drugs.

494

Neurologic dysfunction

More than 2,500 severe strokes per year occur as complications of coronary artery bypass surgery.[1] A substantially larger number of patients experience mild strokes, and more than 10% of patients have prolonged encephalopathy.[1] From the many studies of central nervous system injury after heart surgery, several generalizations can be drawn.[1-5] First, although the incidence of gross motor deficits is low, the incidence of subtle neurologic dysfunction, detectable only by precise testing, is high.[2-3] Second, laboratory evidence of ischemic neurologic damage occurs in an even higher percentage of patients undergoing heart surgery.[4] Third, certain factors, including valvular surgery and advanced age, predispose to a higher incidence of neuropsychiatric morbidity.[1-3, 5, 6]

The cause of postoperative neurologic dysfunction is not completely clear. Both embolic phenomena and inadequate cerebral perfusion have been implicated, but embolic phenomena appear at the present time to be the more important of the two.[7] Most investigators have failed to confirm a relationship between low cerebral perfusion pressure during cardiopulmonary bypass and postoperative neurologic deficits.[8, 9]

In the present case, the patient has a diffuse, nonfocal depression of his level of consciousness 16 hours after bypass surgery. Somnolence in the absence of gross neurologic abnormalities is not a common manifestation of acute stroke. Total ventilator dependence implies absence of adequate spontaneous ventilatory drive. Selective damage to the respiratory center, in the absence of other evidence of focal neurologic lesions, is unlikely. Nor is this pattern characteristic of the type of neuropsychiatric dysfunction that may be demonstrated days to months after open heart surgery, specifically, lack of attentiveness and overall diminution of cognitive skills.[2, 3]

Prolonged Drug Effects

This presentation is much more compatible with prolonged drowsiness due to anesthetic drugs. The patient had received diazepam 10 mg intravenously (IV) and fentanyl 100 μg/kg IV for anesthetic induction and maintenance. This type of anesthetic technique, based upon high-dose fentanyl, has become extremely popular since its introduction approximately a decade ago. The advantages of this technique, in comparison to other anesthetic techniques, are primarily those of increased cardiovascular stability.[10] One disadvantage, however, is that large doses of fentanyl can produce persistent ventilatory depression. Although a few patients having received high-dose fentanyl can be extubated within four hours after the completion of surgery, most require ventilation for 12 to 18 hours after induction of anesthesia.[10] The duration of ventilatory depression depends upon the terminal elimination half-life of fentanyl, and in elderly patients such as this one elimination of fentanyl is markedly prolonged. Bentley et al. reported a terminal half-life of 945 minutes in elderly patients (>60 years old) in contrast to 265 minutes in younger patients (<50 years old).[11] In addition, similar doses of fentanyl produce unconsciousness more predictably in patients older than 60 years.[12]

The additive effects of residual diazepam are difficult to quantitate. Although the dose of diazepam given this patient is relatively small, the elimination half-life of diazepam in the elderly in contrast to that in younger patients is quite prolonged (101 vs. 32 hours).[13] It is reasonable to speculate that some modest residual effect of diazepam is augmenting the residual effects of fentanyl.

Although premedicant or adjuvant drugs are not mentioned in this case report, the potential influence of those agents must also be considered. The majority of patients undergoing coronary artery bypass surgery are sedated before surgery to limit the incidence of anxiety-related angina. The residual effects of diazepam or lorazepam used as a premedicant might also contribute to postoperative drowsiness and ventilatory depression. Cimetidine, which is commonly used preoperatively to reduce gastric acidity, impairs the capacity of the liver to oxidize drugs, thereby prolonging the metabolic clearance of diazepam and of its major metabolite, desmethyldiazepam.[14] Plasma concentrations of diazepam and desmethyldiazepam increase more than 50% when cimetidine is administered concurrently.[14] Although this increase in plasma concentration is not associated with changes in mentation in outpatients, the interaction has not been carefully defined in patients who then undergo anesthesia.

APPROACH TO THE PROBLEM

A patient who has undergone coronary artery bypass surgery while anesthetized with high-dose fentanyl requires no specific therapy for drowsiness during the first 24 postoperative hours. Ventilatory support should be continued as needed until the patient fulfills criteria for extubation (such as easy arousability, intact cough reflex, adequate neuromuscular reserve, and acceptable oxygenation and carbon dioxide elimination) while breathing spontaneously and receiving no more than two mechanical breaths per minute. The last criterion is particularly important, since narcotized patients may meet all of the other criteria, but still have a markedly impaired ventilatory drive that becomes manifest only when mechanical ventilation is withdrawn.

The alternative to patient supportive care is pharmacologic reversal of the residual ventilatory depression from fentanyl, diazepam, or both. We believe that naloxone, physostigmine, and doxapram have limited, if any, usefulness in this situation. Abrupt reversal of narcotic effects with naloxone has been associated with acute hypertension, myocardial ischemia, and acute pulmonary edema.[15,16] The last of those has been reported even in young patients who have received modest doses of naloxone.[17] Physostigmine may reverse drowsiness caused by diazepam but will not reverse the effects of fentanyl. Doxapram is a ventilatory stimulant that increases the elimination of carbon dioxide in narcotized patients without abruptly reversing the narcotic effect; however, doxapram may produce tachycardia, hypertension, and dysrhythmias. Knowing these side effects, we believe it important to emphasize that no reversal of this patient's ventilatory depression is necessary. The problem of residual narcotization will resolve spontaneously without complication if ventilatory support simply is continued until the drug is eliminated.

The management of perioperative neurologic injury, an unlikely diagnosis in this case, is not amenable to any currently available therapy once it is established. The reduction of neurologic deficits is better managed through interventions that limit the likelihood of microembolization during cardiopulmonary bypass or perhaps through specific neuroprotective interventions, such as sodium thiopental, during cardiopulmonary bypass.[18] If a patient has suffered a postoperative stroke, management consists almost entirely of supportive care. Consequently, ventilatory support, continued until the patient meets the criteria for extubation, is the appropriate management for acute neurologic deficits, as it is for residual narcotization. Computed tomography may confirm the diagnosis of focal neurologic injury if it is suspected, but the value of more precise diagnosis should be balanced against the potential risk to the patient of being transported to the radiology suite while receiving ventilatory and cardiovascular support.

DISCUSSION

Following cardiac surgery, most patients are admitted to an intensive care unit where they remain until their cardiovascular, pulmonary, and renal status is stable enough to permit their transfer to a regular nursing unit. Currently, due to steady improvements in surgical technique and myocardial preservation, many patients are hemodynamically stable shortly after the conclusion of surgery. Renal function, in most cases really a measure of cardiovascular stability, is also adequate shortly after a patient's arrival in the intensive care unit. As a consequence, the need for mechanical ventilatory support is likely to be the primary determinant of the duration of time that the patient must spend in a critical care environment.

Patients with prolonged ventilatory depression due to residual narcotization may require ventilation into the early afternoon of the day following surgery. Since it is rare to transfer a patient out of an intensive care area immediately after extubation, most patients will remain in an intensive care environment until the morning of the second postoperative day. It is reasonable to speculate that many stable patients, if they could be extubated within several hours after surgery, would be ready to leave the intensive care unit on the morning after surgery. Consequently, the choice of a high-dose narcotic technique for anesthesia may well commit those patients to an extra day in the intensive care unit. If we assume that the extra day takes the place of a day in a regular surgical unit rather than adding a day to the total stay, it is likely that use of a high-dose narcotic anesthetic will increase the cost of hospitalization by at least $1,000 per patient.

It is not the purpose of this article to debate the merits of various approaches to anesthesia for cardiac surgery. Certainly the popularity of high-dose fentanyl anesthesia attests to its virtues in the eyes of many cardiac anesthesiologists. However, in a day of limited resources, it might be wise to consider whether, in selected patients, alternative anesthetic techniques that permit early extubation might not be preferable. Avoidance of an additional 12 to 24 hours of mechanical ventilation may also serve to decrease some of the iatrogenic sequelae of mechanical ventilation, although there are no controlled studies that compare the morbidity of early versus late extubation in comparable patients. One possible solution to the economic implications of prolonged drowsiness may be the introduction of one of the newer narcotics, such as alfentanil, that provide hemodynamic stability during induction, but permit more rapid postoperative recovery.[19]

SUMMARY

Normal convalescence requires return of consciousness after cardiac surgery. Failure to exhibit a normal consciousness requires diagnosis. If somnolence is due to drug administration, supportive care is indicated. Shorter acting anesthetic drugs may prove valuable in avoiding cases of prolonged drowsiness after cardiac surgery.

REFERENCES

1. Breuer AC, Furlan AJ, Hanson MR, et al: Central nervous system complications of coronary artery bypass graft surgery: Prospective analysis of 421 patients. *Stroke* 1983; 14:682–687.
2. Åberg T, Kihlgren M: Effect of open heart surgery on intellectual function. *Scand J Thorac Cardiovasc Surg* 1974; 8(suppl 15):1–62.
3. Åberg T, Ahlund P, Kihlgren M: Intellectual function late after open-heart operation. *Ann Thorac Surg* 1983; 36:680–683.

4. Åberg T, Ronquist G, Tydén H, et al: Adverse effects on the brain in cardiac operations as assessed by biochemical, psychometric, and radiologic methods. *J Thorac Cardiovasc Surg* 1984; 87:99–105.

5. Slogoff S, Girgis KZ, Keats AS: Etiologic factors in neuropsychiatric complications associated with cardiopulmonary bypass. *Anesth Analg* 1982; 61:903–911.

6. Sotaniemi KA: Brain damage and neurological outcome after open-heart surgery. *J Neurol Neurosurg Psychiatry* 1980; 43:127–135.

7. Furlan AJ, Breuer AC: Central nervous system complications of open heart surgery. *Stroke* 1984; 15:912–915.

8. Kolkka R, Hilberman M: Neurologic dysfunction following cardiac operation with low-flow, low-pressure cardiopulmonary bypass. *J Thorac Cardiovasc Surg* 1980; 79:432–437.

9. Ellis RJ, Wisniewski A, Potts R, et al: Reduction of flow rate and arterial pressure at moderate hypothermia does not result in cerebral dysfunction. *J Thorac Cardiovasc Surg* 1980; 79:173–180.

10. Bovill JG, Sebel PS, Stanley TH: Opioid analgesics in anesthesia: With special reference to their use in cardiovascular anesthesia. *Anesthesiology* 1984; 61:731–755.

11. Bentley JB, Borel JD, Nenad RE Jr, et al: Age and fentanyl pharmacokinetics. *Anesth Analg* 1982; 61:968–971.

12. Bailey PL, Wilbrink J, Zwanikken P, et al: Anesthetic induction with fentanyl. *Anesth Analg* 1985; 64:48–53.

13. Divoll M, Greenblatt DJ, Ochs HR, et al: Absolute bioavailability of oral and intramuscular diazepam: Effects of age and sex. *Anesth Analg* 1983; 62:1–8.

14. Greenblatt DJ, Abernethy DR, Morse DS, et al: Clinical importance of the interaction of diazepam and cimetidine. *N Engl J Med* 1984; 310:1639–1643.

15. Azar I, Turndorf H: Severe hypertension and multiple atrial premature contractions following naloxone administration. *Anesth Analg* 1979; 58:524–525.

16. Flacke JW, Flacke WE, Williams GD: Acute pulmonary edema following naloxone reversal of high-dose morphine anesthesia. *Anesthesiology* 1977; 47:376–378.

17. Prough DS, Roy R, Bumgarner J, et al: Acute pulmonary edema in healthy teenagers following conservative doses of intravenous naloxone. *Anesthesiology* 1984; 60:485–486.

18. Nussmeier NA, Arlund C, Slogoff S: Neuropsychiatric complications after cardiopulmonary bypass: Cerebral protection by a barbiturate. *Anesthesiology* 1986; 64:165–170.

19. Stanski DR, Hug CC Jr: Alfentanil: A kinetically predictable narcotic analgesic, editorial. *Anesthesiology* 1982; 57:435–438.

60

Postmyocardial Revascularization Hypertension

A 55-year-old man was anesthetized with fentanyl 100 μg/kg for coronary artery grafting and weaned from cardiopulmonary bypass without difficulty. He was given nitroprusside (5 μg/kg/minute) in the operating room to treat a blood pressure of ≥150/90 mm Hg. Upon admission to the intensive care unit, the patient's mean blood pressure was 115 mm Hg.

Recommendations by Fawzy G. Estafanous, M.D.

ANALYSIS OF THE PROBLEM

Following cardiopulmonary bypass, the patient experienced an undesirable rise in blood pressure for which he received treatment. Such a rise in blood pressure continued in the postoperative period and required a continuation of blood pressure control. The blood pressure should be treated. [1]

APPROACH TO THE PROBLEM

Adequate treatment depends on correct diagnosis. Wide variations can occur in blood volume, total peripheral resistance, pulmonary vascular resistance, myocardial perfusion, contractility and heart rate, both during and after cardiac surgery. Hence, a correct diagnosis must be based on adequate monitoring and thoughtful interpretation of various hemodynamic indices. These entail close follow-up, using properly calibrated equipment as well as careful monitoring of the filling pressures in the right and left chambers. Determination of cardiac output, systemic vascular resistance, and estimation of fluid balance are important. The most commonly used pharmacologic approach to treatment is use of nitroprusside (see discussion below), but many options exist.

General Measures

Attention to details, thoughtful preparation of the patient, and general measures to avoid pain and vasoconstriction are more important in the prevention and treatment of hypertension than hasty use of antihypertensive agents. Prophylaxis begins long before surgery. In our opinion, antihypertensive therapy including β-adrenergic blocking agents and calcium-channel blockers should be continued until the time of surgery. Hypotension, whether related to antihypertensive therapy or not, can be averted by good monitoring; we believe that in proper circumstances its risks are far less than the deleterious effects of uncontrolled hypertension. During the postoperative period all patients should receive sufficient analgesic and sedative agents when required, in order to ensure that they remain free of pain.[2] Warming blankets should be used when needed to avoid the vasoconstriction provoked by cold.

Unilateral Stellate Block

Unilateral stellate ganglion blockade was effective in our experience[3] for rapid normalization of elevated blood pressure in a large number of patients with hypertension after myocardial revascularization as well as in those with a hypertensive episode immediately after heart valve replacement. We have even found stellate block to be effective when large doses of peripheral vasodilators failed to adequately control the paroxysmal increase in pressure. However, unless this blockade is performed with great care by physicians trained in its use, the incidence of its success rate can be quite low and, more importantly, can be complicated by pneumothorax, hemothorax, or nerve injury.[4] Bilateral stellate block is dangerous because of the possibility of undue cardiac depression. Currently, we do not resort to stellate blockade for control of postmyocardial revascularization hypertension routinely, but only when vasodilation therapy has failed.

β-Adrenergic Blocking Agents

In patients with marked tachycardia, particularly in association with ischemic ST-segment changes, intravenous propranolol or esmolol can be used. In this situation, slowing of the heart rate can be associated with some arterial pressure, especially the systolic level. However, because of its depressing effect on myocardial contractility and its relatively delayed hypotensive action,[5, 6] propranolol is not routinely recommended for postoperative hypertension.

α- and β-Blockers (e.g., labetalol)

These agents have been shown to lower blood pressure effectively without side effects and may be advantageous in controlling postoperative rises in blood pressure. They lower the systemic vascular resistance and, as α-blockers, they also have a direct vasodilator mechanism. As β-blockers, they decrease heart rate and myocardial oxygen consumption. Clinical experience and studies of these agents in the postoperative setting are still needed.

Peripheral Vasodilators

Short-acting peripheral vasodilators that do not overstimulate the heart are the drugs of choice for treatment of hypertension during and after cardiac surgery. They have a rapid onset of action and doses can usually be titrated to achieve the desirable blood pressure level. However, all vasodilators are not equivalent in their spectrum of action; those like diazoxide or hydralazine, which have little effect on veins, may produce undue stimulation of the heart.[7] More appropriate to the conditions of cardiac surgery are vasodilators like sodium nitroprusside, which dilate veins as well as resistance vessels,[7] or nitroglycerin, which has beneficial effects on the coronary circulation.

Nitroglycerin

For the last ten years, we have used different preparations of nitroglycerin perioperatively in open heart surgery.[8] It is a peripheral vasodilator for both resistance and capacitance vessels[9] with beneficial effects on the coronary circulation; in cardiac surgery it has proved useful as a short-acting hypotensive agent.[10] It is used to reduce preoperative angina pectoris and consequent reflex increases in blood pressure; moreover, its routine use may decrease the incidence and degree of hypertension that complicates endotracheal intubation. Because of its venodilating effect and its effect on the pulmonary circulation, we believe it to be the drug of choice for the hypertension associated with right ventricular dysfunction, or with increased pulmonary vascular resistance. However, nitroglycerin is not a very potent antihypertensive agent; therefore, if the use of nitroglycerin does not maintain blood pressure at a desirable level, we resort to sodium nitroprusside.

Sodium Nitroprusside

Sodium nitroprusside is the most consistently effective drug for management of hypertensive crises.[11] In our opinion, it remains the drug of choice for hypertension associated with acute coronary insufficiency and left ventricular impairment.[12–15] Left ventricular stroke work and filling pressure are decreased and left ventricular performance is enhanced.[13–15] Cardiac output could be increased, particularly when the left ventricular filling pressure is initially high and left ventricular function impaired; when left ventricular filling pressure is normal or low, cardiac output might be decreased to a variable extent. Similarly, heart rate is increased in subjects without heart disease, but it is not significantly altered in those with cardiac decompensation.[13]

Moreover, nurses and residents in postoperative intensive care units are currently very familiar with the use of sodium nitroprusside and adjusting its doses to the needs of the patient. This allows the use of sodium nitroprusside as the most common drug to control postmyocardial revascularization hypertension.

DISCUSSION

The therapy described above should be designed to treat the underlying causes of hypertension.

General Causes of Acute Perioperative Hypertension

Hypoxia and Hypercarbia

As sympathetic stimulants, hypoxia and/or hypercarbia in their early stages cause a gradual increase in both heart rate and blood pressure. If left untreated, the rise in blood pressure continues until the vasomotor center fails. Thereafter, bradycardia and hypotension engender a situation that may be irreversible. In a surgical setup, iatrogenic hypoxia and/or hypercarbia have been reported. Postoperatively, variable degrees of hypoxia and hypercarbia can be expected from residual analgesics, anesthetics, and muscle relaxants, and also from surgical interference with the respiratory muscles. Even in a mechanically ventilated patient, hypoxia and hypercarbia may occur from mechanical failure of a ventilator, disconnection of tubing, and tension pneumothorax.[16] Other factors precipitating hypertension include arousal from anesthesia, tracheal and nasopharyngeal manipulations, pain, hypothermia, shivering, poor ventilation, and the use of pressor agents, as well as the waning of antihypertensive drugs.

If unexplained hypertension occurs, the clinician must rule out hypoxia, hypercarbia, and pain as causes of the rise in blood pressure and treat them specifically before initiation of peripheral vasodilatory therapy. The use of peripheral vasodilators to treat hypertension caused by hypoxia and hypercarbia will cause a serious and profound drop in blood pressure, as it counteracts the compensatory vasoconstriction.

Preoperative Hypertension

Preoperatively, hypertensive patients are expected to have a more pronounced rise in blood pressure in response to sympathetic stimulants. [17]

Currently, it is a routine practice to continue antihypertensive medication to the day of surgery. Controlled hypertensive patients are not expected to suffer severe fluctuations in blood pressure with the same frequency or magnitude as untreated or uncontrolled hypertensives. Indeed, results of our studies of more than 200 hypertensive patients, whose antihypertensive therapy was continued until the time of surgery, revealed that the incidence of postoperative hypertension, according to the levels properly defined, was no higher than that for preoperatively normotensive patients. [18]

Apart from the predisposing factors previously mentioned, hypertension related to myocardial revascularization surgery is a well-defined complication. [18]

Intraoperative Hypertension Following Cardiopulmonary Bypass

In this case report, it is assumed that none of the general causes of hypertension described existed: however, the patient still experienced an unexpected rise in blood pressure by the end of surgery, which continued into the postoperative period and required initiation of antihypertensive treatment. This phenomenon is not uncommon, particularly in patients with good ventricular function undergoing myocardial revascularization surgery. [18–20] However, the rise in blood pressure is only one aspect of the hemodynamic changes related to cardiac surgery. [21, 22]

Hemodynamic Alterations Following Cardiopulmonary Bypass

A large number of patients have relatively low blood pressure immediately following termination of cardiopulmonary bypass. Hemodynamic studies at that point demonstrate that such low blood pressure in patients with good ventricular function is mainly due to extremely low systemic vascular resistance in the presence of high cardiac output, which partially compensates for the low systemic vascular resistance. Several factors participate in the pathogenesis of low systemic vascular resistance at this point. These include hemodilution, which decreases viscosity; the rewarming temperature (usually between 39° C and 40° C) that may stimulate the hypothalmus to produce reflex vasodilatation; the effect of bypass in diluting adrenergic components; and the accumulation of metabolic products that may have a vasodilating effect.

An hour or so after termination of cardiopulmonary bypass, most of these factors cease, and the patient's systemic vascular resistance starts to rise. In the presence of an adequate cardiac output, the mean arterial pressure usually can rise significantly, reaching levels culminating in hypertensive episodes. The significant rise of systemic vascular resistance from the postbypass value is remarkable because of the residual hemodilution with its presumed low viscosity.

This hemodynamic pattern, which consists of increasing systemic vascular resistance and blood pressure with practically unchanged levels of cardiac output in the presence of unchanged pulmonary wedge pressure and central venous pressure,[21] resembles the hemodynamic pattern of postmyocardial revascularization hypertension that we initially described.[18, 23]

It is worth reemphasizing that hypertensive episodes may not be experienced in patients with poor ventricular function whose limited cardiac output may be further jeopardized by an increase in afterload.

Postmyocardial Revascularization Hypertension

Clinical Description

Since our original description in 1973, postmyocardial revascularization hypertension is now recognized as a common complication of coronary bypass surgery in the early postoperative period.[18] It occurs in 30% to 50% of patients, which is higher than its incidence following cardiac valve replacement (5% to 10%). This difference can be attributed to fluctuations in blood pressure control, reduced baroreceptor sensitivity, and the frequent hypovolemia in patients with coronary artery disease.[1]

Most investigators have described the following clinical syndrome with typical hemodynamic characteristics. An increase in arterial pressure occurs during the first four hours after operation. The blood pressure increases gradually, but steadily, despite sedation and well-controlled ventilation. The increase in pressure can become severe and exceed initial systolic pressure by 60 mm Hg or more. Despite the increase in pressure, there is no slowing of the heart rate; on the contrary, it can become slightly higher, with occasional premature ventricular complexes.[18] The central venous and left atrial pressures remain within normal limits. Most authors agree that type of anesthetics used,[24–26] duration of cardiopulmonary bypass, and distribution of coronary artery lesions do not significantly influence the incidence of postoperative hypertension. Our impression was that this hypertension occurred more frequently among patients with well-preserved myocardial function.

Possible Causes of Postmyocardial Revascularization Hypertension

Apart from the general causes of hypertension that are already discussed, other causes directly related to myocardial revascularization surgery are involved. Postoperative coronary insufficiency or a myocardial infarction might also raise the blood pressure; signs of cardioadrenergic stimulation are particularly marked following coronary bypass in patients sustaining a postoperative infarction.[27] Hypervolemia is often cited as a possible cause of postoperative hypertension; however, the relationship of fluid overload to increased arterial pressure is a complex one.[28] Compensatory neural mechanisms can adequately buffer sizable blood volume variations[29]; only in the functional absence of such reflexes or with loss of renal excretory function will arterial pressure correlate directly with hypervolemia.[30] On the other hand, marked sympathetic reaction to hypovolemia could be an unrecognized cause of serious hypertension and impaired tissue perfusion.[31]

Patients with arteriographically documented left main coronary artery obstructions of greater than 50% have a higher risk of becoming hypertensive as well. A cardiogenic hypertensive chemoreflex in dogs has been provoked by stimulating the proximal left coronary artery with serotonin.[32] Roberts et al.[32] speculated that trauma during surgery might somehow stimulate coronary chemoreceptors and produce hypertension in man during coronary artery surgery.

However, our studies of postmyocardial revascularization hypertension demonstrated that its incidence is not higher in patients who are preoperatively hypertensive, and it was not accompanied by signs of hypovolemia or hypervolemia, a significant correlation with the site of the obstructed coronary artery, or incidence of perioperative myocardial infarction. The most significant clues about the causes of postmyocardial revascularization hypertension come from studies of the hemodynamic characteristics of this hypertension.

Hemodynamic Characteristics of Postmyocardial Revascularization Hypertension

In all published reports, the increase in blood pressure after coronary bypass surgery was related to a significant increase in total peripheral resistance.[23] Thus, treatment with a vasodilator is the first-line approach. The change in hemodynamic pattern as pressure increased was the same in all patients with no significant change in cardiac output, central venous pressure, or left atrial pressure.

Indeed, these findings helped us to discount hypervolemia as a cause of this hypertension. There were two paradoxical findings associated with the increase in pressure: (1) lack of slowing of the heart rate, and (2) further elevations of the mean rate of left ventricular ejection. This hemodynamic pattern suggested an increased sympathetic drive that in turn helped to explain why cardiac output was not reduced.

Hormonal Changes and Postmyocardial Revascularization Hypertension

Catecholamines.—Mean preoperative levels of plasma norepinephrine were somewhat higher in patients who developed hypertension in comparison with normotensive subjects, but this difference did not reach statistical significance.[23] A possible explanation for this observation is that hypertensive patients have increased sensitivity to catecholamines.[19] Patients who become hypertensive have relatively high levels of circulating epinephrine and norepinephrine in comparison with normotensive control subjects.

Renin-angiotensin System.—Reports by Roberts et al.[19] and other investigators[33–35] emphasize the pathogenic importance of increased plasma renin activity in hypertension following coronary bypass. Although this renin-angiotensin system can be activated during nonpulsatile cardiopulmonary bypass,[36–38] a definite relationship of increased angiotensin II to postoperative hypertension has not, in our opinion, been demonstrated. Furthermore, neither in our experience nor in that of others was it possible to document particularly elevated plasma renin activity in patients in whom hypertension later developed after coronary artery bypass surgery. No correlation was found during the postoperative period between changes in blood pressure and changes in plasma renin activity.[39] Converting enzyme inhibitors was effective in controlling hypertension after bypass surgery,[40] but these results can hardly be considered unequivocal evidence of an angiotensinogenic causation. The very mechanisms by which these inhibitors decrease arterial pressure are themselves debated. These considerations led us to believe that a reflex mechanism must be involved.

The Neurogenic Origin of Postmyocardial Revascularization Hypertension

We postulated as early as 1973 that the sympathetic overdrive was possibly related to activation of pressor reflexes from the heart, great vessels, or coronary arteries. In favor of a reflex mechanism was the paroxysmal nature of the hypertension, its temporal relation to manipulation of the heart and its vessels, and the absence of other obvious hemodynamic factors. The importance of pressor reflexes originating from the heart and great vessels has repeatedly been demonstrated.[41–44]

Our previous experience with stellate stimulation,[45] (as well as the lack of any obvious predilection of postbypass hypertension in operations on any single coronary bed) suggested that of the various possible pressor reflexes, the more important in this context were those that involved sympathetic afferent fibers. We therefore elected to test the effect of unilateral stellate ganglion block in patients with hypertension after coronary bypass surgery. Both in our initial series of 27 patients[46] and in a subsequent larger group, an effective unilateral block resulted in rapid and definitive normalization of arterial pressure in the vast majority of cases. The reduction in blood pressure was rapid, smooth, and related to a decrease in systemic resistance, with no evidence of diminished cardiac performance.[46] These results were interpreted to indicate that the blood pressure response was probably due to interruption of afferent fibers coursing through or relaying in either stellate ganglion.

SUMMARY

Whatever the causes and timing of hypertension, it is a serious complication for patients recovering from open heart surgery. The increase in pressure and in total peripheral resistance increases cardiac work and myocardial oxygen consumption. Previous studies have demonstrated that the endocardial viability ratio as well as the ratio of diastolic to systolic pressure time indexes were lower in patients who had postoperative hypertension than in those who remained normotensive.[19,47] The decrease in those indexes means an increased susceptibility to subendocardial ischemia, which can be further aggravated by the anemia due to hemodilution often used in open heart surgery. Hypertension also increases the risk of cerebral vascular accidents. The incidence and amount of postoperative bleeding in a previously heparinized patient is much greater during hypertension. Therefore, it is evident that every effort should be made to prevent, control, and treat hypertension promptly.

REFERENCES

1. Estafanous FG, Tarazi RC: Systemic arterial hypertension associated with cardiac surgery. *Am J Cardiol* 1980; 46:685–694.
2. Estafanous FG: Management of anesthesia for coronary artery surgery. *Cleve Clin Q* 1978; 45:29–36.
3. Fouad FM, Estafanous FG, Bravo EL, et al: Possible role of cardioaortic reflexes in postcoronary bypass hypertension. *Am J Cardiol* 1979; 44:866–872.
4. Adriani J, Parmley J, Ochsner A: Fatalities and complications after attempts at stellate ganglion block. *Surgery* 1952; 32:615–619.
5. Tarazi RC, Dustan HP: β-Adrenergic blockade in hypertension: Practical and theoretical implications of long-term hemodynamic variations. *Am J Cardiol* 1972; 29:633–640.

6. Whelton PK, Flaherty JT, MacAllister NP, et al: Hypertension following coronary artery bypass surgery: Role of preoperative propranolol therapy. *Hypertension* 1980; 2:291–298.

7. Tarazi RC, Dustan HP, Bravo EL, et al: Vasodilating drugs: Contrasting haemodynamic effects. *Clin Sci Mol Med* 1976; 51(suppl 3):575s–578s.

8. Estafanous FG, Viljoen JF, Loop FD: Anaesthesia for ventricular aneurysmectomy. *Can Anaesth Soc J* 1972; 19:160–172.

9. Mason DT, Braunwald E: The effects of nitroglycerin and amyl nitrite on arteriolar and venous tone in the human forearm. *Circulation* 1965; 32:755–766.

10. Flaherty JT, Magee PA, Gardner TL, et al: Comparison of intravenous nitroglycerin and sodium nitroprusside for treatment of acute hypertension developing after coronary artery bypass surgery. *Circulation* 1982; 65:1072–1077.

11. Gifford RW Jr: Management and treatment of malignant hypertension and hypertensive emergencies, in Genest J, Koiw E, Kuchel O, (eds): *Hypertension*. New York, McGraw-Hill Book Co, 1977, pp 1024–1038.

12. Shah PK: Ventricular unloading in the management of heart disease: I. Role of vasodilators. *Am Heart J* 1977; 93:256–260.

13. Cohn NJ, Franciosa JA: Vasodilator therapy of cardiac failure. *N Engl J Med* 1977; 297:27–31.

14. Chatterjee K, Parmley WW, Ganz W, et al: Hemodynamic and metabolic responses to vasodilator therapy in acute myocardial infarction. *Circulation* 1973; 48:1183–1193.

15. Miller RR, Vismara LA, Zelis R, et al: Clinical use of sodium nitroprusside in chronic ischemic heart disease: Effects on peripheral vascular resistance and venous tone and on ventricular volume, pump and mechanical performance. *Circulation* 1975; 51:328–336.

16. Estafanous FG, Viljoen JF, Barsoum KN: Diagnosis of pneumothorax complicating mechanical ventilation. *Anesth Analg* 1975; 54:730–735.

17. Prys-Roberts C, Greene LT, Meloche R, et al: Studies of anaesthesia in relation to hypertension: II. Haemodynamic consequences of induction and endotracheal intubation. *Br J Anaesth* 1971; 43:531–546.

18. Estafanous FG, Tarazi RC, Viljoen JF, et al: Systemic hypertension following myocardial revascularization. *Am Heart J* 1973; 85:732–738.

19. Roberts AJ, Niarchos AP, Subramanian VA, et al: Systemic hypertension associated with coronary artery bypass surgery. *J Thorac Cardiovasc Surg* 1977; 74:846–859.

20. Chaptal PA, Grolleau-Raoux D, Millet F, et al: Les crises hypertensives dans la chirurgie de l'insuffisance coronarienne: Prevention par le diazepam. *Ann Chir Thorac Cardiovasc* 1975; 14:255–261.

21. Estafanous FG, Urzua J, Yared JP, et al: Pattern of hemodynamic alterations during coronary artery operations. *J Thorac Cardiovasc Surg* 1984; 87:175–182.

22. Kim YD, Jones M, Hanowell ST, et al: Changes in peripheral vascular and cardiac sympathetic activity before and after coronary artery bypass surgery: Interrelationships with hemodynamic alterations. *Am Heart J* 1981; 102:972–979.

23. Fouad FM, Estafanous FG, Bravo EL: Possible role of cardioaortic reflexes in postcoronary bypass hypertension.*Cardiology* 1979; 44:866–872.

24. McIlvaine W, Boulanger M, Maille JG, et al: Hypertension following coronary artery bypass graft. *Can Anaesth Soc J* 1982; 29:212–217.
25. Hess W, Arnold B, Schulte-Sasse U, et al: Comparison of isoflurane and halothane when used to control intraoperative hypertension in patients undergoing coronary artery bypass surgery. *Anesth Analg* 1983; 62:15–20.
26. Hardy JF, Boulanger M, Maille JG, et al: Arterial hypertension following coronary artery surgery: Influence of the narcotic agent used for anaesthesia. *Can Anaesth Soc J* 1983; 30:370–376.
27. Boudoulas H, Lewis RP, Vasko JS, et al: Left ventricular function and adrenergic hyperactivity before and after saphenous vein bypass. *Circulation* 1976; 53:802–806.
28. Tarazi RC: Hemodynamic role of extracellular fluid in hypertension. *Circ Res* 38(suppl II):73–83, 1976.
29. Luetscher JA, Boyers DG, Cuthbertson JG, et al: A model of the human circulation. *Circ Res* 1973; 32(suppl I):84–98.
30. Dustan HP, Tarazi RC, Bravo EL, et al: Plasma and extracellular fluid volumes in hypertension. *Circ Res* 1973; 32(Suppl I):73–83.
31. Cohn JN: Paroxysmal hypertension and hypovolemia. *N Engl J Med* 1966; 275:643–646.
32. Roberts AJ, Niarchos AP, Subramanian VA, et al: Systemic hypertension associated with coronary artery bypass surgery: Predisposing factors, hemodynamic characteristics, humoral profile, and treatment. *J Thorac Cardiovasc Surg* 1977; 74:846–859.
33. Motlagh F, Alavi F, Najmabadi MH, et al: The relation of cardiopulmonary bypass induced hypertension and renin-angiotensin system, abstracted. *Circulation* 1977; 56(suppl III):III–142.
34. Wallach R, Karp RB, Reves JG, et al: Mechanism of hypertension after saphenous vein bypass surgery, abstracted. *Circulation* 1977; 56(suppl III):III–141.
35. Niarchos AP, Roberts AJ, Case DB, et al: Hemodynamic characteristics of hypertension after coronary bypass surgery and effects of the converting enzyme inhibitor. *Am J Cardiol* 1979; 43:586–593.
36. Taylor KM, Morton IJ, Brown JJ, et al: Hypertension and the renin-angiotensin system following open-heart surgery. *J Thorac Cardiovasc Surg* 1977; 74:840–845.
37. Taylor KM, Brannan JJ, Bain WH, et al: Role of angiotensin II in the development of peripheral vasoconstriction during cardiopulmonary bypass. *Cardiovasc Res* 1979; 13:269–273.
38. Bailey DR, Miller ED, Kaplan JA, et al: The renin-angiotensin-aldosterone system during cardiac surgery with morphine-nitrous oxide anesthesia. *Anesthesiology* 1975; 42:538–544.
39. Many M, Soroff HS, Birtwell WC, et al: Effects of bilateral renal artery depulsation on renin levels. *Surg Forum* 1968; 19:387–389.
40. Bravo EL, Tarazi RC: Converting enzyme inhibition with an orally active compound in hypertensive man. *Hypertension* 1979; 1:39–46.
41. James TN, Hageman FR, Urthaler F: Anatomic and physiologic considerations of cardiogenic hypertensive chemoreflex. *Am J Cardiol* 1979; 44:852–859.
42. Malliani A, Pagani M, Bergamaschi M: Positive feedback sympathetic reflexes and hypertension. *Am J Cardiol* 1979; 44:860–865.

43. Malliani A, Brown AM: Reflexes arising from coronary receptors. *Brain Res* 1970; 24:352–355.
44. Peterson DF, Brown AM: Pressor reflexes produced by stimulation of afferent fibers in the cardiac sympathetic nerves of the cat. *Circ Res* 1971; 28:605–610.
45. Liard JF, Tarazi RC, Ferrario CM, et al: Hemodynamic and humoral characteristics of hypertension induced by prolonged stellate ganglion stimulation in conscious dogs. *Circ Res* 1975; 36:455–464.
46. Tarazi RC, Estafanous FG, Fouad FM: Unilateral stellate block in the treatment of hypertension after coronary bypass surgery: Implications of a new therapeutic approach. *Am J Cardiol* 1978; 42:1013–1018.
47. Hoar PF, Hickey RF, Ullyot DJ: Systemic hypertension following myocardial revascularization: A method of treatment using epidural anesthesia. *J Thorac Cardiovasc Surg* 1976; 71:859–864.

61

Postoperative Patient With Decreased Mixed Venous Oxygen Saturation

Three weeks following myocardial infarction, a 73-year-old woman, body surface area 1.55, with a large left ventricular aneurysm and chronic congestive failure underwent a left ventricular aneurysmectomy. An Oximetrix thermodilution continuous-recording mixed venous oxygen saturation (SvO_2) catheter was placed prior to surgery. Her prebypass SvO_2 reflected her impaired cardiac output and was in the range of 55% to 60% (Fig 61–1). Following bypass and ventricular aneurysmectomy her SvO_2 varied between 60% and 75%. Her initial course for the first 90 minutes in the cardiovascular recovery (CVR) unit was satisfactory, with indices of 2.2 to 3.0 L/minute/m^2 and an SvO_2 between 55% and 65% (Fig 61–2). Chest tube drainage increased requiring autotransfusion and supplementary blood and plasma administration to maintain circulating volume and cardiac index. Her SvO_2 gradually declined from 65% to a low of 40% just prior to transfer to the operating room four hours postoperatively. Clinical shivering was noted during the time frame of the bleeding episode (Fig 61–2). Following transfer to the operating room, a dose of pancuronium, 4 mg, was given intravenously. After the onset of neuromuscular paralysis, a dramatic rise in SvO_2 from 40% to 75% followed the onset of neuromuscular blockade and was well maintained throughout the period of surgical hemostasis. The SvO_2 remained at the 70% level following transfer to the CVR unit (Fig 61–3).

Recommendations by John F. Schweiss, M.D.

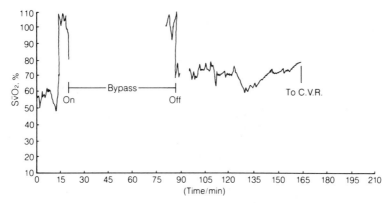

FIG 61–1.
73-year-old woman had a left ventricular aneurysmectomy, following acute myocardial infarction (body surface area, 1.55). Satisfactory SvO2 values prebypass, postbypass, and prior to transfer to the cardiovascular recovery (CVR) unit. (From Schweiss JF (ed): *Continuous Measurement of Blood Oxygen Saturation in the High Risk Patient.* San Diego, Beach International, vol 1, 1983. Used by permission.)

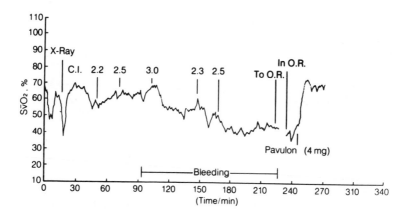

FIG 61–2.
73-year-old woman with decline in SvO2 postoperatively associated with blood loss. Cardiac index maintained with autotransfusion of shed blood. Prompt increase in SvO2 with pancuronium (Pavulon), 4mg. (From Schweiss JF (ed): *Continuous Measurement of Blood Oxygen Saturation in the High Risk Patient.* San Diego, Beach International, vol 1, 1983. Used by permission.)

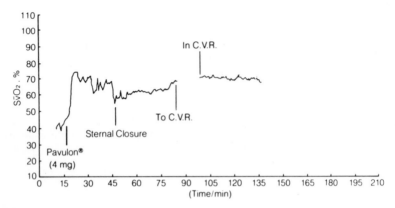

FIG 61–3.
73-year-old woman with SvO₂ increase well maintained in operating room (OR) and cardiovascular recovery (CVR) unit following surgical hemostasis. (From Schweiss JF (ed): *Continuous Measurement of Blood Oxygen Saturation in the High Risk Patient.* San Diego, Beach International, vol 1, 1983. Used by permission.)

ANALYSIS OF THE PROBLEM

This case illustrates the deleterious effects of shivering on the SvO_2. Although low SvO_2 per se is not always indicative of poor perfusion, it may be, and therapy is warranted to treat abnormally low values.

APPROACH TO THE PROBLEM

In this case muscle paralysis with pancuronium was used to treat the shivering related decrease in SvO_2. Muscle paralysis will reduce muscle metabolism and decrease total body oxygen consumption. Small doses of pancuronium given prior to leaving the operating room will generally prevent shivering in the immediate postoperative period.

DISCUSSION

Continuous measurement of mixed venous oxygen saturation (SvO_2) of hemoglobin (Hb) has gained popularity following its introduction in January of 1981 by Oximetrix, Incorporated.[1] Two plastic fiberoptic bundles incorporated into a 7.5 F thermodilution catheter permit red and infrared light impulse transmission to the tip of the catheter positioned in the pulmonary artery through one of the bundles. The light is reflected back via the other fiberoptic bundle to the optical module and the relative proportions of saturated and unsaturated hemoglobin are derived based on reflection oximetry. The percentage saturation of Hb is updated every five seconds. The saturation values are trended on a writer.

Pathophysiology

The normal range of SvO_2 is 60% to 80%, reflecting generally a normal hemodynamic state, and a 5 to 6 volume percent of O_2 uptake by the tissues of the body from each 100 cc of blood. Deviations from this norm are related to either:

1. Anemia (a fall in total Hb per 100 ml)

2. Increased oxygen demand
   e.g., hypermetabolic states, fever, shivering, etc.

3. Decrease in perfusion (reduction in cardiac index)

4. Arterial unsaturation (decreased SaO_2)

A decrease in SvO_2 from normal requires investigation to determine etiology, as a decrease to 50% to 60% is an indication of some decompensation in the cardiorespiratory system. A level of 40% to 50% may precede or warn of an impending catastrophe. A level of 30% to 40% indicates severe compromise. The nature of the decline in this case was elucidated by an arterial blood gas determination that indicated full arterial saturation and acid base normality. Her hemoglobin level of 12 to 14 gm/100 ml provided adequate O_2 carrying capacity and her cardiac index of 2.2 to 2.5 would indicate borderline adequate perfusion. Her left heart filling pressures of 14 to 16 mm Hg were well maintained postoperatively by transfusion. The etiology would appear to have been associated with an increase in oxygen demand.

Case Options

The administration of the neuromuscular blocking drug pancuronium bromide at the time of arrival in the operating room (OR) caused an immediate cessation of shivering and a prompt rise in SvO_2 to 70% from 40%, confirming the role of muscle shivering in reducing SvO_2 levels.

Our concern was that the SvO_2 decline might have been associated with cardiac tamponade as a consequence of blood loss into the pericardium resulting in clot formation in the pericardial sac behind the heart and producing left ventricular compression and compromising left ventricular filling. The patient's filling pressures were slightly elevated at the conclusion of the aneurysmectomy repair on discontinuing bypass. Her indices were above minimal requirements and some restriction of left ventricular filling associated with the operative repair led to the elevation of left atrial and pulmonary artery diastolic pressures to maintain a satisfactory cardiac output.

Minimal clot retention, which was not thought to compromise the filling of the heart as a result of tamponade, was found following mediastinal reexploration of the pericardium. Surgical hemostasis was accomplished and her postoperative course thereafter was associated with SvO_2 levels that varied between 60% and 70%.

As it was in this case, cardiopulmonary bypass with hypothermia to 25° C is frequently associated with a decline in body temperature following discontinuing the bypass, even though nasopharyngeal temperature was restored to 38° C and the pulmonary artery thermistor was 37.5° C at the time of discontinuing bypass and warming at this level of body temperature had been maintained for 15 minutes prior to coming off the bypass. A decline in body temperature to 33.5° to 35.5° C is not an uncommon occurrence in spite of the utilization of a warming blanket at 40° C and the use of warmed humidified gases (38° C) in the inspiratory limb of the anesthesia circle system.

As neuromuscular blockade decreases following transfer to the cardiovascular recovery unit (CVR), visible shivering and/or limb rigidity may be seen. This is usually associated with a fall in SvO_2 and frequently a modest fall in pH to 7.29 and a slight rise in P_{CO_2} to 44 to 46 mm Hg. Oxygen consumption is increased: CO_2 production is increased, and cardiac output is maintained above 2.0 L/minute, but is less than that required to maintain SvO_2 at normal values because of the increase in oxygen demand by the skeletal muscles associated with shivering in response to the decline in body temperature. A further fall occurs associated with the transfusion of blood or fluids whose temperature is below that of the body.

This demand for increased cardiac output (perfusion) to meet oxygen delivery needs may be inappropriate in the immediate postoperative period. The increased myocardial O_2 demand may lead to myocardial ischemia due to an increase in cardiac muscle oxygen requirements in the presence of residual coronary atherosclerosis, since revascularization may not alleviate some areas of relative insufficiency when high work demands are made upon the myocardium.

We have considered this to be as undesirable as hypertension in the early postoperative period and have routinely administered additional pancuronium (average dose, 3 to 4 mg) prior to transfer to the CVR. We have also administered up to 20 mg of apresoline in divided doses of 2 to 4 mg as tolerated to promote arterial vasodilation. This combination of drugs (neuromuscular blocker and vasodilator) appears to reduce or eliminate the decline in $S\bar{v}O_2$ that otherwise accompanies awakening and the early return of motor activity. Occasionally, in spite of this, some shivering develops as neuromuscular blockade wanes in the second and third hours postoperatively, but the profound falls in SvO_2 to the levels of 40% to 50% previously observed are now rarely encountered associated with shivering. Body temperature restores with external warming, heated inspired gases, and the metabolic activities of the body during the first two to three hours postoperatively.

Another disadvantage of the shivering is the increase in intrathoracic pressures (a form of chest wall spasm), which requires an increase in the inflating pressures to maintain tidal volume. The increase in the minute volume of CO_2 produced also requires an increase in alveolar minute volume to maintain CO_2 homeostasis, and result in an increase in mean intrathoracic (airway) pressure, which could potentially reduce cardiac return.

Summary

In summary, shivering with an increase in O_2 demand, CO_2 production, and heart work would appear to be undesirable in the postbypass period. If neuromuscular paralysis is maintained for two to four hours postanesthetically, shivering can be prevented, heart work reduced, and metabolic demands minimized. Artifacts in pressure hemodynamics are reduced, and diagnosis and treatment facilitated.

REFERENCE

1. Schweiss JF (ed): *Continuous Measurement of Blood Oxygen Saturation in the High Risk Patient.* San Diego, Beach International, vol 1, 1983.

62

Atrial Fibrillation in the Immediate Postoperative Period

A 70-year-old man underwent coronary artery surgery uneventfully. Five hours postoperatively he developed atrial fibrillation, with a ventricular response of 130 beats per minute and reduced cardiac index (1.8 L/minute/m^2) and blood pressure 90/65 mm Hg.

Recommendations by Donald C. Finlayson, M.D., F.R.C.P.(C.)

ANALYSIS OF THE PROBLEM

Atrial fibrillation with a rapid ventricular response is common in the perioperative period. The resultant loss of the atrial contribution to ventricular filling and the tachycardia may lead to significant difficulty in patients with compromised left ventricular function and may require urgent treatment. [1]

APPROACH TO THE PROBLEM

The urgency of therapy will depend on the degree of hemodynamic compromise resulting from the loss of the atrial contribution to cardiac output and the assessment of the effect of the tachycardia on myocardial oxygen supply-demand balance. Immediately after surgery, the patients often have a high level of oxygen demand due to shivering as noted above; a poor level of oxygen delivery capacity due to the anemia from the incomplete resolution of the effects of hemodilution; a generalized myocardial insult due to the operation that has not yet been reversed; and a marked increase in myocardial oxygen demand due to the tachycardia and potential increase in filling pressures. The presence of these factors adds a degree of urgency to the need for treatment.

Active treatment should be accompanied by evaluation of oxygenation; CO_2 removal; acid-base balance; electrolytes; and the circumstances in which the arrhythmia occurred. The ventricular pacemaker wires should be rechecked and functioning normally. The atrial wires should have been similarly checked at the end of surgery. With this under way, the clinician may then proceed to drug therapy or immediate cardioversion. Overdrive atrial pacing, although the treatment of choice for atrial flutter, is not useful for atrial fibrillation.

Drug therapy is the first choice, unless severe hemodynamic compromise is present. In the latter instance, cardioversion is indicated. A synchronized countershock in the absence of high blood levels of digoxin has been used by many with few problems. It should be easily done in an anesthetized patient with the resources of the intensive care unit (ICU) available, then followed by appropriate drug therapy.

In the situation described here, with moderate rather than severe compromise present, conservative medical therapy would usually be the treatment of choice rather than cardioversion. The effect of digoxin in a dose of 0.5 mg given over a 10- to 20-minute period should be apparent in an additional 15- to 30-minute period and may be repeated in three to four hours and daily as indicated thereafter. Digoxin is usually accompanied by small doses of either verapamil or propranolol. The use of both together is to be avoided if at all possible and to be used only if adequate pacing capability is assured, since the combination may produce severe bradycardia or even standstill. If pharmacologic therapy does not lead to an adequate improvement, or in the event of further hemodynamic deterioration, cardioversion may still be indicated.

DISCUSSION

In general, most dysrhythmias are due to abnormal impulse formation related to altered automaticity or after-potentials; abnormalities leading to reentry; or both. The sinoatrial (SA) node automaticity has a different ionic basis from that for Purkinje fibers and normally dominates other sites of abnormal impulse generation by depolarizing more rapidly and causing overdrive suppression. [2, 3]

TABLE 62–1.

General Mechanisms for Atrial Tachydysrhythmias

Reentry foci
   Atrioventricular node
   Concealed accessory pathways
   Sinus node
   Intra-atrial sites
Flutter . . . predominantly a reentry problem
Fibrillation . . . fragmentation of flutter
Atrial tachycardia
   Abnormal automaticity
      triggered after-depolarizations

Detailed consideration of the electrophysiologic mechanisms involved are beyond the scope of this discussion, but have been extensively reviewed.[2–6] When dysrhythmias occur, distinguishing disorders of automaticity from those caused by reentry may be very difficult.

The general mechanisms for atrial tachydysrhythmias are listed in Table 62–1.

Although reentry is a more likely cause,[5] the precise mechanisms for atrial tachydysrhythmias are usually obscure, and treatment, therefore, is largely empiric. Nevertheless, a number of predisposing factors are common after open heart surgery (Table 62–2). These should be managed by prevention when possible; searched for aggressively in all patients; and treated equally aggressively when detected.

Intraoperative ischemia is now much less common with the use of better myocardial preservation techniques, but it is still a problem since the right side of the heart is often the first to rewarm and the last to be revascularized. Ischemia results in some degree of disruption of the sarcolemmal membrane and of normal cellular function, with the obvious potential for both abnormal sinus node function and conduction, analogous to the patients reported by Leier and associates.[6]

TABLE 62–2.

Factors Predisposing to Atrial Tachydysrhythmias

Ischemia
Surgical injury, stretch, dilation
Hypoxia
Hypocarbia and hypercarbia
Electrolyte disorders involving potassium,
   magnesium, and calcium ions
Equipment: i.e., PA catheters, pacing wires
Anesthetic and cardiac drug interactions

Atrial injury from manipulation, stretch, and cannulation is an inevitable accompaniment of surgery and may lead to functional disturbances similar to those of ischemia. Dysrhythmias may be caused by varying combinations of depressed SA-nodal function, slowed conduction, and increased degrees of abnormal automaticity with potential reentry.

The effects of disordered electrolyte balance on cardiac function must be assessed in relation to the balance between the intracellular and extracellular ion concentration and may be partly a function of the rate at which the measured change in extracellular fluid has occurred. Long-term moderate hypokalemia in the range of 3.2 mEq clinically appears to be less disruptive to heart rhythm than the same reduction brought about acutely.[7] Acute changes, in contrast, can lead to enhancement of automaticity and excitability.[8] Perioperatively, hypokalemia may result from urinary wasting of potassium due to diuretic use, bypass-induced alterations in aldosterone activity, steroid administration, and hypomagnesemia. Hypokalemia may also result from intracellular shifts caused by intravenous glucose-insulin-potassium, alkalosis, hypothermia, and β-agonist administration.

Increases in ionized calcium within the range that might be seen in the perioperative period, even in the presence of other factors, are rarely of sufficient magnitude to contribute to the risk of atrial fibrillation. Reductions in magnesium levels, however, are very common after open heart surgery, lead to increased automaticity, have been associated with ventricular dysrhythmias, and conceivably might also be associated with atrial fibrillation. Surprisingly, however, the search for magnesium-related atrial dysrhythmias has not been very active or the problem well documented. The concept is supported only by indirect and anecdotal reports.[9, 10] The atrial dysrhythmias actually described with hypomagnesemia have usually been minor disturbances accompanying ventricular ectopy in the presence of digitalis intoxication.

Ventilatory disorders may worsen all of these problems. Hypoxia may be additive to surgical or stretch-induced ischemic injury. Hypocarbia may also acutely affect potassium balance and pH. These problems are common in the early postoperative period, particularly with incomplete rewarming, shivering, and hypercarbia when ventilator settings lag behind CO_2 production.

Atrial dysrhythmias have also been reported with placement of pulmonary artery catheters[11] and with cold fluid injection for cardiac output determination.[12]

Atrial fibrillation is usually seen later rather than early in the postoperative period. When seen later, conversion to and maintenance of sinus rhythm is often difficult. It is often preceded by atrial premature beats. These should elicit a high index of suspicion and a search for the factors noted above. Diagnosis is usually easy. If not, unipolar or bipolar epicardial atrial electrograms using the pacemaker wires in the modified chest lead I or lead II configuration can be used to demonstrate the fibrillatory waves.[13, 14]

SUMMARY

Atrial fibrillation, common after open heart surgery, is often preceded by atrial premature beats. It may lead to severe hemodynamic compromise and usually responds well to conservative medical therapy, although cardioversion may be useful in some circumstances.

REFERENCES

1. Lappas DG, Powell WMJ Jr, Daggett WM: Cardiac dysfunction in the perioperative period: Pathophysiology, diagnosis and treatment. *Anesthesiology* 1977; 7:117.
2. Zipes DP: Genesis of cardiac arrhythmias: Electrophysiologic considerations, in Braunwald E (ed): *Heart Disease,* ed 2. Philadelphia, WB Saunders Co, 1984, p 605.
3. Vassale M: Electrogenic suppression of automaticity in sheep and dog Purkinje fibers. *Circ Res* 1970; 27:361.
4. Wit AL, Weiss MB, Berkowitz WD: Patterns of atrioventricular conduction in human heart. *Circ Res* 1970; 27:345.
5. Hoffman BF, Rosen MR: Cellular mechanisms for cardiac arrhythmias. *Circ Res* 1981; 49:1.
6. Leier CV, Meacham JA, Schaal SF: Prolonged atrial conduction: A major predisposing factor for the development of atrial flutter. *Circulation* 1978; 57:213.
7. Vitez TS, Soper LE, Wong KC, et al: Chronic hypokalemia and intraoperative dysrhythmias. *Anesthesiology* 1985; 63:130.
8. Surawicz B: The interrelationship of electrolyte abnormalities and arrhythmias, in Mandel WJ (ed): *Cardiac Arrhythmias*. Philadelphia, JB Lippincott Co, 1980, p 83.
9. Tilsner V: Beeinflussung von Rhythmusstorungen des Herzen durch Elektrolyte. *Munchen Med Woch* 1968; 110(part 1): Jan-June.
10. Caddell JL: The effect of magnesium therapy on cardiovascular and electrograph changes in severe protein-calorie malnutrition. *Trop Geogr Med* 1969; 21:33–38.
11. Todd MM: Atrial fibrillation induced by the right atrial injection of cold fluids during thermodilution cardiac output determination: A case report. *Anesthesiology* 1983; 59:253.
12. Geha DG, Davis NJ, Lappas DG: Persistent atrial arrhythmias associated with placement of a Swan-Ganz catheter. *Anesthesiology* 1973; 39:651.
13. Zaidan JR, Curling PE: Cardiac dysrhythmias: Recognition and management, in Stoelting RK (ed): *Advances in Anesthesiology*. Chicago, Year Book Medical Publishers, vol 2, 1985.
14. Waldo AL, MacLean WAH, Cooper T, et al: Use of temporarily placed epicardial wire electrodes for the diagnosis and treatment of cardiac arrhythmias following open heart surgery. *J Thorac Cardiovasc Surg* 1978; 76:500.

Index